Adult ADHD

J. J. Sandra Kooij

Adult ADHD

Diagnostic Assessment and Treatment

Fourth Edition

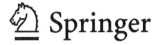 Springer

J. J. Sandra Kooij
VUMc
Amsterdam University Medical Center
Amsterdam
The Netherlands

This fourth edition was translated by Dora Wynchank.

ISBN 978-3-030-82814-1   ISBN 978-3-030-82812-7   (eBook)
https://doi.org/10.1007/978-3-030-82812-7

This Springer imprint is published by the registered company Springer Nature Switzerland AG
The registered company address is: Gewerbestrasse 11, 6330 Cham, Switzerland

Foreword

Sandra Kooij is a leading European psychiatrist who pioneered the development of clinical services for adults with ADHD. She is inspirational in this area, playing a lead role in the development of clinical networks and training programmes across Europe. Her work is built on a background of clinical and epidemiological research that has provided further characterisation of the symptoms, disorders and functional impairments associated with ADHD in adults. This book clearly benefits from this experience and includes many important insights as well as practical guidance on clinical management.

ADHD in adults is one of the most prevalent adult mental health disorders, with an estimated worldwide prevalence of 3–4%. Furthermore, the disorder is associated with the development of numerous comorbid psychopathologies including anxiety, depression, substance abuse and personality disorders. The strong association with addiction and the high rates of ADHD within the criminal justice system highlight the considerable impact of ADHD on some of the most difficult mental health problems facing society. ADHD also affects people in their daily lives due to difficulties in regulating arousal and attention and problems with planning, memory, time-keeping, mood regulation, low self-esteem and poor impulse control. ADHD is highly symptomatic with reports of feeling restless, ceaseless and unfocused thought processes and insomnia often leading to mistaken diagnoses. Yet, ADHD shows highly characteristic responses to both pharmacological and non-pharmacological treatments.

The translation of this book into English is very timely. Recognition and treatment of ADHD in adults has not received sufficient attention, and as a result, many people with ADHD have struggled to obtain the treatment they require. This continues to be a problem leading to persistence of impairments and considerable distress to individuals and their families. There is, however, growing interest in ADHD and its clinical management among adult mental health-care professionals.

This book provides a concise yet detailed summary of the diagnosis and treatment of ADHD in adults. It is no longer acceptable to ignore ADHD as an adult condition or mistake it for other mental health disorders. We now know that correctly targeted treatments for ADHD are effective at improving daily function and quality of life for many people. As such this book is an essential resource for all those engaged in adult mental health.

London, UK   Philip Asherson

Foreword

This book not only serves as an excellent guide for recognising, diagnosing and treating adult ADHD. It also contains fifteen years of history concerning the process leading up to this—a process that I was able to witness at close quarters and that instilled in me a great admiration for the strength and perseverance of psychiatrist Dr. Sandra Kooij, the author of this book.

Sandra referred to research carried out abroad and expressed the ambition to also prove in the Netherlands that ADHD continues into adulthood and brings suffering to a considerable number of people through dysfunctioning and underachievement. But she also pointed out that treatment provides these people with the opportunity to take a different course in life and to develop new certainties and talents. By offering this perspective, Sandra Kooij has become a symbol of hope and new insights for adults with ADHD in the Netherlands.

It did not end there, because, under her supervision, a considerable amount of scientific research has been carried out, there is increasing evidence for the validity of the diagnosis, treatment models have been developed, diagnostic assessment and self-report instruments have been tested and a mental health-care infrastructure in which adults can ask their questions in various locations in the Netherlands was put into place.

Adult ADHD aims to take the next step in the process towards creating a self-evident place for the treatment of adult ADHD in the mental health-care sector. This book provides education programmes with the possibility of including the disorder in their curriculums, so that every psychologist and psychiatrist will eventually know about the seriousness of these problems and their influence on a considerable number of relationships and families. Sandra Kooij concluded in her first study that the adults who came to her department had on average been looking for help for as long as twelve and a half years. The book here before you provides you with an excellent tool for bringing this number down considerably. It is time to start working with it.

Rotterdam, The Netherlands   Arga Paternotte

Preface

The Fourth Edition

Recent research has shown that in the Netherlands adult ADHD is found in 5% of the general population and in approximately 20% of psychiatric and addicted patients. If left untreated, adult ADHD results in impairment of patients, places a burden on the patient's environment and generates higher costs for society as a result of absence, illness and incapacity for work. Effective treatment of adult ADHD is possible and improved drugs are available, but still only a few mental health professionals have been trained in the diagnostic assessment and treatment of this common disorder. This leads to underdiagnosis and undertreatment of adult ADHD, which increases the risk of chronicity.

Now that the diagnostic assessment of adult ADHD has been increasingly validated, it is time to train medical students, psychology students and psychiatry residents. The third edition of this book was written for them as well as for psychologists, psychiatrists, mental health professionals and other interested parties and aims to provide a quick overview of the current state of the science and of the diagnostic assessment and treatment of adult ADHD in clinical practice.

The fourth edition has been thoroughly revised and updated on the basis of the latest scientific research. A lot more is known about the prevalence of adult ADHD in the general population of Europe and the USA as well as in countries such as Lebanon and Mexico. The common patterns of comorbidity in adults with ADHD, including personality disorders, sleep phase disorders, seasonal depression and bipolar II disorder, are discussed in detail. A possible overlap and misdiagnosis among girls and women with ADD or chronic fatigue syndrome is explored using recent research. There is a chapter on the new evidence regarding chronic sleep problems associated with ADHD and the possible consequences for general health (such as obesity, diabetes, cardiovascular diseases and cancer). There are also sections on ADHD and intelligence, sexuality, dyslexia and autism. The section on the neuro-biological background to ADHD, including research into so-called endophenotypes, has been expanded.

New diagnostic tools have been developed: the structured *Diagnostic Interview for Adult ADHD (DIVA-5)*, and an ultra-short and somewhat longer screening tool, all based on the DSM-5 criteria for ADHD. The strategy of the Introduction Group, as used by PsyQ, psycho-medical programmes, has also been included. In this group, new patients with ADHD receive psychoeducation about diagnostic assessment and treatment.

As far as the treatment is concerned, the chapter on psychoeducation has been extended to include tools on how to provide patients with suitable information at various points during the treatment. The long-acting stimulant drugs and other new drugs available for ADHD are discussed, as is the position that the drugs hold with regard to each other, the order of treatment in the case of comorbidity, dosing, effectiveness, side effects and duration of the action and timing of doses over the day, along with the combining of stimulants with each other and with other drugs. The increasing experience with (digital) individual and group coaching and cognitive behavioural therapy has been integrated into the chapter on the psychological treatment of adult ADHD. Finally, a new chapter has been added about the setting up and organisation of a department for adult ADHD with a multidisciplinary team. References, web sites and useful addresses have all been updated.

The Hague, The Netherlands   J. J. Sandra Kooij
May 2021

Contents

1	**Introduction**.	1
1.1	ADHD in Adults	1
	1.1.1 Short history of ADHD	2
	1.1.2 ADHD in Adults in the Netherlands and Europe.	3
	1.1.3 ADHD: A Neurobiological Disorder	4
	1.1.4 Neuroanatomy	7
	1.1.5 Functional Neuroimaging Studies	8
	1.1.6 Biomarkers for ADHD.	9
	1.1.7 Neurophysiology	10
	1.1.8 Neuropsychology.	11
	1.1.9 Continuous Performance Test	12
1.2	Prevalence	12
	1.2.1 ADHD in Older People	14
	1.2.2 Conclusions	14
1.3	Applying DSM Criteria for Children to Adults	14
	1.3.1 How Hard Is the Age of Onset Criterion?	16
	1.3.2 Late-Onset ADHD	17
1.4	Prevention and Presentation of ADHD in Men and Women	18
	1.4.1 Link between ADHD and CFS	19
	1.4.2 ADHD and Comorbidity in Boys and Girls.	19
	1.4.3 ADHD and Comorbidity in Men and Women	20
1.5	Core Symptoms of ADHD.	22
	1.5.1 Attention Problems	23
	1.5.2 Hyperactivity	24
	1.5.3 Impulsivity.	24
1.6	ADHD Seldom Comes Alone: Problems with ADHD and Comorbidity.	25
1.7	Is ADHD a Disorder?.	25
	1.7.1 What Does the Diagnosis of ADHD Mean for the Patient?. .	27
1.8	Morbidity and Mortality in ADHD	28
1.9	Costs of ADHD during the Life Course.	28
	1.9.1 Cost-Effectiveness	29

2   Diagnostics   31
     2.1   Diagnostics: Purpose and Method   31
     2.2   Screening   31
              2.2.1 Ultrashort Screening List for ADHD in Adults   32
              2.2.2 Diagnostics.   33
     2.3   DSM-5 Criteria   33
     2.4   Presentation Types of ADHD.   37
              2.4.1 Prevalence of Presentation Types.   38
     2.5   Age of Onset of ADHD   38
     2.6   ADHD and Intelligence   38
     2.7   Dysfunction in ADHD   40
              2.7.1 ADHD and Driving   41
     2.8   Impact of ADHD on Work, Relationships, and Family Life   42
              2.8.1 ADHD and Work: Being a Jack of all Trades   42
              2.8.2 ADHD and Relationships: Short-Lived and Rapidly
                        Changing   45
              2.8.3 Impact of ADHD on a Relationship.   45
              2.8.4 ADHD and Sexuality   47
              2.8.5 The Impact of ADHD on the Family   48
              2.8.6 Conclusions   49
     2.9   Benefits and Limitations of Recall in History Taking   49
     2.10   Family History   51
     2.11   Additional Information   51
     2.12   Neuropsychological Examination   51
     2.13   A Fashionable Diagnosis and overtreatment?   52
     2.14   Comorbidity and Differential Diagnosis   53
              2.14.1 Comorbidity in ADHD.   53
              2.14.2 ADHD in Other Disorders   54
              2.14.3 ADHD and Health   54
              2.14.4 ADHD and Sleep Disorders.   58
              2.14.5 ADHD and Mood.   61
              2.14.6 ADHD and Anxiety   68
              2.14.7 ADHD and Addiction   70
              2.14.8 ADHD in Personality Disorders   72
              2.14.9 ADHD and Crime   77
              2.14.10 ADHD and Autism Spectrum Disorder   78
              2.14.11 ADHD and Tourette's and Other Tic Disorders.   81
              2.14.12 ADHD and Dyslexia   82
              2.14.13 ADHD and Psychosis   82

3   Diagnostic Instruments.   85
     3.1   Ultrashort Screening list for ADHD in Adults.   85
     3.2   Self-Report questionnaire on Attention
              Problems and Hyperactivity for Adulthood and Childhood.   85
     3.3   Diagnostic Interview for ADHD (DIVA-5) in Adults   86

4 Treatment... 87
  4.1 The Attitude of the Therapist............................... 87
  4.2 Psycho-Education 88
      4.2.1 Online Psycho-Education........................... 89
      4.2.2 Psycho-Education During Treatment.................. 90
  4.3 Important Points for the Practitioner 92
      4.3.1 Possible Answers to FAQs in Psycho-Education......... 92
  4.4 Medication... 94
      4.4.1 Introduction 94
      4.4.2 Stimulants and Addiction Risk 96
      4.4.3 Improvement of Cognitive Functioning................ 97
      4.4.4 Effect of Stimulants on Addiction 97
      4.4.5 Functioning of Stimulants in the Brain 98
      4.4.6 Order of Treating Comorbid Disorders 99
      4.4.7 Medication Available (in The Netherlands).............. 99
      4.4.8 Medication Available in the United States.............. 101
      4.4.9 Drugs in the Pipeline 102
  4.5 Dealing with Alcohol and Cannabis USE Before and
      During Treatment with Medication 102
  4.6 Contraindications to Stimulant Use......................... 103
      4.6.1 Relative Contraindications.......................... 105
  4.7 Measures Prior to and During the Use of Medication 105
  4.8 Instruments for Drug Treatment............................ 106
      4.8.1 Symptom and Side Effects List 106
      4.8.2 ADHD Rating Scale............................... 106
      4.8.3 Example of an Individual Target Symptom List 107
      4.8.4 QbTest 107
  4.9 Prescribing Methylphenidate to Adults 108
      4.9.1 Wearing off of Methylphenidate in the Evening and Its Effect on
            Sleep.. 110
      4.9.2 Short- and Long-term Effectiveness 110
      4.9.3 Differences Between Methylphenidate Preparations....... 112
      4.9.4 Adjusting to the Correct Dosage 113
      4.9.5 Maintenance Treatment with Stimulants 115
      4.9.6 Side Effects 119
      4.9.7 Overdosage 120
      4.9.8 Dexmethylphenidate 120
      4.9.9 Treatment of Physical Conditions During Stimulant Use ... 121
  4.10 Dextroamphetamine...................................... 122
      4.10.1 Starting Dextroamphetamine........................ 123
  4.11 Pregnancy, Lactation, and the Stimulants 123
  4.12 Driving While Using Stimulants 124
  4.13 Travelling Abroad 124
  4.14 Atomoxetine... 124
      4.14.1 Starting Atomoxetine.............................. 125

4.15 Guanfacine XR. 126
4.16 Long-Acting Bupropion. 127
4.17 Other Antidepressants: Tricyclic Antidepressants, Venlafaxine,
       Duloxetine, and Reboxetine. 128
4.18 Modiodal 128
4.19 Drug Treatment of ADHD in the Elderly. 129
       4.19.1 Methylphenidate 129
       4.19.2 Methylphenidate in the Elderly with Depression and
                Dementia 131
4.20 Combining Stimulants with Treatment for Comorbidity. 132
       4.20.1 Combining Stimulants with Antidepressants. 132
       4.20.2 Low Mood Associated with Stimulant Use 133
       4.20.3 Combining Stimulants with a Mood Stabilizer 133
       4.20.4 Stimulants in ADHD with Psychosis. 136
       4.20.5 Stimulants in ADHD and Cluster B Personality Disorder. . . 137
       4.20.6 Stimulants in ADHD and Addiction 138
       4.20.7 Stimulants and Sexuality 140
4.21 Treatment with Melatonin in Delayed Sleep Phase Disorder 141
       4.21.1 Delayed Sleep Phase 141
       4.21.2 Melatonin for Delayed Sleep Phase. 141
       4.21.3 First, Sleep Hygiene. 143
       4.21.4 Side Effects and Protective Effects of Melatonin 145
       4.21.5 Melatonin as a Sleep Aid 145
       4.21.6 Melatonin Resets the Clock. 146
       4.21.7 Instructions to the Patient. 147
       4.21.8 Tips and Tricks. 147
       4.21.9 Light Therapy for the Delayed Sleep Phase and
                Possibly for ADHD 148
4.22 Alternative Treatments for ADHD. 148
       4.22.1 Gaming and Exercise in Young Children with ADHD 149

5 Treatment: Coaching of Adults with ADHD. 151
5.1 What Is Coaching?. 151
5.2 Similarities and Differences in Cognitive Behavioral
      Therapy in ADHD and Other Disorders 152
5.3 Rationale of the Treatment. 152
5.4 Who Should Provide the Coaching? 154
5.5 (Contra) Indications for Coaching. 154
5.6 Motivation for Treatment. 156
      5.6.1 What Is Motivation all about? 156
      5.6.2 Where Does Motivation Begin?. 157
5.7 Attitude and Tasks of the Coach 158
      5.7.1 Active Structuring 158
      5.7.2 Acceptance. 159
      5.7.3 Information 159

      5.7.4   Motivation 159
      5.7.5   Case Management 159
      5.7.6   Giving Insight 160
      5.7.7   Supporting 160
      5.7.8   Changing Role of the Coach 160
      5.7.9   Relationship between Individual Coaching and Group
              Treatment....................................... 161
      5.7.10 Cooperation with the Doctor 161
      5.7.11 Digital Coaching 162
      5.7.12 Cooperation with External Organizations 162
5.8   The Structure of Coaching............................... 162
      5.8.1   Patient Expectations............................... 162
      5.8.2   Duration and Frequency of the Coaching Sessions 163
      5.8.3   Duration of Treatment 163
      5.8.4   Use of a Session Agenda 163
      5.8.5   Common Treatment Objectives 163
      5.8.6   Setting Targets 164
      5.8.7   Dealing with Being Late 164
      5.8.8   Dealing with no-Show............................. 165
5.9   Structure of the Treatment 165
      5.9.1   Acceptance....................................... 166
      5.9.2   Coaching for Comorbidity.......................... 167
      5.9.3   ADHD skills...................................... 169
5.10 Pitfalls and Tips for the Coach............................ 179
      5.10.1 The Coach Is Too Active 179
      5.10.2 The Coach Is Too Passive 179
      5.10.3 The Coach overestimates the (Intelligent) Patient......... 180
      5.10.4 Tips for the Coach 180
      5.10.5 Handy Questions to Ask............................ 180
5.11 Patient Characteristics 181
      5.11.1 Impatient and Enthusiastic.......................... 181
      5.11.2 Complaints that Cause Minimal Distress................ 181
      5.11.3 I Have no Problem (but Others Have a Problem with me) .. 182
5.12 Problems in the Treatment................................ 182
      5.12.1 The List of Problems Is Overwhelming................. 182
      5.12.2 Resistance to Structure............................. 182
5.13 Cognitive Behavioral Therapy 183
5.14 Schema therapy for Adults with ADHD 184
5.15 Mindfulness 184
5.16 Relationship Therapy.................................... 185
5.17 Prevention of Relapse 186
5.18 Conclusion.. 186
5.19 Aftercare 186
5.20 Contact with Fellow Experience Experts..................... 187

6   Set up and Organization of an Outpatient and Life
     Course Clinic for ADHD. 189
     6.1   Introduction 189
           6.1.1   Starting a Life Course Clinic for ADHD 190
     6.2   Employees 191
           6.2.1   Tasks and Responsibilities of Treatment Staff. 191
     6.3   Inclusion and Exclusion Criteria 192
     6.4   Intake 192
     6.5   Staff Discussion 193
     6.6   Range of Treatment 194
           6.6.1   Minimum Treatment 194
           6.6.2   Treatment Objectives and Plan 194
           6.6.3   Groups 197
     6.7   Evaluation and Impact Measurement. 198
           6.7.1   Objective of the Evaluation 198
           6.7.2   Evaluation of the Treatment Plan. 198
           6.7.3   Discussion of Evaluation in Patient Consultations 199
     6.8   End of Treatment 199

Appendix A: Instruments for Diagnostic Assessment 201

Appendix B: Instruments for Treatment Medication and Coaching 205

Appendix C: Introduction Course. 211

Internet Sites 225

Useful Addresses 227

References 229

Index. 271

About the Author

J. J. Sandra Kooij is a psychiatrist and researcher on ADHD in adults. She initiated the Department and Expertise Center Adult ADHD at PsyQ in the Hague, the Netherlands. She is a professor of adult ADHD at the Department of Psychiatry at Amsterdam University Medical Center, location VUmc in Amsterdam, the Netherlands. She is president of the DIVA Foundation and the European Network Adult ADHD and a *board member of* Eunethydis, ADHD-Europe and APSARD. She publishes articles, books, websites, newsletters, webinars and podcasts, is a speaker at (inter)national congresses and is involved in educational activities such as courses, webinars and podcasts on ADHD in adulthood.

Sandra Kooij is also the author of:

- Kooij, J.J.S. (2006). *ADHD in adults: clinical studies on assessment and treatment. Thesis*, Radboud Universiteit Nijmegen, the Netherlands. ISBN 978 90 265 1793 8.
- Kooij, J.J.S. (2008). *Over medicatie voor volwassenen met ADHD*. Den Haag: PsyQ en Impuls.
- Kooij, J.J.S. (2017). ADHD bij volwassenen. Diagnostiek en behandeling. 4th ed. Pearson Assessment and Information. Amsterdam. ISBN 978 90 265 1850 8.
- Kooij, J.J.S. & Otten-Pablos, S. (2013). *Hyper Sapiens. Praktische gids voor mensen met ADHD*. Houten: Uitgeverij Spectrum/Unieboek. ISBN 978 90 003 4751 3.
- Kooij, J.J.S. & Paternotte, A. (2001). *In kort bestek. ADHD bij volwassenen*. Bilthoven: Vereniging Balans. ISBN 978 90 806 6741 9.
- Schuijers, F. & Kooij, J.J.S. (2007). *ADHD'ers voor elkaar. Lotgenotenproject*. Uitgeverij patiëntenvereniging Impuls. ISBN 978 90 888 4002 9.

1.1   ADHD in Adults

Adults with ADHD suffer from distractibility, poor planning and organization, mood swings and anger. They seek tension and risk in order to concentrate better, often use drugs and alcohol, and are impulsive and restless. In addition, they almost always have comorbid disorders, such as anxiety, depression, addiction, sleep, bipolar, or personality disorder. Together, these cause problems in functioning at school, at work, and in relationships. People with ADHD therefore often have a history of underperforming at school, and at work. Furthermore, they are more likely to have (car) accidents, are often ill and underproductive, due to chronic physical complaints. Behind this multitude of problems lurks ADHD, but without a diagnosis, there is no treatment. The advantage of a diagnosis is that the disorder is highly responsive to treatment. But in adulthood, there is a long journey until the treatment stage: all the contributing factors need to be analyzed, understanding why one feels different from others and does not function at one's own level. Health care providers may be ill-equipped to treat adult ADHD, as they were not exposed to this relatively new diagnosis during their training.

More and more adults with ADHD are describing their lives with the disorder. One of them is nineteen-year-old Hannah Buenting, who wrote about her experiences in *Hyper: Up and down with ADHD*. In witty anecdotes and confessions, she shows what an ADHD life really looks like, emphasizing "not only little boys are hyperactive." At the age of thirteen years, it became clear that "something" was going on with her. She was "completely thrown by deadlines" and could not perform simple practical tasks (wash or clean up). She was recommended to attend a technical high school, but thanks to her parents' insistence, she continued within an academic stream. She coped easily with the academic demands, but not with the homework obligations. In class, her overenthusiasm and constant talking made her a disturbance. At the age of sixteen years, she was diagnosed with ADHD. At first, she was "angry" about it, as it was not a temporary illness and she had to defend herself constantly against people who think that ADHD is a trendy label. On the

© The Author(s), under exclusive license to Springer Nature   1
Switzerland AG 2022
J. J. S. Kooij, *Adult ADHD*, https://doi.org/10.1007/978-3-030-82812-7_1

other hand, she was happy that the chaos in her head could now improve. Suddenly, there were treatment guidelines, including the drug methylphenidate. She writes about that chaos before treatment, the painful and funny situations that resulted from it. About forgetfulness, being gifted, using drugs, and what it is like to fall in love while having ADHD.

Jacob Klompstra, who was only diagnosed with ADHD at the age of 58 years, also published a book: *Fireworks on the Brain!* After his diagnosis, all kinds of problems from the past fell into place. Not only could he better understand his own behavior, but also life-long conflicts with authority, his physical complaints, burn-out, and the attitude of his family members. His grandfather always commented about him: "How busy that boy is." A life with ADHD turns out to be a busy, turbulent life, from primary school to middle age. Klompstra describes the period after the diagnosis, his "second life," as if he was reborn. By telling his story, he aims to shorten the search for peace and recognition for others with the same disorder (www.watisdiejongendruk.nl).

1.1.1   Short history of ADHD

ADHD symptoms in children were first described by George Still in 1902 (Martinez-Badía & Martinez-Raga, 2005). He named the cluster of inattention, learning difficulties, hyperactive behavior, and impulsivity a "defect of moral control." Even then, he described a chronic course for these symptoms. When Bradley, in 1937, published the positive impact of the stimulant benzedrine on the behavior and learning performance of hyperactive children, it was considered a breakthrough (Strohl, 2011). However, only in the 1960s was there more interest in children with attention deficit and hyperactivity (Sandberg, 1996). The predecessors of Attention-Deficit/ Hyperactivity Disorder (ADHD) include the terms Minimal Brain Damage and Minimal Brain Dysfunction, Hyperkinetic Reaction of Childhood (DSM-II), Hyperkinetic Disorder (ICD-10), and Attention-Deficit Disorder with and without Hyperactivity (ADDH and ADD) (DSM-III). The description of the disorder in classification systems such as the Diagnostic and Statistical Manual of Mental Disorders (DSM) of the American Psychiatric Association (APA), and the International Classification of Disease (ICD) of the World Health Organisation (WHO) improved in response to new insights from research. The reference to an organic cause was omitted when EEG research did not show clear abnormalities. Subsequently, the name changed from Minimal Brain Damage to a description of the characteristic symptoms.

The DSM-IV (APA, 1994) has eighteen criteria for ADHD, nine for attention deficit and nine for hyperactivity/impulsivity. By definition, ADHD begins in childhood and can continue into adolescence and adulthood, possibly with fewer symptoms than in childhood. The cut-off point for ADHD in children is six of the nine criteria for attention deficit, or hyperactivity/impulsivity, or both. In the current diagnostic manual, DSM-5, the cut-off point for adults has been reduced from six to five of the nine symptoms; the age of onset of symptoms has also changed from before the seventh year to before the twelfth year. For more information on the DSM-5 and the changes in the Diagnostic Interview for ADHD (DIVA-5), see Sect. 3.3.

1.1.2 ADHD in Adults in the Netherlands and Europe

Although ADHD in children attracted growing interest from the 1960s onward, it was not until 1993 that a first publication appeared in The Netherlands about the problems of children with ADHD when they reached adulthood (Compernolle, 1993). After these children had outgrown the child psychiatric services, their disorder appeared to persist, but they did not receive treatment in adult psychiatry. ADHD was unknown, there was no experience with stimulants and the fear of addiction to these drugs was high. Patients thus fell between child and adult psychiatry. In 1996, the first publications in Dutch appeared on the validity of the diagnosis and treatment of ADHD in adults (Herpers & Buitelaar, 1996; Kooij et al., 1996). Since then, internationally, the number of publications on ADHD in adults has increased enormously. The author of this book began diagnosing and treating ADHD in adults in 1995. Shortly thereafter, the association Balans, for the parents of ADHD children, referred many adults with ADHD for help, from all over the country. Balans had 10,000 members at the time. This necessitated the establishment of a national network of professionals in 1998, so that patients could be referred back to a practitioner in their own region after treatment. These clinicians were interested in more information about diagnostics and treatment. Courses were developed for them, research was started, and publications appeared (Boonstra et al., 1999; Middelkoop et al., 1997; Kooij et al., 1999, 2001). In 2010, the Network ADHD in adults merged with the Paediatricians' Network ADHD, to form the "ADHD Network" that brought together approximately 700 professionals involved in the care of children and adults with ADHD in The Netherlands. The work of this independent foundation is supported by the contributions of the participants and a number of mental health institutions. For more information about the Network please visit www.adhd-netwerk.nl.

In 2001, the patient association for adults with ADHD and related disorders, Impuls, was founded (www.impulsenwoortblind.nl). In 2002, the first multidisciplinary outpatient department for adults with ADHD was established, at Parnassia in The Hague. This department developed coherent and protocol-based instruments for diagnosis and treatment of ADHD. Simultaneously, the Adult ADHD Expertise Centre, a hive of research and training, was created. This focused on developing, disseminating, and implementing knowledge in Dutch mental health care facilities. Teams and departments were also set up in other locations of Parnassia to treat ADHD in adults. In 2004, the Trimbos Institute in Utrecht developed the first protocol "ADHD in addiction" and invested in training employees of five major addiction care institutions.

This was followed in 2003 by the establishment of the European Network Adult ADHD (www.eunetworkadultadhd.com), which aims to unite researchers and practitioners of adult ADHD in Europe, collaborate in research, disseminate knowledge, improve diagnosis and treatment, and promote access for patients to adequate care in Europe. Similar interest and research activity have emerged in several countries (Asherson et al., 2004; Krause et al., 1998; Rasmussen et al., 2001; Toone & Van der Linden, 1997; Van der Linden et al., 2000). As a result of the establishment of the European Network, the US-based pharmaceutical industries became aware of an interest in treating ADHD in adults in Europe. This was important because patients in most European countries could only be treated with short-acting methylphenidate at the time, and had no alternative medication. At that time, the United States already had ten or so pharmacological treatment options approved. The United States is still at the forefront of the knowledge and development of new and improved drugs, but registration studies in Europe for long-acting medications have led to the licensing of medications that have been specifically studied and tested for effectiveness and safety in adults with ADHD.

1.1.3 ADHD: A Neurobiological Disorder

ADHD is the abbreviation of *Attention-Deficit/Hyperactivity Disorder* and is known as a childhood psychiatric disorder that often persists in adulthood. ADHD occurs in 4–8% of children (Faraone et al., 2003). ADHD used to be known as Minimal Brain Damage because at the time it was assumed that a minor brain damage, which could occur at birth due to lack of oxygen, for example, was the cause. Nowadays, heredity is regarded as the most important risk factor for ADHD. Twin, adoption, and family research demonstrate these findings. 60–80% of the variance for ADHD is explained by genetic factors, as repeatedly shown in research on monozygous twins (Faraone et al., 2005). In identical twins, the concordance is also increased compared to the incidence in the general population (30%), as much as in siblings (Gilger et al., 1992; Sherman et al., 1997). ADHD often runs in families and the cause may be explained both by genetic and by environmental influences, as well as their interaction. Perinatal, short-term hypoxia alone explains the occurrence of ADHD in 2% of cases (Buitelaar, 2002). Unfavorable prenatal factors, such as prolonged oxygen deficiency due to blood loss or a malfunctioning placenta, smoking, and alcohol consumption by the mother during pregnancy, may influence the development of ADHD (Milberger et al., 1997).

Low birth weight, preterm birth, and congenital hypothyroidism are also associated with ADHD (Botting et al., 1997; Millichap, 2008). There is increasing interest in the effect of nutrition on behavior in psychiatric disorders (Lakhan & Vieira, 2008).

Indications for diet therapy may include: insufficient effect or too many side effects of medication, patient preference, and change from an unhealthy diet high in fat and sugars to a healthy diet. An unhealthy diet with an irregular eating pattern is very common in practice. Iron and zinc can be supplemented in case of a proven deficiency, and can increase the effectiveness of treatment with stimulants (Millichap et al., 2012).

The question is often asked whether sugar can cause or exacerbate ADHD. A diet in which sugar is omitted is not, in controlled pediatric studies, associated with a decrease in ADHD symptoms (Arnold, 2001). Another hypothesis is that in children, adolescents, and adults with ADHD, the uptake of nutrients, in particular omega 3, 4, and 6 fatty acids, is different from that in normal controls, or is inadequate. There is some evidence for this faulty uptake. Therefore, even with a healthy diet, a person with ADHD does not absorb enough of these fatty acids (Antalis et al., 2006; Colter et al., 2008; Young et al., 2004). Whether fatty acid supplementation does indeed reduce the symptoms of ADHD has not yet been conclusively shown (Busch, 2007). An extensive Cochrane review of the effects of unsaturated fatty acids in ADHD shows no significant differences between omega 3 and omega 6 fatty acids and placebo (Gillies et al., 2012). A small number of studies do show the effect of the combined omega 3 and 6 fatty acids. More solid research is needed to confirm this. On the other hand, some researchers claim that the omission of certain components from the diet (the so-called elimination diet) has a beneficial effect on ADHD symptoms (Pelsser et al., 2009).

Dutch research in one hundred children with ADHD (and ODD) aged 4–8 years who either received the elimination diet, or continued with their own diet plus healthy dietary advice, showed promising results (Pelsser et al., 2011). In the elimination diet, more and more foods were phased out during the first three weeks, after which the restricted diet had to be maintained for four to nine weeks. If the diet had no effect on ADHD symptoms during the first three weeks (in 41%) it was further restricted to only rice, turkey, vegetables, pear, and water. In 64% of the children ($n = 32$) who followed the study diet strictly, both ADHD and ODD symptoms decreased significantly. The children in the control group with an ordinary healthy diet did not improve. A second phase followed, in which certain foods that were suspected of inducing relapses in ADHD symptoms, were added. Relapse in ADHD/ODD symptoms did in fact occur in nineteen out of thirty children (63%). Some of the children who responded well to the diet also used less medication.

Strengths of the study were the large sample size, the study design, and the fact that several research centers participated. A weak point of the study was that it was uncontrolled: patients and researchers knew who was receiving the elimination diet, which may have increased the placebo response in the group of respondents. Moreover, the research group of motivated parents did not reflect clinical practice. An intriguing scientific question is how exactly food influences the genetically determined disorder of ADHD? For the time being, the direct applicability of the diet is limited for groups other than those studied: small children with highly motivated parents (and teachers). The diet has been described as "complicated and burdensome" and is difficult to maintain for older children and adults with ADHD, where parents play a smaller role. Another problem is the availability of the diet. Replication of the study results in an average patient population compared with a control group, is necessary to determine the added value of the diet. The elimination diet was discussed in a review (Stevenson et al., 2014) and in a meta-analysis of non-pharmacological treatment methods for ADHD, where there were strict inclusion criteria (Sonuga Barke, 2013). These authors found that unblinded research, such as in the elimination diet study, ultimately did not hold up statistically. This implies that the requirements for non-pharmacological research should be as stringent as those for medication studies.

An increasing number of controlled studies in children with ADHD show much lower ferritin levels than controls. This is related to the severity of the disorder(s) (Juneja et al., 2010; Oner et al., 2010, 2012; Donfrancesco et al., 2013; Tan et al., 2011). Ferritin is needed for dopamine metabolism, which could explain the connection with ADHD. There also appears to be overlap between ADHD, Restless Legs Syndrome (RLS), and ferritin levels (Oner et al., 2007). Low ferritin levels in children with ADHD may be related to their sleep problems (Cortese et al., 2009). Iron supplementation in children with ADHD and low ferritin levels appears to promote the effect of stimulants (Calarge et al., 2010). In addition, iron deficiency is associated with cardiovascular problems, and iron supplementation could protect against cardiovascular side effects of stimulants in high-risk groups. However, more research into this is needed (Parisi et al., 2012). In MRI studies, iron levels were also found to be lowered in the left and right thalami in children with ADHD compared to controls (Cortese et al., 2012). The significance of iron and ferritin levels for the pathophysiology of ADHD and comorbidity, as well as for treatment with medication, will have to be elucidated in future research.

Heredity is the most convincing risk factor for ADHD. So-called linkage studies in families with ADHD focus on DNA markers in affected and unaffected family members. Genome wide linkage has been demonstrated repeatedly for chromosomes 5p13, 6q, 7p, 9q, 11 q, 12q, and 17p (Hebebrand et al., 2006) and new links are continually being found (Mick & Faraone, 2008). Molecular genetic research focuses on dysfunction of the dopaminergic and noradrenergic systems in ADHD. Dopamine is believed to stimulate inhibition in ADHD. A genetically controlled, hypodopaminergic neurotransmission is thought to be responsible for the expression of ADHD, possibly in interaction with as yet unexplained environmental factors such as hypertension, smoking, and alcohol consumption in pregnancy. Although the exact genetic transmission is not known, there is increasing clarity about the association of the following genes with ADHD: the dopamine-4 receptor (DRD4, the dopamine-5 receptor (DRD5), the dopamine transporter (DAT1), the dopamine beta-hydroxylase gene (DBH), the serotonergic transporter (5-HTT), the serotonergic receptor (HTR1B), and the synaptosomal associated protein, 25 kDa (WW-25) (Faraone et al., 2005). Each gene contributes only a small part to the risk of the disorder. Genome wide association studies (GWAS) in ADHD have so far found 12 loci with significant associations with ADHD (Demontis et al., 2019). ADHD is a.o. associated with genes for motor problems, such as Restless Legs (Franke et al., 2009; Fliers et al., 2012). Furthermore, so-called rare copy number variants (CNVs), which occur in less than 1% of the population, were compared in children with ADHD and controls. In ADHD, CNVs occurred significantly more frequently, and at the same loci as in autism and schizophrenia (Williams et al., 2012; Stergiakouli et al., 2012).

Current molecular genetic research focuses on the so-called endophenotypes, also known as non-clinical markers of genetic risk. Endophenotypes are at the level between genes and behavior, such as neuropsychological, neuroimaging, or neurophysiological abnormalities with genetic associations (Crosbie et al., 2008; Doyle et al., 2005; 2005; Rommelse et al., 2008).

Deviations in working memory, in the so-called *default-mode network* (DMN) (deactivation or resting state of the brain during tasks), and the dopamine transporter (DAT1) are seen as possible endophenotypes for ADHD. These systems are interrelated. By combining genetic and imaging research with working memory tasks, it became clear that the DAT1 9R allele is associated with adult ADHD compared to controls.

The so-called *dual pathway model* partly explains the neuropsychological heterogeneity in ADHD, i.e., cognitive and motivational deficits can be distinguished that occur in some, but not all, patients. A third factor also seems to play a role: *temporal processing*, but this has yet to be confirmed by more research (Sonuga-Barke et al., 2010).

Genetically controlled, hypodopaminergic neurotransmission is thought to be responsible for the manifestation of ADHD, possibly in interaction with not yet fully clarified environmental factors, such as hypertension, smoking, and alcohol consumption during pregnancy.

1.1.4 Neuroanatomy

Neuroanatomical differences have been found between controls and patients with ADHD. When compared at group level, in children with ADHD, the total brain volume is 4.7% lower than controls, especially in those areas involved in executive function dorsolateral prefrontal cortex, caudate, globus pallidus, and cerebellum (Castellanos et al., 2002; Seidman et al., 2005). In cross-sectional research, boys with ADHD have larger brain volumes than girls with ADHD, but the brain volume of both is below the standards for gender and age. This difference appears to be constant during the development of children between 5 and 19 years of age. Brain size correlates significantly with the severity of ADHD (Castellanos et al., 2002; Castellanos & Tannock, 2002). Boys and girls with ADHD have the same abnormalities in the frontal cortex, basal ganglia, and cerebellar vermis (Castellanos et al., 2001). ADHD children have an inverse asymmetry of the caudate nuclei compared to normal controls: the right part is larger than the left, while normally the left part is larger. This asymmetry is most striking in boys with ADHD and is caused by a smaller left caudate nucleus (Hynd et al., 1993).

The ENIGMA study, comparing brain differences between around 2000 children, adolescents, and adults with ADHD and controls however showed lower surface areas in children, but in the adolescent or adults groups with ADHD no longer surface area nor thickness differences were found (Hoogman et al., 2017). Explanations for this difference between children with ADHD, and adolescents and adults are subject of new research.

Since a smaller basal ganglia volume has been found in both patients with ADHD and in unaffected family members, this finding is thought to be associated with an increased family risk for the disorder. In other research, only boys with ADHD had smaller cerebellar volume, and not their unaffected relatives. This means that the volume of the cerebellum may be directly associated with the pathophysiology of the disorder (Castellanos, 2002; Durston et al., 2004).

1.1.4.1 Neural Connectivity in ADHD

The term connectivity refers to the neural networks between different brain areas. These connections are either increased or decreased in certain brain areas in ADHD compared to controls (Tomasi & Volkow, 2012). There is increased connectivity in the regions involved in reward and motivation, and decreased connectivity in the areas of the default mode network and the dorsal attention networks. This explains why in ADHD, there is limited interaction between control and reward. Research into the myelination and micro-organization of the white matter shows differences between children with and without ADHD: especially in the fronto-striatal area. In this region, changes in the micro-organization may be related to the attentional (dys) function (de Zeeuw et al., 2012).

Structural changes in the volume of different brain areas after treatment with methylphenidate could not be demonstrated in a recent mega-analysis (Hoogman et al., 2017).

1.1.5   Functional Neuroimaging Studies

SPECT and PET studies in children and/or adults indicate hypoperfusion and functional disorders (reduced glucose metabolism) of the prefrontal and premotor cortices and the striatum (Lou et al., 1989; Zametkin et al., 1990). In fMRI-research of eight adults with ADHD compared to controls, the anterior cingulus did not activate bilaterally during a so-called Counting Stroop-task, which measures distractibility. In ADHD patients, another brain area was activated, which correlated with poorer performance on the task (Bush et al., 1999). Furthermore, fMRI research has shown that during a "working memory" task in adults with ADHD, there is reduced neuronal activity compared to normal controls, especially in cerebellar and occipital brain areas (Valera et al., 2005).

In SPECT studies of adults with ADHD, the dopamine transporter (DAT) density in the striatum was 70% higher than in controls (Dougherty et al., 1999; Krause et al., 2000). This may fit the hypothesis of hypodopaminergic neurotransmission in ADHD. This dopamine transmission density appears to be reduced by treatment with methylphenidate—medication for ADHD (Castellanos & Tannock, 2002; Kelly et al., 2007).

In a meta-analysis of 55 fMRI studies in children and adults with ADHD versus controls, dopaminergic hypoactivation was found in ADHD, especially in systems involved in executive functioning (fronto-parietal network) and attention (ventral attention network). Hyperactivation was found in the default, ventral attention and somatomotor networks. In adults, there was also hyperactivation in the visual networks (Cortese et al., 2012).

A review of all MRI studies in children and adults with ADHD compared to controls, shows that in ADHD there are several functional and structural neural network abnormalities, especially fronto-striatal, but also fronto-parietal temporal, fronto-cerebellar, and in the fronto-limbic networks (Rubia et al., 2014a, b). Longitudinal research shows a delayed maturation of the brain in ADHD, abnormalities in the connections between brain parts (connectivity) and in the basal ganglia (Rubia et al., 2014a, b). In the future, these findings may be applied in clinical practice for diagnostic and prognostic classification and/or for "neurotherapy" to adjust abnormalities in brain functions.

In a cross-sectional mega-analysis of neuroimaging studies of 1713 participants with ADHD and 1529 controls aged 4–63 years, where subcortical and intracranial brain volume were analyzed, it was found that brain volumes of the following structures were smaller in ADHD than in controls: nucleus accumbens, amygdala, caudate, hippocampus, putamen, and intracranial volume. Both treatments with ADHD medication or psychiatric comorbidity did not influence these findings (Hoogman et al., 2017).

1.1.5.1   New Neuroimaging Techniques

Structural and functional MRI scans can be used to develop a potential diagnostic test for ADHD. Based on pattern recognition, patients with ADHD can be distinguished from controls or for instance autistic patients. By calculating the number of voXEls in the white and gray matter, ADHD can be accurately differentiated from controls at individual level, in more than 90% of cases. Similar results were also found using this method in schizophrenia, Alzheimer's disease, and depression (Christakou et al., 2013; Klöppel et al., 2008; Koutsouleris et al., 2009; Mwangi et al., 2012). Research with VoXEl Based Morphometry (VBM) of the gray matter has shown that boys with ADHD have a significantly smaller right posterior cerebellum volume than both controls and boys with autism spectrum disorder. This abnormality seems to be able to differentiate ADHD from both other groups (Lim et al., 2014).

If this method is indeed reliable enough to be used as a (differential) diagnostic test, the next question will be the financial feasibility of an individual diagnostic MRI test in clinical practice.

In summary, in ADHD, various brain abnormalities have been found compared to controls: in volume, the degree of activity during certain tasks, connections, and in brain maturation.

1.1.6   Biomarkers for ADHD

The literature contains many experimental studies searching for a biomarker for ADHD. These putative markers range from brain scans, EEGs, neuropsychological tests, the amount of iron in the brain, blood cortisol levels, and heart rate variability. The last two are reviewed here.

1.1.6.1 Cortisol

Cortisol is produced in the adrenal cortex under stress and excreted in the saliva. Cortisol levels show a circadian rhythm. Children with ADHD have a lower level of morning cortisol than children without ADHD. This may be due to a disturbance of the hypothalamic–pituitary–adrenal axis (HPA axis), or to a phase shift (delay) of the circadian rhythm of cortisol release. Stressful events in the fetal or preterm period did not appear to be related to this (Isaksson et al., 2012, 2013). Treatment with methylphenidate or atomoXEtine for six months had no clear influence on the cortisol level (Wang et al., 2014). The relationship between cortisol and expressed parental emotion was compared in children with ADHD and oppositional defiant disorder, and controls. When parents showed negative reactions to an emotionally provocative task, the cortisol level increased in children with ADHD (Christiansen et al., 2010). It appears that cortisol has a different function profile in ADHD children. Less research has been conducted in adults with ADHD: while one study showed no difference in the cortisol response to stress in adults with ADHD compared to controls (Corominas-Roso et al., 2015), another study showed a stronger physiological response to stress in ADHD patients than in controls (even though the baseline values of cortisol did not differ) (Raz et al., 2015).

1.1.6.2 Heart Rate Variability

Heart rate variability in children with ADHD who are as yet unmedicated was compared with controls. The heart rate was higher in children with ADHD than in controls, especially in the afternoon and at night. There seems to be an imbalance of the autonomic nervous system related to the circadian rhythm in ADHD. The increased heart rate could not be explained by activity or comorbidity (Imeraj et al., 2011). In other studies, heart rate variability in children with ADHD compared to controls suggests an increase in parasympathetic nervous system activity (De Carvalho et al., 2014). Heart rate asymmetry also changed in children with ADHD compared to controls (Tonhajzerová et al., 2014). Further research may show the impact of these findings on cardiac health in adulthood, as well as the influence of stimulant treatment on these parameters.

1.1.7 Neurophysiology

Neurophysiological and Event-Related Potential (ERP) studies indicate abnormalities in children with ADHD compared to controls. ERP studies show a smaller N2 and P3 amplitude in both children and adults with ADHD compared to controls. These differences may fit the theory that ADHD is a disorder of inhibition. Methylphenidate normalizes parietal P3 during certain tasks. Attention is also an important factor in ADHD and is necessary for successful inhibition (Bekker et al., 2004, 2005).

ERP research is increasingly focusing on certain executive functions and whether they produce an abnormal ERP response in ADHD. In adults with ADHD, the ERP process of learning, working memory, but also of facial versus non-facial stimuli in the visual oddball task is different from that of controls (Stroux et al., 2016; Thoma et al., 2015; Raz et al., 2015).

In a meta-analysis of EEG research, ADHD has been associated with a relative increase in theta and delta waves, and a decrease in alpha and beta waves. This may fit the idea of underarousal in ADHD and other externalizing disorders. With *higher-density* EEGs and new three-dimensional imaging measures, diagnostic heterogeneity and neurophysiological differences between patients with AD(H)D, and between ADHD and controls can be better distinguished (Loo et al., 2013; Jeste et al., 2015; Rudo-Hutt et al., 2015).

1.1.8   Neuropsychology

Historically cognitive abnormalities in ADHD were primarily regarded as a result of inattention. Other theories describe ADHD as a disorder of motivation, reward, behavioral inhibition, working memory, and overly slow processing of cognitive responses. The variability of performance at different times and in various contexts was also described (Banaschewski et al., 2005; Roessner et al., 2004; Sonuga-Barke, 2002). In recent years, ADHD has increasingly been understood as a disorder of executive function. Executive functioning (EF) is the ability to generate adequate problem-solving capacity in order to achieve a future goal (Pennington & Ozonoff, 1996). There are five domains of EF: *inhibition* (the ability to inhibit or interrupt one's own actions), *set shifting (the ability to* switch to another action or solution to a problem if necessary), *fluency (the ability to generate* different solutions to a problem), *planning (the ability to* plan the steps needed to solve a problem), and working memory (the ability to consult information while performing a task) (Barkley, 1997a).

Executive function cannot explain the full clinical picture of ADHD, and not all individuals with ADHD have executive function disorders, so EF measures are not yet sufficiently reliable as diagnostic tests (Seidman, 2006; Willcutt et al., 2005). In addition, executive dysfunction is not markedly different in ADHD and other psychiatric populations (Boonstra et al., 2005). However, in pediatric research, children with ADHD have EF patterns that distinguished them from children with reading disorders (Marzocchi et al., 2008). Pharmacological studies with methylphenidate in children with ADHD show an improvement in certain executive functions, such as vigilance, short-term memory, reaction time, cognitive impulsivity, and learning (Faraone, 2005).

What is the significance of research into cognitive functions for the diagnosis of ADHD? This question has occupied researchers and clinicians for decades. So far, research has yielded a miXEd picture with varying outcomes. Although at group level, patients with ADHD differ from controls in terms of cognitive functioning, there is no special cognitive test or test profile that is useful for the diagnosis of ADHD. However, a benefit of neuropsychological research is that it can provide a precise description of certain cognitive problems in individual patients prior to treatment. Furthermore, this research can contribute to endophenotyping or bio-marker research in ADHD. At present, neuropsychological research has no specific added value in the diagnosis of ADHD (Lange et al., 2014).

1.1.9 Continuous Performance Test

Various Continuous Performance Tests (CPTs) are available that can objectively measure impulsivity and concentration problems (so-called *commission* and *omission errors*) in ADHD. These include the MOXO, TOVA, CPT, and QbTest. The only test that also measures the hyperactivity of ADHD is the Quantified Behaviour Test (QbTest which uses an infrared camera to record movements of the head during the test (Vogt et al., 2011; Reh et al., 2015). Individual test results are presented visually and compared with standard data. The QbTest can be used as an additional test for the diagnosis and for the evaluation of the medication response and response prediction. The US FDA has recognized the standardized QbTest in 2014 for use in children and adults with ADHD. Research with the QbTest in the elderly with ADHD is ongoing (Bijlenga et al., in preparation). The adult version of the QbTest has a positive predictive value of 84%, a sensitivity of 86%, and a specificity of 83%, as measured in a group of adults with ADHD compared to a norm group from the general population (Edebol et al., 2013). Comparison of scores on the ADHD Rating Scale with the results of the QbTest before and after treatment with medication for ADHD shows that the correlation between both measures is weak. The objective QbTest is significantly more sensitive to medication effects than the Self-report questionnaire (Bijlenga et al., 2015). It seems useful to add a CPT to the therapeutic arsenal for the evaluation of the pharmacological treatment, and possibly for optimal dose titration.

1.2 Prevalence

The prevalence of ADHD in children is estimated at 4–8% (Faraone et al., 2003). Until 1995, ADHD was only diagnosed in child and adolescent psychiatry. It was assumed that ADHD would be outgrown by adulthood. Follow-up studies of children with ADHD have shown that this is usually not the case (Weiss et al., 1985). In a number of patients, the severity of the symptoms did decrease (especially the outward hyperactivity), but in 60% the symptoms remained annoying and in 90% there was still dysfunction in adulthood (Biederman et al., 2000). It seems that ADHD, a genetically determined disorder, does not simply end, but that in adulthood one learns to deal with it more or less successfully. Predictors for an unfavorable chronic course are where ADHD is combined with aggressive behavior at a young age, low intelligence and/or additional learning problems, a positive family history for ADHD, family problems, and poor relationships with peers. In contrast, high intelligence, low comorbidity, and a stable home situation seem to influence the prognosis positively (Biederman et al., 1996, 1996).

The prevalence of ADHD in adults is estimated at 2.5–5%. These figures are based on Dutch population research, research in the United States and research in 20 other countries (Murphy & Barkley, 1996; Kessler et al., 2005, 2006; Kooij et al., 2005; Ten Have et al., 2006; Fayyad et al., 2017). A meta-analysis reported a mean prevalence of ADHD of 2.5% in adults (Simon et al., 2009).

Epidemiological studies among the adult Dutch population using a self-report questionnaire showed that symptoms of ADHD cluster on an individual level, i.e., ADHD symptoms are interrelated. ADHD symptoms were significantly correlated with dysfunction, even after controlling for dysfunction caused by other comorbid disorders. In this study, a conservative estimate of the prevalence of ADHD in adults in The Netherlands came to 1% at a cut-off point of six current criteria and to 2.5% at a cut-off point of four current criteria. ADHD was present until an advanced age (75 years) (Kooij et al., 2005). The cut-off point of four current DSM-IV criteria for ADHD in adulthood proved, after checking for dysfunction and comorbidity, to be the best to differentiate between cases and non-cases. The prevalence figure of 2.5% is therefore probably the most realistic. These data are reasonably similar to those of the ESEMeD study (Ten Have et al., 2006). This study used a new version of the structured interview, the CIDI, which includes a section for retrospective diagnosis of ADHD in adults. An ADHD diagnosis was defined as six symptoms in childhood, and "symptoms still causing significant distress" in adulthood. The prevalence of ADHD in childhood was estimated at 2.9%, and of ADHD in adulthood at 1%. The lower prevalence in adults may have resulted from no cut-off point being for adulthood ADHD.

The first American data were collected by Murphy and Barkley in 1996. Using self-report questionnaires, among a sample of 720 adults renewing their driving license, they found the ADHD prevalence to be 4.7% (Murphy & Barkley, 1996). In 2006, the *National Comorbidity Survey Replication* (NCS-R) among 3199 American respondents aged 18–44 years, found a similar ADHD prevalence of 4.4%. This study had a two-stage design: self-report followed by a structured interview. ADHD was correlated with male gender, divorced status, and unemployment, as well as significant comorbidity, dysfunction, and work absenteeism. Most people with ADHD had not been treated, although they had received help for their comorbid disorders and addictions (Kessler et al., 2005, 2006).

The prevalence of ADHD in children is estimated at 4–8%, and in adults at 2.5–5%.

In epidemiological studies in ten different countries, the prevalence of ADHD in adults was 1.2%-7.3% (average 3.4%). A prevalence of 5% was found in the Netherlands (Fayyad et al., 2007). The last two studies used a self-report questionnaire as well as a structured interview. The results of such studies are probably more reliable than those with self-reporting alone, because of the greater chance of underreporting.

In a US telephone survey of 966 randomly selected adults from the general population, two definitions for ADHD were used: *narrow* (according to DSM-IV criteria) and *broad* (with fewer symptoms than in DSM-IV). The prevalence of narrow ADHD was 2.9% and of broad ADHD 16.4%. Having any form of ADHD was associated with a lower level of education and work. The conclusion was that ADHD symptoms are common and lead to dysfunction, even in those who do not (or no longer) meet all the formal criteria (Faraone & Biederman, 2005).

1.2.1   ADHD in Older People

ADHD is a chronic disorder. As both children and adults with ADHD experience problems, it is to be expected that the elderly population may also suffer from the disorder. In Sweden, the first study on ADHD in older people was conducted 3% had ADHD symptoms in childhood, and they continued to have difficulty with functioning later in life (Guldberg-Kjär et al., 2009). The Dutch population survey (LASA, VUmc Amsterdam) showed that in the elderly over the age of 65 years, ADHD occurs at a prevalence of 2.8–4.2%. The cut-off point used was six out of nine or four out of nine *current* symptoms, and six out of nine symptoms *in childhood* (Michielsen et al., 2012). Elderly people with ADHD had higher levels of loneliness, depression, and anxiety symptoms compared to controls, and poorer physical health. The cognitive differences between elderly with ADHD and controls were mainly due to comorbid depression, not ADHD (Semeijn et al., 2015). Furthermore, the elderly with ADHD were more often divorced and had a lower income. Despite clear dysfunction due to ADHD, most older ADHD patients indicated that they were less disrupted by their ADHD symptoms in old age, because the pressures from work and family life had diminished (Michielsen et al., 2018). An increasing number of older people with ADHD are now seeking help. The next step is to assess the wishes of elderly people with ADHD with regard to treatment, and to focus treatment recommendations on these wishes. The first proposal for a treatment protocol for ADHD in the elderly has been published (Kooij et al., 2016), see also sect. 4.18.

1.2.2   Conclusions

Epidemiological research on ADHD in adults has increased and ADHD is now recognized in the general adult population across several continents. The prevalence varies on the instruments used, cut-off points, and research methods (questionnaire or interview). The consensus prevalence rate is 2.5–5% in adults. ADHD is associated with considerable comorbidity and dysfunction in untreated persons, as is the case in clinical populations. People with a subclinical form of ADHD also function less well. ADHD in adults is underdiagnosed and under-treated in the United States, where most research into this disorder has been done. It is likely that this situation applies equally to other countries.

1.3   Applying DSM Criteria for Children to Adults

The formulation of the criteria for ADHD in the DSM-IV (APA, 1994) posed a problem in determining the prevalence of ADHD in adults, and in the diagnosis of individual patients. These criteria were researched and developed for children aged

4–16 years. It was understandable that criteria that mentioned "climbing excessively" were inappropriate for adults, even though adults with ADHD still report internal restlessness. Since the formulation of the ADHD criteria was specific to children, the chance of underdiagnosis of adults increased. A problem of possible overdiagnosis emerged in children younger than 4 years of age. For them, the criteria were possibly not stringent enough, so that active toddlers could be diagnosed with ADHD too readily (Barkley, 1997b). Adults are in a different life with other demands, compared to children. As a result, attentional difficulties predominate in adulthood. These include disorganization, poor planning, inability to sustain focus, and purpose on tasks, indecision, difficulty with being punctual, tidying up, and prioritizing. Hyperactivity in adults may be rechanneled, compensated for, or internalized. For example, because of extreme restlessness, meetings, where one has to sit still for lengthy periods, are avoided. This inner agitation is compensated for by excessive sports or a hectic job full of variety. Other ADHD adults keep themselves calm by using cannabis, alcohol, or tranquillizers. ADHD adults often attempt to hide their inner restlessness. Symptoms of adult hyperactivity include pressured speech, speaking loudly, or a dominant social presence (Kooij et al., 2001; Millstein et al., 1997). The decrease in outwardly conspicuous hyperactivity with increasing age probably gave rise to the outdated hypothesis that ADHD is outgrown in adulthood.

The person assessing the presence of the DSM criteria also has impact on the diagnosis. Is this an observer report or self-report by the patient? The DSM criteria are intended to assess the behavior of a child by collateral observers, i.e., the parents, teachers, or researchers. When adult patients use the same criteria to evaluate their own behavior (self-report), this can produce a distorted picture. In a group of adolescents who had been diagnosed with ADHD as children, only 3% met the DSM-IV criteria for ADHD using a self-report questionnaire (as investigated by Barkley). When the wording of the questionnaire was adjusted to their age (19 years), this percentage increased to 28%. However, when the same questionnaire was completed by their parents, 58% of the adolescents now met the criteria! Adolescents tend to underreport their symptoms when using the DSM-IV criteria in self-report (Barkley, 1997b). This may also be the case for adults, due to the above-mentioned problems with the formulation of the criteria.

Determining how often the DSM criteria occur may also generate ambiguity in questionnaires. The frequency based on the DSM has been formulated as "rarely or never," "sometimes," "often," and "very often." It would be preferable if the frequency were quantifiable and verifiable, for example, formulated as "once a week" or "daily."

Then there is the problem of the definition of remission of ADHD. In the DSM-IV, the cut-off point for ADHD symptoms in childhood was six out of nine characteristics of either attention deficit or hyperactivity/impulsivity, or both. For adolescence and adulthood, no clear conclusion was given about the cut-off point. However, it was stated that there could be fewer than six symptoms and that the diagnosis "ADHD, partly in remission" could be made. This lack of clarity generated uncertainty and doubt about the diagnosis in adult patients and practitioners. Adults could therefore have fewer symptoms than children, but how much less was not defined. Based on scientific research, the cut-off point for adolescents and adults in the DSM-5 was lowered from six to five out of nine for the current symptoms (Biederman et al., 2000; Kooij et al., 2005; Faraone et al., 2000; 2006b; Barkley, 1997a, 1997b).

In Dutch epidemiological studies using a DSM-IV self-report questionnaire for ADHD (*n* = 1800), adults were found to experience significantly more dysfunction from the cut-off point of four symptoms than from three and fewer symptoms. This cut-off point applied to both attention problems and hyperactivity/impulsivity, for different age groups and for both seXEs. Even after monitoring for dysfunction, for example, due to comorbid anxiety or depression, the cut-off point of four ADHD symptoms remained significantly correlated with dysfunction (Kooij et al., 2005). Also in clinical trials with the same DSM-IV self-report questionnaire, the cut-off point of four criteria identified most patients diagnosed with ADHD (Kooij et al., 2008). The self-report questionnaire for attention problems and hyperactivity applied in Dutch research can be found in see section "Instruments for Screening" in Appendix and can be used for screening purposes. The recommendation is to maintain the cut-off point for the retrospective determination of ADHD in childhood at six of the nine characteristics of either attention deficit or hyperactivity/impulsivity, or both; for adulthood a cut-off point of five of the nine DSM-IV criteria has been established on the basis of the DSM-5. Internationally, there is the validated 6-item World Health Organisation Adult ADHD Self-Report Scale (ASRS) (Adler et al., 2006; Kessler et al., 2007), which contains the six best predictive DSM-IV criteria for diagnosing ADHD in adults. The questionnaire has been translated into twelve languages and published on the Internet (www.hcp.med.harvard. edu/ncs/asrs.php). Another questionnaire is Barkley's 9-item questionnaire, which mainly measures executive functions and is not based on the DSM-IV criteria (Barkley et al., 2007).

Researchers advocate not only determining the number of symptoms, but also at the level of dysfunction when diagnosing ADHD. This does justice to the definition of a disorder: even if there are symptoms, a disorder cannot be said to exist without dysfunction. In adults with ADHD, fewer symptoms do not appear to be associated with better functioning (Biederman et al., 2000).

1.3.1   How Hard Is the Age of Onset Criterion?

Doubts existed both about the reliability of hindsight memories. How valid is determining the exact age of onset of the symptoms and how important is it for the validity of the diagnosis (Applegate et al., 1997; Barkley & Biederman, 1997; Faraone, Biederman, Doyle et al., 2006; Faraone, Biederman & Mick, 2006; Faraone, Biederman, Spencer et al., 2006)? The DSM-IV stated that the symptoms of ADHD must have started in childhood, and that "some symptoms were present before the age of seven." This required onset before the seventh year was never validated in research. It was included in the criteria because it allowed the most hyperactive children to be identified for scientific research (hyperactivity begins early). However, in studies of children with an age of onset before and after the seventh year, there appeared to be no difference in severity, course, or response to medication (Applegate et al., 1997; Barkley & Biederman, 1997; Hesslinger et al., 2003). Moreover, the criterion erroneously excluded 43% of patients with only attentional problems (ADD) who were diagnosed only later, because of dysfunction in the context of high school and homework (Willoughby et al., 2000). In comparison, the percentage of missed diagnoses was 18% for the combined type of ADHD. In other studies, differences and similarities were investigated between 127 adults with early-onset ADHD (before age of 7 years) and in 79 cases, later-onset ADHD (after age seven, but before age of 12 years). Both groups had similar patterns of psychiatric comorbidity, dysfunction, and ADHD symptoms in the family history, confirming the validity of a later age of onset. The conclusion is that the DSM-IV criterion that "some symptoms (be) present before the seventh year" is too stringent (Faraone et al., 2006c). For adults, who had to be diagnosed retrospectively, the criterion led to underdiagnosis due to difficulty recalling childhood symptoms. For this reason, in the DSM-5, the age of onset of symptoms has been extended to the twelfth year (www.dsm5.org).

1.3.2   Late-Onset ADHD

Three recent longitudinal population studies have shaken the foundations of the ADHD diagnosis, in particular the criterion of age of onset in childhood. There appears to be a form of ADHD with a later onset, *after* the twelfth year. First, a cohort study followed more than 1000 children from New Zealand for 38 years. As was expected, ADHD occurred in 6% of the children, particularly in the boys. ADHD was associated with comorbidity, neurocognitive problems, genetic predisposition, and limitations in adult functioning. In adults, as expected, ADHD occurred in 3% (in equal numbers of men as women). ADHD in adulthood was associated with substance abuse, functional disability, and treatment interventions. What was unexpected is that the group with childhood-onset and the adult ADHD group hardly overlapped: 90% of adults with ADHD did not have onset in childhood. The adult group had no evidence of neurocognitive problems in childhood or adulthood, and there appeared to be no polygenic risk for ADHD in childhood (Moffitt et al., 2015).

The second study comes from England, in which 2232 twins were followed for more than 20 years. Two-hundred and forty-seven persons had ADHD as children; of these, 54 (21.9%) still had ADHD at the age of 18 years. Persistent ADHD was associated with greater severity of ADHD and lower IQ. At the age of 18 years, this group had more limited functioning in various areas, more generalized anxiety and behavioral disorders, and dependence on cannabis than those who no longer met the criteria for ADHD. 112 out of 166 persons (67.5%) with adult ADHD did not meet the criteria for ADHD at any time during childhood and appeared to be a late-onset group. They had fewer behavioral problems and a higher IQ in childhood compared to the group with persistent ADHD. However, in adulthood, their symptoms of

ADHD, disability, and comorbidities were similar to those of the group with early-onset ADHD (Agnew-Blais et al., 2016).

The third study is from Brazil. It followed more than 5000 children until the age of 19 years. Almost 9% had ADHD at the age of 11 years, and 12% at the age of 18 years, but this group did not have a childhood onset. Childhood-onset ADHD was more common in boys, while young adults with ADHD were more likely to be women. Both groups were dysfunctional, for example, had more accidents, criminal activity, convictions, suicide attempts, and comorbidities. Seventeen percent of children with ADHD were diagnosed as adults, and only 13% of young adults with ADHD were also diagnosed in childhood.

In these studies, ADHD tends not to persist after childhood onset. There appear to be at least two different syndromes with their own developmental path. ADHD may have a much more heterogeneous course than previously assumed. Further research into genetic differences and treatment response is needed (Caye et al., 2016). If the data turn out to be reliable and applicable to clinical populations, this might change our view of ADHD as a neurodevelopmental disorder. However, since the DSM-5 has changed the age of onset from some symptoms before age of 7 years, to several symptoms before age of 12 years, many individuals may no longer qualify for this "late-onset ADHD." On the other hand, there might be a small group in whom late onset is applicable (Chandra ea. 2021).

1.4   Prevention and Presentation of ADHD in Men and Women

Epidemiological research in adults indicates an equal gender distribution in ADHD (Kooij et al., 2005; Murphy & Barkley, 1996; Ten Have et al., 2006) or a small predominance for men (Kessler et al., 2005). This is different from population research among children, where boys are in the majority (Buitelaar, 2002). In clinical populations, boys are referred for help more frequently than girls. Girls are probably underdiagnosed. Explanations for this are that ADHD in girls is less well known to GPs and other care providers, and that girls are relatively more likely to have the inattentive presentation, with only attention problems (also known as ADD). This form causes less disruption and is, therefore, less commonly referred for treatment. The third explanation is that girls have a different pattern of comorbidity, with anxiety and depression at the forefront, while boys show more oppositional and aggressive behavioral disorders (Biederman et al., 1999, 1994, 2002; Ratey et al., 1995). The behavioral disorders in boys are so disruptive that teachers and parents are more inclined to seek help for boys, as opposed to the quiet, withdrawn girls with attention problems.

The inattentive mode of presentation (ADD occurs twice as often in girls as in boys, although the combined mode of presentation ADHD is most frequently observed in girls (Biederman et al., 2002). The diagnosis "ADHD, inattentive presentation mode" is missed in 50% of the cases in children, while only 5% of the hyperactive presentations are missed. Attention problems alone tend not to cause dysfunction until puberty, when the demand for school and homework require increased attention and concentration. In addition, attention problems alone produce a vaguer clinical picture, namely learning difficulties and general underperformance. These children are described as "having the know how inside, but it doesn't come out." A boy with only attention problems is referred for treatment less often than a boy with the hyperactive variant of ADHD, but still more often than a girl with ADD. The reason that boys with ADD are recognized more often than girls may be related to higher societal expectations of boys (Quinn & Nadeau, 2004; Quinn & Wigal, 2004). As long as teachers, parents, and social workers are not familiar with the more subtle presentation of girls with ADHD, the diagnosis will continue to be missed and girls will not receive timely help.

1.4.1 Link between ADHD and CFS

Research into chronic fatigue syndrome (CFS), which occurs four times more frequently in girls than in boys, has revealed a possible link between ADHD and ADD. Girls with CFS have brothers with ADHD significantly more often and perform just as poorly as their brothers on certain attention tasks (Van de Putte, 2006). One explanation is that having chronic attention problems is extremely tiring because of the continuous mental effort that is necessary for daily tasks. As ADHD runs in families, the chronic fatigue in the sisters of boys with ADHD can also be interpreted as a consequence of long-standing attention problems.

A patient who reports a primary complaint of fatigue to the GP, is usually investigated for a somatic cause, where CFS can be diagnosed. It is possible that chronically tired girls with attention problems end up here, instead of in child psychiatry. The mothers of these girls are more likely to report the fatigue to the GP, rather than the more subtle attention problems. More research into this hypothesis is needed: if these girls indeed have AD(H)D, a new treatment option may be appropriate for them.

In a group of 158 adults with CFS, 30% received an ADHD diagnosis in childhood, and another 20% as adults. Those with ADHD and CFS had more and more severe anxiety and depression, and a higher risk of suicide. Their fatigue was more severe than the average in CFS (Sáez-Francàs et al., 2012).

In a study of adult CFS patients, about 20% responded well to a trial treatment with methylphenidate (Blockmans et al., 2006; Valdizán Usón & Idiazábal Alecha, 2008; Young & Redmond, 2007).

1.4.2 ADHD and Comorbidity in Boys and Girls

Research in 140 boys and 140 girls with ADHD compared to controls, showed no difference in ADHD severity between boys and girls.

Girls with ADHD differed as much from control group girls like boys with ADHD differed from male controls. Although girls, like boys, usually had the

Table 1.1 Differences in comorbidities in girls and boys with ADHD (Biederman et al., 2002)

	Girls (n = 140)	*Boys (n = 140)*	
Any behavioral disorder	36%	66%	$(p < 0.001)$
• Conduct disorder	8%	21%	
• Oppositional defiant disorder	35%	66%	
Depressive disorder	15%	29%	$(p = 0.001)$
Multiple anxiety disorders	33%	28%	
Substance abuse or dependence	6%	2%	$(p = 0.004)$
Tic disorder	15%	16%	
Enuresis	25%	32%	
Anorexia	1%	0%	
Bulimia	1%	0%	

combined presentation ADHD, girls were more than twice as likely to have the ADD presentation. Compared to boys with ADD, the ADD girls were less likely to have behavioral and depressive disorders and learning difficulties. Girls were slightly more likely to have comorbid anxiety disorders (particularly panic disorder) and significantly more likely to have substance abuse or dependence. The latter was an unexpected finding (Biederman et al., 2002). See also Table 1.1.

1.4.3   ADHD and Comorbidity in Men and Women

In a study of 128 adults with ADHD (78 men and 50 women) and controls, patients with ADHD were found to have more comorbidities than controls. Patients with ADHD also had a lower socioeconomic status than their peers. The patterns of comorbidity and cognitive functioning in adults with ADHD were similar to those of children with the disorder. The comorbid disorders in men and women with ADHD were similar. However, women were less likely to have behavioral disorders than men, just as is found in girls and boys with ADHD. Women and men with ADHD had similar prevalences of substance abuse, dependence, anxiety, and depression. Both were found to have the same levels of dysfunction: psychosocial (more often divorced), cognitive, and academic (learning problems, needing tutoring, failing the year more often). However, men had received special education more often, probably caused by the higher prevalence of behavioral disorders (Biederman et al., 1994). These data are broadly consistent with the patterns of comorbidity in boys and girls with ADHD and support the validity of the diagnosis in adults.

Dutch research in a population of 141 adults with ADHD performed at a general psychiatric outpatient clinic found double the number of men compared to women. Their presenting complaints, ADHD symptoms, functioning in work and relationships and axis I and axis II DSM-IV diagnoses were recorded. There were more similarities than differences between the men and women with ADHD (Table 1.2). ADD, (or ADHD, predominantly inattentive presentation type) was present in 10% of both seXEs. With respect to the differences, men had a higher prevalence of perinatal complications, previous childhood diagnosis of MBD, or ADHD, repeating a

Table 1.2 Clinical characteristics and gender differences in a population of adults with ADHD ($n = 141$)

	% Women	% Men
Psychiatric history	90%	90%
Help seeking in childhood	50%	50%
Depression	70%	70%
Anxiety disorder	80%	60%
Substance abuse	8%	30%
Perinatal complications	24%	42%
Motor clumsiness in childhood	60%	60%
MBD diagnosis in adolescence	2%	19%
Bullied at school	50%	50%
Repeating a grade at school	20%	38%
Sexual abuse by a family member	25%	1%
Work problems	50%	50%
Relationship problems	60%	60%
Presentation type of ADD	10%	10%
Comorbid disorder on axis I	78%	78%
Comorbid disorder on axis II	40%	40%
Antisocial personality traits/disorder	2%	42%
Borderline personality traits/disorder	28%	3%

grade at school, substance abuse, and antisocial personality disorder. Childhood sexual abuse, concomitant anxiety, and borderline personality disorder were more common in women. In both men and women, it took an average of 12.5 years before the diagnosis of ADHD was made (Kooij et al., 2001).

With respect to the differences, men had a higher prevalence of perinatal complications, previous childhood diagnosis of MBD or ADHD.

Underdiagnosis of girls has far-reaching consequences for their development into adulthood. Untreated girls live with their symptoms for longer. This increases their chance of a lower level of education and job grade than for boys, who receive treatment. Women tend to have low self-esteem because of their many work and relationships failures. Their difficulties with executive function make them more dependent on others: first on teachers, later on their partners. The combination of work, family, and household is often too difficult for them to manage Chronic underperformance in the workplace increases the chance of being fired or retrenched. Women with untreated ADHD often have a negative memory of their youth (Quinn & Wigal, 2004). Women in the family tend to be the organizational hub, so ADHD symptoms such as difficulty with organization and planning may lead to chaos in the household with consequences for all family members.

Boys and men with ADHD are hyperactive and impulsive, behavior that is immediately noticed and disruptive to the environment. Comorbidities in boys and men are externalizing behaviors, in the form of oppositional defiant and aggressive disorders; later the cluster B personality disorders. This behavior is often a reason for referral and treatment. Men with ADHD may have the advantage of external scaffolding, in the form of a secretary at work or a supportive partner at home. Owing to differences in socialization between men and women, these men are relieved of the responsibility of household administration, housework, childrearing, and maintaining social contacts.

1.5   Core Symptoms of ADHD

The core symptoms of ADHD are inattention or poor concentration, hyperactivity or (inner) restlessness, and impulsive behavior. See Table 1.3 for examples. In adults, attentional and organizational problems are usually more prominent than in

Table 1.3 Core symptoms of ADHD in adults

Core symptoms	Appearance
ATTENTION ISSUES	Quickly distracted and bored
	Difficulty finishing things
	Moving from one activity to another
	No overview of main and side issues
	Poor ability to plan, organize and make choices
	Only be able to read for a short time, can concentrate only when the subject is of great interest
	Difficulty listening, absorbing information
	Losing oneself in detail or being overly precise
	Endless procrastination
	Difficulty filling in forms, understanding instructions, remembering things
	Doubtfulness
	Forgetfulness
	Losing possessions often
	Being chaotic
	Temporary overconcentration or hyper-focus
HYPERACTIVITY	Difficulty sitting still
	Always busy
	Always having to move around
	A feeling of inner restlessness
	Fidgeting
	Not being able to relax in a quiet way
	Incessant talking
IMPULSIVENESS	Blurting things out
	Interrupting others
	Being impatient
	Doing things without thinking (spending too much money, gambling, stealing, impulsive eating, etc.)
	Impulsively starting or breaking relationships and jobs
MOOD CHANGES AND TANTRUMS	A "short fuse"
	Rapidly changing moods in the event of a setback, up to 5 times a day
	(for mood changes, see also Sect. 2.14.5.1)

children. In children, hyperactive and impulsive behavior is particularly noticeable. Adults are expected to be able to manage their own agenda, appointments, time, and money, in contrast to children. Support is more often provided to children by parents and teachers. Many intelligent children with ADHD only present clinically when their external structure disappears, they move out of home and become independent. Then "suddenly," their lack of overview and difficulty with planning lead to problems. Such a presentation may be explained by latent AD(H)D.

Many children and adults with ADHD also suffer from mood changes and irritability. Approximately three-quarters of patients have one or more disorders in addition to ADHD, particularly behavioral, sleep, anxiety, and mood disorders. These, too, often have a lifelong course.

1.5.1   Attention Problems

There is some confusion about the nature and course of the attention problems in ADHD. It is not true that a person with ADHD can never concentrate. Attention can be maintained in the short term when starting a new or interesting task (hobby, computer game, important conversation). Poor attention predominates in boring or routine tasks that require prolonged concentration, such as administration, reading instructions or mail, filling in forms or tax returns, organizing the household, planning tasks, or the time necessary for travel.

People with inattention (but no hyperactivity or impulsivity) are often slow in thinking and formulating ideas. After all, this requires attention and therefore effort. Their cognitive style may be broad and associative in nature. During the diagnostic examination, they are indecisive when answering questions. For example, they cannot decide whether or not a symptom is present, or what is most common. They tend to lose themselves in irrelevant details and cannot see the big picture. They may focus on the rare moments when they are productive and ignore the glaring problem. This problem in having an overview appears to be part of the attention disorder and can make it difficult to make the diagnosis.

Investigating inattention requires patience on the part of the researcher. If the investigator insists on a brief and concise reply, the patient replies that this is impossible. The answer can only be given in one way: telling the whole story with its ramifications. Without this, it would seem that the patient would lose the storyline. Some patients show irritation when interrupted. The clinician should mention in advance that interruptions may be necessary from time to time.

1.5.1.1 Hyper-Focus
In ADHD there is also a form of overconcentration or "hyper-focus," where people cannot be distracted from a task. This phenomenon occurs mainly during activities that the patient finds very interesting, such as computer work or surfing on the Internet. It is then possible to continue for hours at a time without a break, in a highly concentrated manner. It is possible that the dynamic Internet environment stimulates hyper-focus and maintains. ADHD is therefore characterized by both a

lack of attention and periodic overconcentration. The concentration problem in ADHD seems to involve the inability to focus and to give attention appropriately.

The problem is not that a patient with ADHD cannot concentrate, but that he/she cannot concentrate when he/she needs to.

Those around the patient notice the difference in concentration during various activities, but do not understand the cause. This often leads to incomprehension from family, colleagues, and professionals. Patients are accused of being lazy or unmotivated. Or told, "you can do it, if you want to!" Unfortunately, this is incorrect; simply wishing it is not enough to stimulate and sustain concentration.

1.5.2   Hyperactivity

The degree and form of hyperactivity in adults is also misunderstood, because adults are not restless in the same way as children. Agitated and hyperactive adults with ADHD do exist, but for a large group, restlessness is more subtle and takes other forms. Examples of hyperactivity may include: fidgeting, rocking on a chair, frequently getting up from a chair, being unable to sit still for more than five or ten minutes, pacing, talking incessantly, fiddling with everything within reach, finding an office job intolerable due to restlessness, throwing things around or knocking them due to excessive movements, and finally, restless sleep.

If an adult patient sits quietly (and attentively) during the examination interview, many novice professionals do not consider ADHD. This is incorrect. Targeted questions will reveal how the patient usually feels and behaves. A first impression should not be decisive.

Sitting quietly during the examination interview does not rule out hyperactivity.

Hyperactivity in adults manifests as inner restlessness, a feeling of continuous agitation, not being able to relax or needing alcohol or drugs to relax or sleep (Weisfelt et al., 2001). Hyperactivity can always be compensated for by eXErcise, up to five times a week. Strain injuries may result as the body does not have time to recover. If this outlet valve for the restlessness disappears, the hyperactivity often becomes more obvious and annoying. Hyperactivity also manifests as endless talking, an inability to stop activities, or rambling on or on. ADHD is also described as a condition where "the brake is off." This is recognized by many patients with hyperactivity.

1.5.3   Impulsivity

Together, hyperactivity and impulsivity form one symptom domain in the DSM-IV; the attention problems belong to the other domain. Restlessness and impulsivity often occur together in the same person, but this is not always the case. Attention problems and impulsivity may also be more prominent. Impulsive behavior means doing something without thinking. It manifests as blurting things out, spending too much, diving into projects, suddenly quitting jobs, starting relationships rapidly, and not being able to postpone self-gratification. This behavior has consequences for intimate relationships, at work with employers, as well as financially. Blurting things out creates conflict. Tact and diplomacy are usually not the strong points of the impulsive person Impulsive eating binges may be a technique to counter agitation or result from an inability to delay gratification. This explains the overweight status in ADHD. Some patients admit to eating sugar to promote concentration (transiently).

Impulsivity is the inability to inhibit an unwanted action, so it has also been termed inhibition deficiency.

Closely related to impulsivity is "sensation seeking" or "novelty seeking," the search for excitement. This manifests itself in the need for new experiences with intense emotional sensations, variety, and thrill. Concrete examples include: being drawn to accidents or fires, speeding, taking risks in traffic or with sexual contacts, starting fights, creating an environment with excitement and variety, often changing jobs or partner. Some sensation seekers choose professions that provide this, for example, journalism, start-up business, or a job that requires frequent travelling.

Interestingly, this trait appears to be genetically determined and is associated with the so-called 7-repeat allele of the dopamine-4-receptor gene, also involved in ADHD.

1.6   ADHD Seldom Comes Alone: Problems with ADHD and Comorbidity

Someone who has had ADHD since childhood has to deal with the consequences on their schooling, emotional development, performance, promotion prospects, and relationships with others. In addition, a child with ADHD is more likely to experience anxiety, depression, substance abuse, and behavioral disorders than average. This pattern continues in adults. Depression, anxiety disorders, substance abuse, sleep problems (Bekker et al., 2008; Gau et al., 2007), and personality disorders occur more frequently in adults with ADHD (Biederman et al., 1993; Wilens et al., 1994).

In three-quarters of patients with ADHD, one or more other psychiatric disorders are comorbid. In 33% of ADHD adults, two other diagnoses will be made, in addition to ADHD (Kooij et al., 2001). For problems associated with ADHD and typical patterns of comorbidity, see Table 1.4.

1.7   Is ADHD a Disorder?

Regularly, the question is asked whether ADHD is a disorder or whether can also confer benefits, both for the person concerned and for the society (Hartmann, 2010).

People with ADHD are impulsive, like to start something new and creative. People who possess these characteristics to a limited extent, function well in society. A society devoid of such people would be stifled by over regulation, leaving no

Table 1.4 Problems and patterns of comorbidity associated with ADHD

Problems

- Learning difficulties, lower level of education, training not completed
- Difficulty with social contacts, bullied at school
- Financial problems, gambling
- Compulsiveness, perfectionism (often as a coping style for forgetfulness and chaos)
- Accidents, increased mortality (Scott et al., 2017; Dalsgaard et al., 2015)
- Behavioral problems: aggressive behavior, oppositional behavior or conflicts with authority, self-mutilation, suicide attempts
- Sensation seeking: needing excitement (e.g., driving too fast, taking risks, quarrelling, and dangerous sports)
- Violence (Wymbs et al., 2015; Buitelaar et al., 2015)
- Criminal behavior, contact with police or justice (Young et al., 2015; Gaïffas et al., 2014; Dalsgaard et al., 2013)
- Relationship problems (not keeping appointments, forgetful, chaotic)
- Work problems (pace too slow, careless mistakes, conflicts)
- Sleeping problems (late to bed, restless sleep, difficulty getting up) (Kooij et al., 2001b; Van Veen et al., 2010; Kooij & Bijlenga, 2014)

Common comorbidities

- Anxiety (25–40%) (Biederman et al., 1993; Kessler, 2007; Kooij et al., 2001a)
- Depression (20–40%) (Amons et al., 2006; Biederman et al., 1993; Kessler, 2007; Kooij et al., 2001a; Levitan et al., 1999)
- Drug and/or alcohol abuse (9–45%) (Wilens et al., 1994; Wilens et al., 1997; Wilens et al., 2004a, 2004b)
- Behavioral or personality disorders (25% of ADHD children develop a cluster B personality disorder) (Fossati et al., 2002; Weiss et al., 1985; Winkler & Rossi, 2001; Young & Gudjonsson, 2006)

chance for new initiatives. However, for those seeking help in the mental health sector, it is precisely the suffering from the symptoms and a lifelong pattern of failure that stands out. Here, the negative consequences of ADHD dominate and this leads to the request for treatment.

Concentration problems, restlessness, and impulsivity are commonly found in society. The question is repeatedly asked whether identifying such symptoms in large groups of people could lead too easily to the diagnosis of ADHD and the use of stimulants (Buitelaar, 2001). Here, the diagnosis of ADHD is regarded as the medicalization of problems that are due to the demands of our hectic, Western lifestyle. It is suggested that when we return to a "natural" lifestyle with sufficient calm and relaxation, such complaints would disappear by themselves.

Although stress and pressure are likely to increase the symptoms of ADHD, this does not mean that they are also the cause of the disorder. Nor does it mean that if there is no stress (which is impossible), the symptoms would disappear. So, can ADHD symptoms be distinguished from "normal" reactions to stress? Is there an identifiable disorder? Scientific research, especially in child and adolescent psychiatry, has brought more clarity to this question over the past 25 years (Buitelaar and Kooij, 2000).

ADHD is a disorder with symptoms that everyone recognizes from time to time in themselves. For those with ADHD, these symptoms persist for life and they never get a grip on them. The symptoms lead to demonstrable underperformance and dysfunction, something that does not occur in someone with transient symptoms. ADHD is therefore a dimensional disorder where the degree to which the complaints occur determines whether there is a disorder. Epidemiological research has shown that although symptoms of ADHD often occur among the general population, they are not severe enough to diagnose a disorder in that large group. As expected, serious symptoms occur in a minority (Kooij et al., 2005).

On the other hand, applying a broader definition of ADHD (with subclinical symptom levels) in a telephone population survey showed that the group meeting the broad definition had a lower level of education and work, similar to those who met all the ADHD criteria. ADHD symptoms, both subclinical and not, occurred in 16.4% of the group surveyed (Faraone & Biederman, 2005).

In psychiatry, there is no hard division between normal and abnormal behavior. The transition is often gradual. ADHD is also a dimensional disorder. It is not like pregnancy or diabetes, where a simple blood test determines pregnant or not, diabetic or not. In psychiatric disorders, the symptom severity and the suffering they cause can vary. One's work situation, a supportive environment, and compensation by one's partner also determine whether decompensation will occur. For some people suffering from depression, the illness is mild, for others, severe. This also applies to ADHD. Help is only sought where the patient or the support system suffers a great deal from the symptoms. Specifically, there must be evidence of dysfunction.

In general, a psychiatric disorder cannot be said to exist if functioning remains intact. Someone who suffers from concentration problems, but without problems at school or work, is unlikely to have a disorder, including ADHD.

Of course, it is important that the diagnostician has knowledge of the different manifestations of ADHD, the modes of presentation, comorbidities, and the most common forms of dysfunction in ADHD. It is necessary that the clinician inquires carefully in order to make the best possible assessment. Ultimately, it is this knowledge, together with the information given by the patient and family, that determines whether or not the diagnosis can be made.

Some degree of subjectivity is inevitable in making a diagnosis. Does this present a problem? There is currently no litmus test to demonstrate or rule out any psychiatric disorder with certainty. A combination of the history, the course of the symptoms, the degree of dysfunction, and the family history provides the information that leads to the diagnosis. Perhaps, as knowledge about genetics and brain imaging in various psychiatric disorders increases, diagnostic tests for ADHD will become available in the future.

1.7.1   What Does the Diagnosis of ADHD Mean for the Patient?

People with ADHD have had the symptoms all their lives, by the time of diagnosis, the symptoms have become commonplace Those who suffer from the symptoms may experience the diagnosis as a huge relief. They recognize that they are not "crazy, lazy, unmotivated or stupid," but limited by a disorder that was unrecognized and untreated. Others find it difficult to accept that what they considered an (idiosyncratic) personality trait turns out to be part of a disorder. They may feel hurt by this. Hence paying attention to self-esteem and acceptance of the diagnosis are central in treatment. Experience shows that the positive aspects of ADHD only surface with acceptance of the diagnosis and treatment of the symptoms. After all, it is frustrating to be bursting with ideas, but never finish anything. If medical treatment provides a better overview and planning, this creativity will finally blossom. Such a positive experience stimulates self-esteem and self-confidence the most.

1.8   Morbidity and Mortality in ADHD

Morbidity and mortality are both increased in ADHD. As discussed in sect. 1.6, ADHD is frequently accompanied by other psychiatric disorders. Physical conditions that are more common in ADHD include asthma, allergies, and injuries due to accidents (e.g., dog bite injuries, burns, road traffic accidents). Lifestyle also makes a significant contribution (e.g., the consequences of a fast paced, impulsive life: smoking, alcohol and drug abuse, irregular eating and sleeping habits, poor dental hygiene, sexually transmitted diseases, teenage pregnancies, abortion, avoiding timely health check-ups) (Mitchell et al., 2003; Leibson et al., 2001; Nielsen et al., 2017). The risk of suicide is increased in ADHD, especially in the combined presentation, which is probably related to impulsivity (Murphy et al., 2002). Furthermore, in the case of a comorbid mood disorder, addiction, or antisocial personality disorder, the risk of suicide is increased (Barkley & Fischer, 2005; Biederman et al., 2008; Semiz et al., 2008; Young et al., 2003).

In a large population cohort study, after correction for behavioral and substance abuse disorders in children, adolescents, and adults with ADHD, the risk of premature death. It was striking that the risk was higher for girls and women with ADHD than for boys and men (Dalsgaard et al., 2015).

As ADHD runs in families, adults with ADHD may have children with the same condition, so that the risks and problems multiply.

1.9   Costs of ADHD during the Life Course

The social and health care costs of children with ADHD are estimated to be twice as high as those of children without a disorder (Leibson et al., 2001; Chan et al., 2002). These costs are based on significantly more outpatient treatments, admissions, and first aid visits. Undiagnosed and untreated ADHD leads to inefficient use of health care and to less favorable outcomes. As a result, failure to make a diagnosis contributes to an increase in costs. The costs of ADHD in adolescents and adults are increasingly being investigated. Research focuses on the toll of incomplete education, psychosocial problems, addiction, needing psychiatric help and risk-taking behavior. These problems affect work performance, absenteeism, medical visits, traffic and other accidents, and crime (Bernfort et al., 2008; Birnbaum et al., 2005; Matza et al., 2005).

Adults with ADHD appear to graduate less often than controls, to work full-time less frequently (34% versus 59%), and to earn significantly less. Based on these findings, the cost of lost work productivity associated with ADHD was estimated at $67 to $116 billion (Biederman & Faraone, 2006).

In studies of the insurance claim registers, children, adolescents, and adults with ADHD are 1.7 times more likely to have accidents than controls. In adults especially, the costs of these claims have increased (Swensen et al., 2004). Research has estimated the costs treated ADHD to be $31.6 billion. These costs include: medication, absenteeism reduced productivity, and the impact of ADHD on family members $31.6 billion. Of this amount, $1.6 billion was for the treatment of ADHD, $12.1 billion was for their other health care costs, $14.2 billion was for the health care costs of family members, and $3.7 billion was for the loss of labor productivity of both patients and their families (Birnbaum et al., 2005).

The health economic impact of ADHD was calculated among employees of a large company. ADHD occurred in 1.9% of employees. The employees with ADHD worked 4–5% less due to absenteeism, were sick twice as often and had accidents at work twice as often. The estimated costs of this were more than $4000 per employee with ADHD, per year. Only a small proportion of these employees were in treatment. It would be interesting to conduct studies into the cost-effectiveness of the treatment of ADHD (Kessler et al., 2008).

1.9.1   Cost-Effectiveness

Cost-effectiveness focuses on the relationship between the benefit that a treatment brings to the patient and its cost. From a societal point of view, pharmacotherapy is cost-effective, i.e., there is a proven good efficacy at a relatively low cost (Faraone et al., 2010; Frederiksen et al., 2013). In children and adolescents, there is evidence that pharmacological treatment is cost-effective compared with no treatment or behavioral therapy, in adults there is yet limited evidence (Gilmore et al., 2001; Frederiksen et al., 2013; Ornoy et al., 2019; King et al., 2006; Narayan et al., 2004; Zupancic 1998; Donelly et al., 2004; Wu et al., 2012). It is complex to create a single model of cost-effectiveness because of the varying pharmacotherapies, their dosages and costs; different health care systems in the countries studied; and because inclusion criteria for costs differ amongst studies.

Research among Dutch children with ADHD (average age 11 years) shows that the social, medical, and non-pharmacological costs are lower for medicated child responders than for non-responders (Van der Kolk et al., 2015). This means that treatment response has considerable societal benefits. Conversely, not treating ADHD generates enormous costs for society (Maia et al., 2015; Le et al., 2014).

Diagnostics

2

2.1 Diagnostics: Purpose and Method

The diagnostic phase aims to determine whether the following DSM-5 criteria for ADHD are met:

- Started in childhood (before the twelfth year)
- Are sufficiently serious
- Have been lifelong
- Have caused longstanding dysfunction

The impression a patient makes during the diagnostic interview does not confirm or invalidate the diagnosis The results of mental state examination are also not definitive. Adults with ADHD can transiently show increased alertness and focus because of the stress caused by the diagnostic interview. A thorough clinical history gives a definite answer as to whether the criteria for ADHD are met.

When diagnosing ADHD in adulthood, if possible, the patient's partner, parents, or family members are interviewed in addition to the patient. The diagnosis is based on the patient's and collateral description of the current symptoms, (dys)function in education, work, and relationship(s). All sources should be questioned about the symptoms and functioning in childhood.

2.2 Screening

People who wish to know whether they have ADHD symptoms or possibly meet the criteria for the diagnosis, can fill in a short screening list online and receive feedback about the risk of ADHD. A more extensive screening tool (self-report questionnaire for attention problems and hyperactivity) has been used in epidemiological and clinical research in the Netherlands and is included as an appendix at the end of this book (see section "Self-report questionnaire on attention problems and

© The Author(s), under exclusive license to Springer Nature Switzerland AG 2022
J. J. S. Kooij, *Adult ADHD*, https://doi.org/10.1007/978-3-030-82812-7_2

hyperactivity for adulthood and childhood" in Appendix) (Kooij et al., 2004; Kooij et al., 2005). Research has shown that this self-report questionnaire has comparable validity to two of the most commonly used American screeners, the Conners Adult ADHD Rating Scale (CAARS) and the Brown Attention Deficit Disorder Scale (BADDS) (Kooij et al., 2008). Short and longer versions of the CAARS, which measures the DSM-IV criteria, and versions for patients and family members are available (Conners, Erhardt, & Sparrow, 1999). The BADDS does not measure the DSM criteria, but rather, executive function in attention and organization. A disadvantage of the BADDS is that there are no items for hyperactivity/impulsivity (Brown, 1996). The six-item Adult ADHD Self-Report Screener (ASRSv1.1) developed by the World Health Organization (WHO), has been validated and is available online in several languages (www.hcp.med.harvard.edu/ncs/asrs.php) (Adler et al., 2006; Kessler et al., 2007). Russell Barkley developed a nine-item screening tool for ADHD in adults, based on executive dysfunction (Barkley, Murphy, & Fischer, 2007).

A screening instrument is very useful when ADHD is suspected, to determine whether further investigation is necessary. However, screeners are not diagnostic tools, which is why further questioning is always advised when results are positive.

2.2.1   Ultrashort Screening List for ADHD in Adults

General practitioners and other care providers who wish to examine a patient briefly for the core symptoms of ADHD can ask the following four questions:

1. Do you generally feel restless?
   (e.g., *rushed, fidgety, have difficulty in sitting still, doing excessive sports, or being agitated*)
   Yes/No
2. Do you generally do things first and then think about the consequences?
   (*e.g., blurting things out, overspending, or being impatient*)
   Yes/No
3. Do you generally have concentration problems?
   (*e.g., easily distracted, not finishing things, rapidly becoming bored, forgetful, or chaotic*)
   Yes/No
   If the answer to question 1 and/or 2 and/or 3 is yes:
4. Have you always had this?
   (*as long as you can remember, or for most of your life*)
   Yes/No

If the answer to question 4 is yes, further consider the diagnosis of ADHD.

This questionnaire has not been validated in research, but does cover the DSM-5 criteria for the diagnosis: the three core symptoms of restlessness/ hyperactivity, impulsivity, and concentration/ attention problems. A symptom should have been present from childhood, not simply intermittently. These 4 questions cover the 3 clinical presentations of ADHD. The screener demonstrates that the core of ADHD is its chronicity, not so much the presence of one or more symptoms.

The core of ADHD is not so much the presence of one or more symptoms as its chronicity.

The diagnosis of ADHD can be confirmed using the Self Report Questionnaire for attention problems and hyperactivity in childhood and adulthood (see section "Self-report questionnaire on attention problems and hyperactivity for adulthood and childhood" in Appendix) and/or the Diagnostic Interview for ADHD (DIVA).

2.2.2   Diagnostics

The diagnosis of ADHD can be confirmed using the semi-structured Diagnostic Interview for ADHD (DIVA-5, formerly DIVA 2.0) (Kooij & Francken, 2007a) (see also Sect. 3.3). While DIVA 2.0 was based on the DSM-IV criteria, the updated DIVA-5 is based on the DSM-5 criteria. DIVA 2.0 was validated in Spanish and Swedish studies (Pettersson et al., 2017; Ramos-Quiroga et al., 2016), and DIVA-5 is increasingly used in research.

The DIVA-5 gives concrete examples of each DSM-5 criterion, both for childhood and for adulthood. This makes it easier for the patient and family to recognize the symptoms in the different stages of life. Like the Conners Adult ADHD Diagnostic Interview (CAADID), the DIVA is based on the DSM criteria in adulthood and childhood (Epstein, Johnson, & Conners, 2001; Epstein & Kollins, 2006). As a result, the structure of the DIVA resembles that of the CAADID. However, the examples of each criterion in both phases of life and the extensive discussion of dysfunction in five areas, giving concrete examples, diverge from the CAADID. No DSM-5 version of CAADID has yet been published. The DIVA has been translated into several languages and can be downloaded at minimal cost from www.diva-center.eu.

If the diagnosis of ADHD is made, further research into possible comorbidity should follow, as well as treatment advice.

2.3   DSM-5 Criteria

According to the DSM-5 (APA, 2013), the diagnosis of ADHD requires:

- Several symptoms (not necessarily all) started before the twelfth year.
- As a child, six of the nine attention problems *and/or* six of the nine hyperactive/ impulsive characteristics were met. This *and/or* means that there are three possible ways of presenting ADHD: with six of the nine characteristics of attention deficit only, with six of the nine characteristics of hyperactivity/impulsivity only and with six of the nine characteristics of both attention deficit and hyperactivity/ impulsivity.

- Dysfunction at home, at school or at work, with friends or family, in other activities.
- A continuous persistent pattern of symptoms and dysfunctions until the present.
- Five of the nine characteristics of attention deficit and/or hyperactivity/impulsivity must be met in adolescence or adulthood.

The DSM-5 was published in 2013. Compared to DSM-IV, the most important changes in the ADHD criteria are:

1. The requirement that the complaints should start before the seventh year of life was found to be too restrictive for adults, as these symptoms are only diagnosed after childhood. The onset of the complaints is now before the age of 12 years.
2. Certain symptoms and limitations are appropriate for children, but not older patients. The profile of symptoms changes with age. In adults, inattention predominates and symptoms of hyperactivity are often internalized or compensated for by frequent exercise and/or use of alcohol and drugs. Therefore, more examples of typical behavior have been added to the criteria for all ages.
3. The symptoms must be present in two or more areas, and there are extensive examples given: at school, at work, with friends, acquaintances, or elsewhere.
4. Autism is no longer an exclusion criterion for the diagnosis of ADHD, in line with research into the frequent comorbidity of the disorders.
5. The subtypes of ADHD remain the same but are now called "presentation types."

DSM-5 Criteria for ADHD (APA, 2013)
Attention-deficit/hyperactivity disorder

A. A continuous pattern of inattention and/or hyperactivity/impulsivity that interferes with functioning or development, characterized by (1) and/or (2).

1. *Inattention.*
   Six (or more) of the following symptoms of inattention have been present for at least six months to an extent not appropriate to the level of development and which has a direct negative impact on social and school/professional activities. N.B. The symptoms are not merely an expression of oppositional behavior, unmanageability, hostility or inability to understand tasks and instructions. Older adolescents and adults (≥17 years) should have at least five symptoms.
   - Often fails to pay sufficient attention to details or makes careless mistakes in schoolwork, at work, or during other activities (e.g., looks over details or misses them, delivers sloppy work).
   - Often finds it difficult to keep focus on tasks or game activities (e.g., has difficulty staying focused during a lesson or conversation, or when reading a long text).
   - Often does not seem to listen when addressed directly (e.g., seems absent, even if there is no clear distraction).

- Often does not follow instructions and often fails to complete schoolwork, chores, or tasks at work (e.g., starts with a task but quickly gets distracted).
- Often has difficulty organizing tasks and activities (e.g., has difficulty completing a series of tasks in a row; finds it difficult to store supplies and belongings in place; the work is sloppy and disorderly; has difficulty organizing time; fails to meet deadlines).
- Often avoids, has an aversion to, or is unwilling to engage in tasks that require prolonged mental effort (e.g., school assignments or homework; for adolescents and adults: prepare a report, fill in forms, or go through long articles).
- Often loses things needed for tasks or activities (e.g., materials for school, pencils, books, tools, wallet, keys, papers, glasses, and mobile phone).
- Is easily distracted by external stimuli (in older adolescents and adults it may be thoughts of something else).
- Is often forgetful during daily activities (e.g., chores, shopping; in older adolescents and adults, e.g., call back, pay bills, keep appointments).

2. *Hyperactivity and impulsivity.*
   Six (or more) of the following symptoms of hyperactivity and impulsivity have been present for six months to an extent inconsistent with the level of development and which adversely affects social, school, or occupational activities. N.B. The symptoms are not merely an expression of oppositional behavior, unmanageability, hostility, or an inability to understand tasks and instructions. Older adolescents and adults (≥17 years) should have at least five symptoms.
   - Often moves restlessly with hands or feet, or turns in his or her chair.
   - Often gets up in situations where you are expected to stay in your seat (e.g., gets up from his or her seat in the classroom, office or other workplaces, or in other situations where you need to stay in your seat).
   - Often runs around or climbs up everywhere in situations where this is inappropriate (N.B. In adolescents or adults, this may be limited to feelings of restlessness).
   - Can hardly play quietly or engage in relaxing activities.
   - Is often "busy" or "trotting on and on" (e.g., is unable to sit still for a long time or feels uncomfortable, such as in a restaurant, during a meeting; others may find the person concerned restless or difficult to keep up with).
   - Talk excessively often.
   - Often throws out the answer before a question is finished (e.g., finishes other people's sentences; cannot wait for his or her turn during a conversation).
   - Often finds it difficult to wait for his or her turn (e.g., waiting in a queue).
   - Often interferes with or intrudes on others (e.g., interferes in conversations, games, or activities; uses another person's belongings unsolicited and without permission; in adolescents and adults: intrudes on or takes over other people's activities).

B. Several symptoms of inattention or hyperactivity/impulsivity were present before the twelfth year.

C. Several symptoms of inattention or hyperactivity/impulsivity are present in two or more areas (e.g., at school or work, with friends or family members; during other activities).
D. There is clear evidence that the symptoms interfere with, or reduce the quality of social, school, or professional functioning.
E. The symptoms do not occur exclusively in the course of schizophrenia or another psychotic disorder and cannot be better explained by another psychological disorder (e.g., mood disorder, anxiety disorder, dissociative disorder, personality disorder, and withdrawal syndrome).

Coding based on presentation type:

- **314.01 Combined presentation type** If both criteria A1 and A2 have been met during the last six months.
- **314.00 Predominantly inattentive presentation type**. If criterion A1 has been met during the last six months, but not criterion A2.
- **314.01 Predominantly hyperactive/impulsive presentation type.** If criterion A2 has been met during the past six months, but not criterion A1.

Specify
In partial remission: If all criteria have been met in the past, but less than all criteria have been met in the last six months, and the symptoms still cause limitations in social, school, or professional functioning.

Indicate Current Severity

- Light: Hardly any more symptoms than those required for classification are present, and the symptoms only lead to mild impairment of social or occupational functioning.
- Mild: There are symptoms or functional limitations between "mild" and "severe."
- Severe: Many more symptoms than required for classification are present, or several particularly severe symptoms are present, or the symptoms result in obvious impairment of social or occupational functioning.

314.01 Other specified attention-deficit/hyperactivity disorders: If all the criteria are not met (e.g., with too few symptoms of inattention).
314.01 Unspecified attention-deficit/hyperactivity disorder: If all criteria are not met, without further specification.
DSM-5 criteria for ADHD (APA, 2013, 2014).[1]

---

[1] Reproduced and made public with permission of Boom publishers Amsterdam from the *Handbook for the Classification of Mental Disorders (DSM-5)*, © 2014 American Psychiatric Association p/a Boom Publishers, Amsterdam.

2.4   Presentation Types of ADHD

Three presentation types of ADHD are distinguished:

A. *ADHD, combined presentation type.* This is ADHD with all three symptom clusters: Attention deficit, hyperactivity, and impulsive behavior. The combination is the most common in clinical populations. Attention deficit and impulsive behavior seem to change the least over time. Hyperactivity may be present in childhood, but may decrease or become more manageable over time. Many patients without overt hyperactivity still experience continuous inner turmoil or agitation. This restlessness can often be transiently channelled by playing intensive sports.

B. *ADHD, predominantly inattentive presentation type.*
   This is ADHD with only the attention problems, and is also called Attention-Deficit Disorder (ADD). These dreamy, introverted adults are often absent minded. They may be slow, rigid, and doubtful. Sometimes they are perfectionistic or compulsive. They are easily distracted, suffer from fear of failure, and may panic when they lose control. They are not agitated or impulsive. ADD appears to be more common in girls. These patients are unlikely to be diagnosed during childhood. Intelligent patients with ADD can often compensate for their attentional problems for many years.

   High intelligence allows for rapid comprehension of a topic and prolonged periods of concentration are not necessary. This ability can mask underlying ADHD. Only when there are long texts to read or memorize, when the level and pace increase, does the difficulty become apparent. At the university level, the structure of the parental home also falls away, so these people decompensate. It may seem as if the problems with concentration are suddenly emerging and causing new dysfunction. However, careful investigation shows that these problems were previously present.

   A high IQ or a completed university education do not exclude AD(H)D. However, attention problems can be masked for a long period of time by high intelligence.

   Attention problems often seem to be absent during the diagnostic interview. This may be related to the tension that such an interview evokes. It is known that tension or arousal can (temporarily) improve concentration. In AD(H)D patients, "sensation seeking," i.e., looking for excitement and sensation, generates a form of arousal that reduces symptoms.

C. *ADHD, predominantly hyperactive/impulsive presentation type.* This is ADHD with only hyperactivity/impulsivity, and was first described in the DSM-IV. They present as busy impulsive people without attention problems. In clinical samples, this group is the least common. As yet, there is little data on the validity of this presentation type. There may be overlap with the oppositional defiant and antisocial personality disorders. In epidemiological studies, this presentation type is the most common in adult populations (Murphy & Barkley, 1996; Kooij et al., 2005).

2.4.1 Prevalence of Presentation Types

The combined presentation type occurs in a clinical adult population ($n = 141$) in 82%, ADD or the inattentive presentation type in 11% and the hyperactive/impulsive presentation type in a small minority (Kooij et al., 2001a). In children, the combined presentation type is most common in clinical populations (Lahey et al., 1994). Epidemiological populations show a different distribution, where in children, the inattentive presentation is most common (Buitelaar, 2002). It is possible that in clinical populations children with the inattentive presentation type are underrepresented because they are less well recognized. In many cases, hyperactive, disruptive children are more likely to be reported for help by their parents than dreamy children with only attention problems. In epidemiological studies in adults, the hyperactive/impulsive presentation type is most common (Kooij et al., 2005; Murphy & Barkley, 1996).

2.5   Age of Onset of ADHD

The DSM-5 states that ADHD must start before the twelfth year with at least several symptoms of attention deficit and/or hyperactivity/impulsivity, and at least six of nine current symptoms of inattention and/or hyperactivity/impulsivity until age of 17 years. The age of onset criterion "before the seventh year with some symptoms" from the DSM-IV has been abandoned on the basis of research showing that there is no difference in severity of symptoms, dysfunction, or comorbidity with onset before and after the seventh year (Barkley, 1997b; Applegate et al., 1997). Age of onset before 12 years does justice to people with the inattentive form of ADHD, in which dysfunction often only becomes apparent in adolescence, where academic demands are increased. Where the age of onset is later, retrospective recall of childhood symptoms is also more accurate.

Three recent longitudinal studies in children with ADHD followed until the ages of 20–40 years, show that there is also a "late-onset ADHD," starting after the age of 12 years. Here, the symptoms, comorbidity, and dysfunction are similar to the classic childhood-onset ADHD, but there is different cognitive and genetic profiles (see also Sect. 1.3.2). Remarkably, in these longitudinal studies, the majority of adults with ADHD had an onset after the twelfth year.

2.6   ADHD and Intelligence

ADHD occurs in persons with low, normal, and high intelligence (Antshel et al., 2008; Antshel, Phillips, Gordon, Barkley, & Faraone, 2006). Research among adults with an IQ above and below 110, showed that the gifted group experienced fewer problems with executive function, and seemed better able to compensate. When diagnostic tests for executive function are used in a highly gifted group, this may lead to underdiagnosis of ADHD (Milioni et al., 2014). In a large population study of five-year-old twins, IQ and ADHD symptoms were measured. The diagnosis of ADHD was negatively correlated with IQ, and ADHD children had an average IQ that was 9 points lower than control children. This association implies a shared genetic profile, which should be mapped out further (Kuntsi et al., 2004).

There is still relatively little research into similarities and differences between people with ADHD with varying levels of intelligence. The DSM-5 ADHD criteria do not provide any guidance for application to people with a low or high IQ. When diagnosing children, ADHD symptoms should be compared with those of peers with the same developmental level, such as classmates. In the case of intellectual disability, cognitive abilities are not comparable to those of classmates or peers, which makes it difficult to identify attention problems. For this reason, when examining a child with low IQ, hyperactivity, and impulsivity are better guides to diagnosis than inattention.

Hyperactivity in children with mental retardation is one of the main reasons for referral to mental health care. In clinical populations of mentally retarded children, the prevalence of ADHD is 42% (Hardan & Sahl, 1997). A large study of low IQ children in special education showed a prevalence of ADHD of 15% (Dekker & Koot, 2003). Various hereditary syndromes associated with hyperactive behavior occur in patients with intellectual disabilities, such as neurofibromatosis, Angelman syndrome, fragile X syndrome, Noonan syndrome, velocardiofacial syndrome, and Williams syndrome (Simonoff, 2007). However, these hereditary syndromes contribute only a small amount to hyperactivity in children with low IQ. Furthermore, ADHD is comorbid with behavioral disorders in children with intellectual disability and in those with normal IQ.

In low IQ children, as in ADHD in the presence of average IQ, comorbidity is common, particularly behavioral disorders (Dekker & Koot, 2003). Hyperactivity persists in two-thirds of follow-up studies. This subgroup of children with ADHD are more frequently expelled from school, have problems with police/judiciary (Aman, Armstrong, Buican, & Sillick, 2002).

Diagnosing individuals with low intelligence should include information from parents and teachers, physical and laboratory tests, and the use of questionnaires for ADHD and other disorders. The "DIVA-5-ID" has been developed to diagnose people with intellectual disability, see www.divacenter.eu.

Treatment with stimulants in children with low IQ and ADHD is effective, but less so than in normal and gifted children with ADHD. This may be due to the fact that gifted children express their difficulties more easily, whereas these may be missed in the evaluation of low IQ children. In addition to a more complex diagnostic process, there may be comorbidities, so reaching a clinical conclusion may be difficult (Aman et al., 2002; Aman, Buican, & Arnold, 2003). Poor efficacy of stimulants in ADHD with low IQ may be related to underdosage (Simonoff, 2007). A great deal of research is therefore needed in people with intellectual disability and ADHD.

Although high intelligence is usually an advantage, it does not prevent dysfunction in ADHD. Research demonstrates that highly intelligent people with ADHD had more fines for speeding, more arrests and accidents, more dysfunction at work and in relationships, and a lower quality of life than highly intelligent people without ADHD. They also had more depression, anxiety, and compulsivity. ADHD was more common in their family members. Their profile was therefore very similar to that of people with ADHD of average intelligence (Antshel et al., 2008). Diagnosing the highly gifted person with ADHD is complicated by the fact that the patient and collateral sources may deny dysfunction because he/she performs better than average. However, this does not mean that the patient is performing at his/her optimal capacity. Furthermore, chronic underperforming is exhausting and only sustained through willpower and excessively long working hours. The work these highly intelligent people perform may provide an insufficient intellectual challenge. Gifted patients with ADHD cannot sustain attention on tasks, their chaotic disorganization and their need for prolonged time to complete tasks do not match their level of intelligence and results in underperformance. Some claim that a high IQ alone can mimic ADHD. As far as we know, this claim has not been substantiated by research. Although it is conceivable that under-stimulation of gifted children at school can lead to boredom and behavioral problems, it is difficult to imagine that gifted adults without any comorbid disorder experience in their development.

2.7   Dysfunction in ADHD

What is dysfunction in ADHD? It is important that the clinician has knowledge of the typical problems that patients with ADHD deal with. Dysfunction in adults with ADHD includes:

- Educated below one's intellectual level or has not completed training.
- Underperforming at work (see Sect. 2.8).
- Frequent changing of job or work functions, due to conflicts or rapidly becoming bored.
- Relationship difficulties due to being unreliable and irresponsible, irritability, needing variety with many (sexual) partners in a short time (see Sects. 2.8.2 and 2.8.3).
- Social problems or isolation due to fear of failure, social anxiety, shame, poorly developed social skills.
- Inability to organize daily life, keep finances under control and keep the household in order.
- Speeding and more frequent accidents (see Sect. 2.7.1).
- Increased risk of premature death.
- More teenage pregnancies.
- Starting earlier with alcohol and drug abuse.

Two phases of poor performance may be seen where ADHD is presenting in a person with normal to high IQ: once at school, resulting in a lower level of education; and then at work, where disorganization, poor concentration, and conflicts limit promotion. The result is that patients often end up in an unsatisfactory work environment where they do not feel comfortable.

Danish research among 151 adults with ADHD shows that for 51%, the highest level of education was a primary or lower secondary school diploma; 65% were unable to support themselves. Criminal behavior occurred in more than half, 16% lost their driving licenses and 37–51% showed risky sexual behavior. Comorbidity did not worsen the risk of a low educational level or risky behavior, underlining the importance of treating ADHD (Soendergaard et al., 2015).

Some patients believe that they are not dysfunctional, while careful research reveals that they are. A reason for this discrepancy is that they have adapted their lives to the disorder. For example, administration and maintaining social contact are taken over by the partner. The patient may cope at work because the job is of a low level, with variety and space so that restlessness remains manageable.

High intelligence can also offer some compensation because it shortens the concentration needed to complete tasks. It is important to establish whether the patient is functioning at his/her own level and whether they are satisfied. Situations that cost effort are often avoided and this has its price. The patient may become accustomed to the current (low) level of functioning and is unaware of how things could be done differently. As a result, relying solely on the patient's report wrongly suggests that there is no dysfunction. Determining dysfunction, therefore, requires further questioning, often with the help of the partner.

2.7.1 ADHD and Driving

ADHD appears to create danger on the road. This emerges from American research where adolescents with ADHD had four to five times as many accidents, more speeding fines, and driving disqualifications, compared to controls (Barkley & Cox, 2007; Barkley, Guevremont, Anastopoulos, DuPaul, & Shelton, 1993; Barkley, Murphy, & Kwasnik, 1996). Adults with ADHD also appear to have had more accidents than controls. In research using a simulated driving test, the accidents in the ADHD group were most frequent in the morning, when compared to controls. ADHD drivers tired more rapidly during driving than controls; possibly because of the lack of visual stimulation during long car journeys (Reimer, DíAmbrosio, Coughlin, Fried, & Biederman, 2007). Simulated driving test and questionnaire research showed that adults with ADHD had more speeding fines and accidents compared to controls. They drove faster, had less control over their vehicle and were easily provoked by the behavior of fellow road users. They drove recklessly when crossing or taking an exit. Similar results came from Dutch questionnaire research in which the driving behavior of 330 patients with ADHD was compared with the same number of controls: the ADHD group had significantly more fines, car accidents, and unsafe driving behavior (Bron et al., submitted Bron et al., 2017).

ADHD characteristics and research findings overlap: when driving, adults with ADHD are rapidly distracted, by every billboard (or moving object). Sensation seeking promotes overtaking other cars in risky situations. ADHD adults frequently describe themselves as "speed freaks," because high velocity improves their attention and concentration. Heightened arousal or excitement can indeed stimulate concentration. Another symptom of ADHD is impatience, difficulty awaiting one's turn, which can play a role in traffic jams, for example. This can lead to tailgating and other annoying driving behavior. Finally, attention problems prevent timeous anticipation of dangerous traffic situations, so evasive action is taken at the last minute.

2.8   Impact of ADHD on Work, Relationships, and Family Life

2.8.1   ADHD and Work: Being a Jack of all Trades

People with ADHD do not reach their potential owing to chronic turmoil, distractibility, and concentration problems at school, further studies and work. They underperform, change course in education and in jobs which results in a pattern of "much potential, little success."

Dutch research among 54 adults with ADHD aged 18–56 years showed that they had worked for an average duration of fifteen years. Twenty-seven percent were receiving unemployment. Half of them described losing interest in their workplace or work function. For 60%, the shortest job duration was under 6 months, and for 70% it was under a year. The *longest job duration was* less than five years for 50% of those studied. More than 40% had had more than nine jobs or positions (see Table 2.1). In addition to rapidly tiring of a job, other reasons for change included conflicts and dysfunction in the workplace. Almost 40% had been dismissed, and in almost a third this had occurred more than four times (Table 2.2). More than 50% had resigned from jobs, of which more than 20% had done so more than four times (Table 2.3).

Half of the study participants worked below their educational level (Table 2.4). In this study, for 60%, underperformance began early in the form of learning problems in childhood and 30% had repeated an academic year at least once. About 50% of parents of the ADHD subjects had sought academic support. This included homework support, remedial teaching, private tutoring, or special education. From the literature it is known that compared to controls, adolescents with ADHD are less likely to complete their studies, be suspended (6% versus 18%), or expelled from school (13% versus 5%), obtain lower grades and finish secondary school with a diploma (5% versus 35%) (Weiss & Hechtman, 1993; Mannuzza, Klein, Bessler, Malloy, & Hynes, 1997).

The fact that almost half of the people in this study work below their educational capacity indicates that a decline in functioning can occur twice in people with ADHD: once during the school period, and again when finding suitable work. This underperformance causes a lot of suffering for people with ADHD; it takes a lot more effort for them to get to a place where they can develop without the appropriate qualifications. This often fails, and it is conceivable that under-stimulation will more easily lead to job hopping, conflict, and dismissal.

Table 2.1 Number of jobs

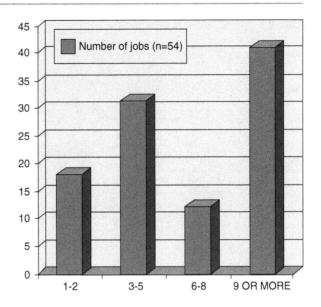

Table 2.2 Number of times fired from a job: 39% (n=54)

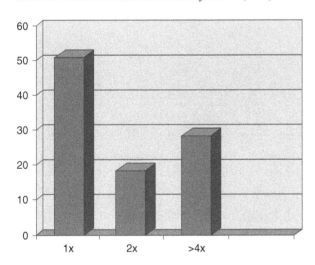

By underperforming in this way, someone with ADHD will earn less than they would have without the disorder. The tendency to change jobs frequently means that growth, development, and promotion are not achieved. The changes themselves entail additional risks of loss of income (diminishing pension etc.).

Research on the work performance of adults with ADHD in ten countries showed that they missed 22 days per year extra compared to controls, regardless of profession, education, age, gender, or partner status. Research in a large company showed a correlation between ADHD and a 4–5% decline in work performance. In this

Table 2.3 Number of resignations (n=54)

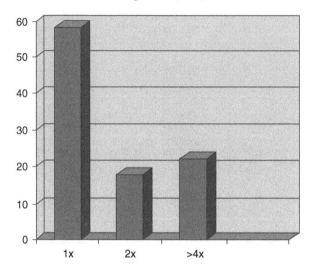

Table 2.4 Work level in relation to educational level (n=54)

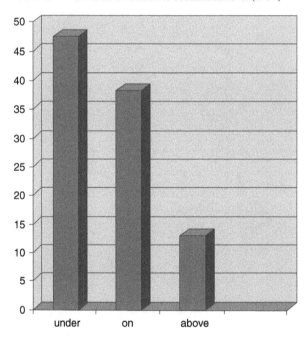

study, absenteeism due to illness and workplace accidents both occurred twice as frequently in adults with ADHD. The costs associated with decreased work performance in ADHD were over $4000 per employee in the year prior to the study. Only a small number of adults with ADHD were in treatment (Kessler, Lane, Stang, & Van Brunt, 2009). On the basis of these findings, when combined with the under-treatment of ADHD in most countries, there are improvements to be made in terms of performance at work, both for people with ADHD and for their employers.

2.8.2   ADHD and Relationships: Short-Lived and Rapidly Changing

Problematic patterns can also be discovered in the area of relationships. Of the 54 adults with ADHD between the ages 18 and 56 years, 38 had a relationship (70%). In 78% of the relationships, there were problems (Kooij, 2002). In 68%, the relationship lasted longer than five years. The relationship was described as "good" by 45% of the patients and as "moderate to (very) bad" by 55%. The partner was even more negative about the relationship. Reasons cited for the problems were: conflicts about insufficient communication and intimacy; not keeping appointments, not taking responsibility for family and household; alcohol or drug abuse; aggressive behavior. Most relationship problems were related to a combination of the conflicts mentioned here.

Before the current partner, there had been several other relationships. Thirteen patients had not had a partner (24%), sixteen had one to four partners (30%), eight patients had five to ten partners (14%), and seventeen had had more than ten partners (32%). Thirty to forty short-term relationships were no exception in the latter group. The duration of most relationships (excluding the current ones) fits a pattern of short-term relationships with rapid changes (Table 2.5).

The duration of most previous relationships was less than a year for almost half of the patients, and less than six months for more than 35%. This pattern of short-term relationships that change rapidly is usually not a problem for adolescents, who generally experiment with relationships at this age. It begins to cause problems when people feel the need to settle down. Ultimately, people with ADHD do not manage to find and keep a steady partner.

2.8.3   Impact of ADHD on a Relationship

The influence of ADHD affects the duration and rapid turnover of relationships. The quality of the relationship suffers if one of the partners has ADHD. Robin (2002) conducted research with the "Marital Impact Checklist" (34 questions) on eighty couples, one of whom had ADHD. He interviewed 35 men (44%) and 45 women (56%) with ADHD, and their partners. The average age was 42 years.

Table 2.5 Length of previous relationships

Duration of previous relationships	n = 53	%
<0.5 years	19	35,8
0.5–1 years	7	13,2
1–5 years	6	11,3
5–10 years	9	17,0
N/A	12	23,6

The most problematic areas for both partners were:

- Poor communication, problems with time management and with emotional self-regulation.
- Forgetting things that had previously been discussed.
- Saying things without thinking.
- Not paying attention during conversations.
- Struggling to deal with frustration.
- Trouble starting tasks.
- Misjudging time needed for tasks.
- Leaving a mess.
- Not completing tasks.

The questions that were answered were:

1. How many items do both partners indicate as annoying?
2. How severe is the feeling of being unloved by the partners?
3. What is the negative impact of this behavior on the relationship, according to both partners?

The ADHD partner scored higher on the number of items, the feeling of being unloved and feeling the negative impact of the behavior on the relationship. There was no difference in scores between men and women with ADHD. The scores of each partner in a couple showed moderate to high correlation. For the partners without ADHD, the men scored higher than the women on the number of items, the feeling of being unloved and the negative impact of the behavior on the relationship. In summary, this research showed that:

- The ADHD partners experience most of the burden and impact.
- The partner of a woman with ADHD is much more dissatisfied with the relationship than the partner of a man with ADHD.
- The gender role and associated expectations may partly determine the impact of ADHD behavior on the relationship.
- Therapists should pay more attention to communication, acceptance, and understanding among male partners of women with ADHD.

In recent years, more has been elucidated concerning about partner violence in the relationships of people with ADHD. Young women with ADHD are more likely to experience partner violence in intimate relationships (Guendelman et al., 2016; Snyder, 2015). Young men with ADHD are more likely to treat their partners aggressively, both verbally and physically, especially if there are also personality disorders (Wymbs et al., 2012; Fang, Massetti, Ouyang, Grosse, & Mercy, 2010). Hardly any thought has yet been given to treatment or prevention of these problems, but this seems necessary.

2.8.4   ADHD and Sexuality

In addition to the effects of treatment, the well-known MTA study looked at the sexual maturation of adolescents with ADHD (10–14 years) compared to controls, and at the impact of the use of stimulants on sexual maturation. The ADHD group did not differ from the controls, nor did sexual maturation differ between groups that had never, occasionally, recently or inconsistently been treated with stimulants (Greenfield, Hechtman, Stehli, & Wigal, 2014).

Sexuality in Adolescents with ADHD has been studied more often than in adults. Striking findings are that on average, they are sexually active one year earlier than their peers (15 and 16 years, respectively) and exhibit more risky sexual behavior (more partners, one-night stands, less use of contraception). This results in more sexually transmitted diseases (17% versus 4%) and a higher percentage of teenage pregnancies (38% versus 4%), when compared to peers without ADHD (Barkley, Fischer, Smallish, & Fletcher, 2006; Flory, Molina, Pelham Jr., Gnagy, & Smith, 2006).

So far, little research has been done into the sexual experiences of adults with ADHD. It is known from clinical practice that certain sexual problems can be related to ADHD symptoms: for example, when attention problems, poor concentration, or distraction, occur during sex, this can cause problems with ejaculation. Partners who go to bed at different times commonly have less opportunity for sexual contact. This can be caused by poor planning, but also by the late sleep phase that occurs in the majority of adults with ADHD, so that partners are unlikely to go to bed at the same time. There are also indications that some adults with ADHD have an increased libido. Frequent masturbation in someone with ADHD, for example, can serve to combat the continuous inner restlessness. Other biological factors may also contribute.

In questionnaire research into sexual dysfunction and disorders in 136 adults with ADHD, about 40% of both men and women had a sexual dysfunction, and a further 17% and 5%, respectively, had a sexual disorder. These dysfunctions included: no desire for sex/sexual aversion, negative emotions during sex, too little excitement, and difficulty with ejaculation. The sexual disorders concerned were: hypersexuality, sadomasochistic fantasies, transvestism, pedophilic fantasies, and ambivalent gender identity, strikingly enough especially in women (Bijlenga et al., 2017). All of these disorders were significantly more common in the ADHD group than in the general population. Similar findings regarding gender identity emerge from research among children with ASD and ADHD: about 5% of parents reported gender identity problems in their child, while this percentage was only 1.7% in control children (Strang et al., 2014). Further research will have to show whether these problems have a biological or psychological background.

In other adult studies, those with the combined presentation type of ADHD were slightly more likely to be bisexual than controls, but not homosexual. There were no more sexual problems or disorders in ADHD compared to controls (Barkley et al., 2007).

There are indications in the literature that those with the combined presentation type have a higher sex drive than the inattentive presentation (Canu & Carlson, 2003). Sexual problems that appear to be directly related to ADHD, such as restlessness, tension, impatience, rapid distractibility, and poor planning, can also lead to less interest in sex; these problems were equally distributed across the sexes.

2.8.4.1 Traumatic Sexual Experiences

In a Dutch study, 35 of 120 adult ADHD patients reported traumatic sexual experiences (29.4%), 27 women and 8 men (Kooij, 2002). The experiences were registered and then categorized. Two types of traumatic sexual experiences were distinguished (41 in total): rape (27) and sexual assault/abuse (14). Among the 22 perpetrators were: eight family members, eleven acquaintances, and three strangers. All but one of the perpetrators were male. There was a blood relationship with seven perpetrators. In five of the offenders who were related to the victim, there was impulsive and aggressive behavior, restlessness or hyperactivity, and concentration problems. Although these perpetrators who were biologically related to the victim are a small group, their symptoms resemble ADHD with comorbid behavioral disorders.

Sexual Abuse

Sexual abuse was reported by 22 out of 120 patients (18.3%). Nineteen women and three men were involved. In 18 (82%), the abuse took place during childhood or adolescence. The difference between sexual abuse and unpleasant sexual experiences was that the unpleasant experiences took place later in life and were more often once-off. Seventeen patients were abused several times (Kooij, 2002).

2.8.5   The Impact of ADHD on the Family

In the Dutch study of 54 adults with ADHD, 31 had one or more children (59%) (Kooij, 2002). Of these, 24 experienced problems with parenting their children (77%). The reasons given were: having a child with ADHD symptoms, learning or behavioral problems ($n = 18$; 58%), and conflicts with the partner about parenting styles ($n = 14$; 45%). Six patients reported other problems. What was striking was the high percentage of children with problems. This proportion is in line with the results of family research by Barkley (1997a), who found a 50% risk of ADHD in children where a parent had the disorder.

Comparable data emerged in Canadian research. In this study, families with and without a parent with ADHD were compared (Minde et al., 2003). Children with an ADHD parent had more psychological symptoms than children without an ADHD parent. Children with ADHD also had other disorders more frequently than their siblings. Family and marital relationships were affected, regardless of the gender of the ADHD parent. Children without ADHD who had one psychologically healthy parent and another parent with ADHD, did well. However, the behavior of children with ADHD was always problematic. This behavior was not associated with the mental health of the parent(s). This study confirms the strong genetic predisposition to ADHD. From these results, it is recommended that the functioning of the partner without ADHD be closely monitored; this partner has a great deal of influence on the well-being of children without ADHD.

2.8.6 Conclusions

In summary, families with ADHD have a hard time: due to underperformance in education and work, a person with ADHD will change jobs more often, have less financial security and earn less than they would have without ADHD. Then there are additional risks to physical and mental health related to an ADHD diagnosis. These create higher costs for society and health care structures. In addition, the relationship with partner is also problematic (in 78% of cases) as well as with the upbringing of children, which is complicated by the presence of ADHD symptoms, learning or behavioral problems in 58% of cases. Children without ADHD are also at risk as they are exposed to parents with a chaotic lifestyle Together, these conditions give rise to conflict, and if the affected parent is not treated, there is little chance for structure or problem-solving skills to succeed. As a result, the parent without ADHD may be faced with the almost impossible task of keeping the family financially and emotionally afloat, and seeking help for everyone who needs it. It seems time that more attention is paid to the important role of the partner of adults with ADHD, both within the family and by health care workers.

2.9 Benefits and Limitations of Recall in History Taking

Research raises questions about the reliability of self-reporting in adolescents with ADHD where the condition is frequently underreported (Barkley, 1997a). Adults, too, do not always have good insight into their own functioning. It is difficult for someone with lifelong symptoms of ADHD to compare their own functioning to that of someone without ADHD.

Therefore, it may be useful to ask a family member for collateral information concerning childhood symptoms. The partner is asked to report on the current symptoms. The diagnosis of ADHD can be made without collateral sources of information. For example, in the case of a patient who indicates that he or she had lifelong ADHD symptoms, who can give examples with associated dysfunction, the diagnosis can be made reliably. Collateral history is desirable if the patient's recall of adolescent behavior is inadequate, or if there are doubts about the reliability of the history (e.g., in addiction care).

Questionnaire research shows that the patient is the best informant compared to parents and partner; i.e., the patient's reporting of symptoms is closest to that of the clinical investigator (who rated the information of all informants at intake). The partner and parents recognize the outer characteristics better than the internal manifestations of ADHD, such as concentration problems. Therefore, the patient's story should be used as a guideline. The patient reports most accurately about him/herself, but tends to underreport compared to the clinical diagnosis. The collateral history adds information about the frequency and severity of symptoms (Kooij et al., 2008).

Sometimes it is not possible to obtain a collateral history immediately because the family relationships are problematic. It often helps to explain that it is very important for the diagnosis to gather as much information as possible and that the family can help. After the intake, problems in the family may resolve when it becomes clear that ADHD played a role in causing the difficulties. Some therapists refer to "clashing personality styles and avoid attributing blame." The explanation that follows the diagnosis is often enlightening for the patient, family, and partner. Many events from the past are better understood and this can contribute to improved relationships within the family.

A common difficulty when taking a collateral history in ADHD is that the family members do not agree among themselves about certain symptoms or the cause of events. Contradictory information can cause confusion for the clinician and it predicts a worse prognosis in families with ADHD (Ferdinand, Van der Ende, & Verhulst, 2004). Because of the hereditary nature of ADHD, multiple individuals in the family may have ADHD, which can lead to bias in the form of underreporting of severity, or to denial of the presence of symptoms. ("If that is ADHD, we all have it"). Although more information is sometimes required to arrive at an accurate diagnosis, collateral history does not always provide the desired certainty.

In the semi-structured Diagnostic Interview for ADHD (DIVA) (see section "Self-report questionnaire on attention problems and hyperactivity for adulthood and childhood" in Appendix) the collateral history is taken at the same time as the patient interview, so that questions only need to be asked once. Patient, family, and partner always report the presence or absence of each symptom in childhood or adulthood. This gives an overview of the reporting on the symptoms by all parties, after which the clinician decides on the score for each DSM-5-CRITERION. This procedure aims to simplify the process of diagnosis.

In the past, family relationships were often disturbed by conflicts and ignorance about the existence of ADHD. Diagnostic research and psycho-education post diagnosis can provide a different perspective for all parties, without the need to apologize for ADHD.

It is not uncommon for a family member who has recognized the ADHD symptoms to request help. Other family members may reject the diagnosis because the symptoms are so common: "Everybody's agitated, he's not even the worst." Some parents experience the diagnostic examination as an accusation, as if it was their fault. ADHD is not primarily caused by a troubled upbringing, although this can make the symptoms worse. For this reason, at the start of the interview, parents are reassured and informed that the diagnostic process aims to obtain information about the functioning of their son or daughter in childhood, not to pass judgment on their upbringing. It is often apparent that the parents did a good job by providing safety and structure. Their efforts may have prevented more serious dysfunction.

2.10   Family History

ADHD is often familial (Faraone et al., 2000a). Heredity is therefore considered to be the most important risk for ADHD. A family history focusing on ADHD symptoms and additional psychiatric disorders can provide information on the hereditary aspects. Comorbid anxiety, depression, alcohol and/or drug abuse, impulsive, and aggressive behavior are also more common in families with ADHD. This information can support the diagnosis.

2.11   Additional Information

When in doubt about the lifelong presence of the ADHD symptoms, previous psychological and psychiatric tests and primary school reports can be requested. Reports of previous testing rarely contain a diagnosis of ADHD. However, the symptoms will often be described. In this way, the chronic presence of the symptoms is demonstrated.

Sometimes school reports aptly describe childhood behavior in a way that supports the diagnosis, for example, "poor concentration, easily distracted, can do much better, many carelessness mistakes, talks too much." Good grades on a primary school report without comments on the behavior do not exclude the diagnosis.

2.12   Neuropsychological Examination

Despite decades of research, the neuropsychological profile in ADHD is mixed and the outcomes of different studies vary. Patients with ADHD clearly differ from controls at group level in terms of cognitive functioning, but there is no special cognitive test profile for the individual diagnosis of ADHD. At group level, executive functioning shows abnormalities in visuo-spatial, verbal working memory, inhibition control, vigilance, and planning. Patients with ADHD make suboptimal decisions by overestimating the extent of the immediate reward, rather than considering the delayed rewards. ADHD patients also show differences in timing, speech and language, memory, speed, and response time. Patients with ADHD may have abnormalities in several cognitive areas, or in none at all. The conclusion is that cognitive functioning does not sufficiently reflect behavioral symptoms. Neuropsychological research, therefore, has no added value in the diagnosis of ADHD (Fuermaier et al., 2015). However, it may be useful to map cognitive functioning for other purposes. Neuropsychological research in adults with ADHD is carried out for differential diagnosis of comorbidity, when investigating IQ, or to gain more insight into the personality or coping style of the patient.

Changes in scores on tests of executive function can demonstrate the effect of medication in clinical practice (Bron et al., 2014). The Continuous Performance Tests (CPT) objectify significant effects of pharmacological treatment. The

Quantified Behaviour Test (QbTest) measures inattentiveness, impulsivity, and hyperactivity using a computer-mounted infrared camera. As a result, all ADHD core symptoms can be measured before and after treatment. A study showed that the objective QbTest proved to be more sensitive to the medication response than subjective self-report questionnaires. In 54% of patients, the test detected a response to medication that had not been reported by self-report questionnaire (Bijlenga, Jasperse, Gehlhaar, & Kooij, 2015). However, the QbTest does not correlate well with clinical symptoms.

Biological endophenotypes describe the relationship between genes and behavior. In this new area of research, neuropsychological, neurophysiological, genetic, and neuroimaging measures are combined in order to understand the pathophysiology of various disorders, and ultimately to develop objective measures for diagnosis (Crosbie, Perusse, Barr, & Schachar, 2008; Doyle et al., 2005).

2.13   A Fashionable Diagnosis and overtreatment?

In the press, ADHD is often dismissed as a trendy diagnosis. Lazy parents are accused of wishing to improve their children's poor school performance while adults are accused of eliminating study and job-related difficulties with a pill. The fact that academic and work-related underperformance is a standard consequence of ADHD is overlooked. This does not do people with ADHD justice. The media also question whether ADHD is a reliable diagnosis even though it is based on the DSM-5 criteria: an onset of symptoms in childhood (six out of nine); a chronically persistent course until adulthood with a validated cut-off point of five out of nine symptoms; and long-term dysfunction due to the symptoms in two or more areas of life. Psychiatric diagnoses are established by means of diagnostic interviews; biological tests are lacking so far. Is there a hype, as is often claimed, and does this lead to medicalization and overtreatment? Again, the answer is no. The increase in ADHD diagnoses in children, including previously undiagnosed girls, adults and elderly is related to increased knowledge and treatment options. The image of ADHD as a disorder of hyperactive boys is outdated. This development is positive because groups that were previously underdiagnosed—adolescents, girls, ethnic minorities, adults, the elderly—can now be recognized and helped.

Dutch figures for the prescription of ADHD medications (brands and generics) in 2016 show an average of 65,100 prescriptions per month for adults (QuintilesIMS, 2016). Assuming one prescription per person per month (the maximum duration of a scheduled prescription), an estimated 65,100 adults were prescribed ADHD medication. This number reached only 14% of the prevalence of ADHD (4% of 12 million adults, an estimated 480,000 people). On the basis of these estimates, there does not appear to be overtreatment of adult ADHD in The Netherlands.

Over- and underdiagnosis of ADHD in adults can only be combatted by training the mental health services in the disorder.

2.14   Comorbidity and Differential Diagnosis

In the diagnostic phase, in addition to identifying ADHD, comorbidity should also be evaluated. ADHD is almost always accompanied by one or more additional disorders and the diagnosis of ADHD cannot be made without demarcating other disorders. Instruments that can be used in the diagnosis of comorbidity, include the SCID I and II (Van Groenestijn et al., 2006; Weertman, Arntz, & Kerkhofs, 2006).

2.14.1   Comorbidity in ADHD

ADHD is associated with one or more additional psychiatric disorders in three-quarters of outpatients. The average number of comorbid disorders in referred patients with ADHD is three (Biederman et al., 1993; Kooij et al., 2001a, 2004). The National Comorbidity Survey Replication (NCS-R) in the general population of the United States found a similar pattern of comorbidity in non-referred patients. The presence of three comorbid disorders increased the risk of ADHD in the general population 8.3 times (Kessler, 2007). This means that ADHD is not innocuous, but may be present, undiscovered, in patients who have already sought help for other complexes, potentially therapy-resistant problems. According to the findings of the study, untreated, active ADHD may lead to chronic comorbid disorders. This was particularly the case with mood disorders, including bipolar disorder, post-traumatic stress disorder (PTSD), generalized anxiety disorder, panic disorder, and drug dependence. The risk of ADHD with a mood disorder was 20%, with an anxiety disorder 17% and with addiction 18%. Conversely, mood disorders occurred in 31% of those with ADHD, anxiety disorders in 51%, and addiction disorders in 14% (see Table 2.6).

In epidemiological studies with 26,000 respondents in 20 countries ranging from the United States to Peru, the Netherlands, and China, ADHD was often comorbid with other psychiatric disorders: the odds ratio for a comorbid disorder was 3, for two disorders 6, and for three or more disorders 9. The risk for depression in the past year was 8% in the presence of ADHD: 8%, for bipolar disorder 15%, for anxiety disorders 9%, for alcohol abuse 9% and for drug abuse 16%. Conversely, in the ADHD group, depression was present in 15%, anxiety in 34%, alcohol abuse in 5% and drug abuse in 2.7% (Fayyad et al., 2017).

The pattern and frequency of comorbidity in adults and children with ADHD are remarkably consistent. Like adults, children with ADHD often have comorbid mood, anxiety, and behavioral disorders (the precursors of later personality disorders), as well as tics and autism spectrum disorders (Elia et al., 2008). Similar percentages of these comorbid disorders in childhood and adulthood indicate an early onset of many of the disorders in childhood.

Three-quarters of ADHD is associated with comorbidity; an ADHD patient has an average of three comorbid disorders.

2.14.2 ADHD in Other Disorders

In populations of patients with disorders associated with ADHD, such as depression, bipolar, anxiety, sleep, personality disorders, and addiction, the risk of ADHD is thus increased. This has been demonstrated in research. In a population of depressed patients, 16% also appeared to have ADHD (Alpert et al., 1996) and in a population with anxiety disorders, the prevalence of ADHD was 23–33% (Fones, Pollack, Susswein, & Otto, 2000; Van Ameringen, 2008). A conservative estimate of the prevalence of ADHD among alcohol and/or drug addicts, both in the Netherlands and in the United States, is around 20–30% (Van de Glind, Kooij, Van Duin, Goossensen, & Carpentier, 2004; Van Ameringen, 2004, 2008; Goossensen et al., 2006; Schubiner et al., 2000; Wilens et al., 1994, 2007; Wood, Wender, & Reimherr, 1983). In German research among 118 women with borderline personality disorder, it appeared that 41% of the women had a history of ADHD in adolescence and that 16% still had ADHD. In this patient group, childhood ADHD was correlated with emotional abuse in childhood, with more comorbidity on axis I and II, and with more severe borderline symptoms (Philipsen et al., 2008). Similar results were found in Italian research (Fossati, Novella, Donati, Donini, & Maffei, 2002). In a Dutch study of 103 patients with borderline personality disorder, 33% also had ADHD (Van Dijk et al., 2011).

The conclusion is that the percentage of ADHD where there are comorbid disorders is at least around 20%. This means that one in five psychiatric or addicted patients who report for treatment could also have ADHD. This high number has consequences for the organization of patient care and training of professionals in mental health care (see also Sect. 2.13).

One in five psychiatric patients could also have ADHD.

Untreated ADHD can contribute to the chronicity of comorbidity.

2.14.3 ADHD and Health

2.14.3.1 ADHD, Eating Binges, and Obesity

Children with ADHD are found to be overweight significantly more often than average, despite the hyperactivity associated with the disorder. In population studies, children who are not treated with medication for ADHD have an increased risk of being overweight, while treated children are more likely to be underweight (Holtkamp et al., 2004; Waring et al., 2008). Stimulants used in the treatment of ADHD inhibit appetite, reducing the intake of calories, especially from fatty foods (Liu, Li, Yang, & Wang, 2008).

In children and adults with ADHD, a systematic review and meta-analysis showed a significant association with overweight and obesity after control for confounders such as depression (Cortese et al., 2016). The risk of obesity increased with age. Individuals taking stimulants did not have an increased risk of obesity, which may be associated with increased control of behavior by the medication, and the side effect of appetite suppression. Obesity is associated with type II diabetes,

Table 2.6 Occurrence of comorbid disorders in ADHD

	Clinical research adults	Epidemiological studies on adults	Clinical research children
Some comorbidities	75%	66%	66%
Average number of comorbid disorders per patient	3	Chance of ADHD 8.3 times increased in three comorbid disorders	–
Depressive disorder	25–66% (of which 60% with seasonal pattern)	31%	20–25%
Bipolar disorder	10% (most type II)	Probability of bipolar disorder 6.2 times increased in ADHD	20%
Anxiety disorder	25–63%	51%	15–25%
Addiction	25–55%	14%	10–25%
Smoking	40%	Each ADHD symptom contributes to an earlier onset of smoking, and to more smoking	20–30%
Sleep disorder (particularly delayed sleep phase)	80%	–	73%
Behavioral or personality disorder	6–25% cluster B	–	45–50% ODD or CD
Eating disorders (particularly bulimia)	9%	–	4%
Autism spectrum disorder	–	–	22%
Tic disorder	11%	–	50%

References: Amons, Kooij, Haffmans, Hoffman, & Hoencamp, 2006; Biederman, Newcorn, & Sprich, 1991; Biederman et al., 1993, 2002, 2005; Brown, 2000; Elia, Ambrosini, & Berrettini, 2008; Gau et al., 2007; Kessler, 2007; Knell & Comings, 1993; Kollins, McClernon, & Fuemmeler, 2005; Kooij et al., 2001a, 2004, 2005, Kooij, Boonstra, Huijbrechts, & Buitelaar, 2006; Ronald, Simonoff, Kuntsi, Asherson, & Plomin, 2008; Spencer, Wilens, Biederman, Wozniak, & Harding-Crawford, 2000; Van Ameringen, 2008; Van der Heijden, Smits, Van Someren, & Gunning, 2005; Van Dijk, Lappenschaar, Kan, Verkes, & Buitelaar, 2011, 2012; Van Veen, Kooij, Boonstra, Gordijn, & Van Someren, 2010; Weiss, Hechtman, & Milroy, 1985; Wilens, Biederman, Spencer, & Frances, 1994; Wilens, Upadhyaya, Faraone, & Biederman, 2007

cardiovascular disease, and cancer. The question is which factors drive obesity in ADHD, and thus how the development of chronic associated diseases can be prevented.

The ADHD symptoms of impulsivity and poor planning can contribute to irregular eating patterns (e.g., skipping breakfast), eating binges, unhealthy food preferences, and lack of exercise. In addition, a late sleep phase, which is associated with sleep deprivation, is very common in ADHD (see Sect. 2.14.4) (Bijlenga et al., 2013; Kooij & Bijlenga, 2013). This dysregulates the appetite hormones, leptin and ghrelin, resulting in an increase in appetite, especially for carbohydrate-rich foods (Copinschi, Leproult, & Spiegel, 2014). A similar effect comes from a seasonal mood disorder (winter depression) that is three times more common in ADHD than in controls: in winter there is an increase in intake of carbohydrate-rich foods and an increase in weight (Wynchank et al., 2016). Furthermore, the literature mentions the addictive aspects of eating, behavioral disorders, and genetic influences (Cortese & Tessari, 2017).

In one study, 60% of adults aged 18–56 years with ADHD (*n* = 120) suffered from eating problems, particularly binge-eating or eating binges. Most patients described their eating behavior as "impulsive" or "to calm down." In almost 40% of patients, eating binges occurred once or several times a day, in 40% at least once a week and in the rest, at least once a month. Patients also remarked that they forgot to eat or did not plan their meals adequately (Kooij, 2001). Almost 40% of the patients had weight fluctuations, for 22%, weight varied between 10 and 20 kg, and in more than one-third of the group it varied more than 20 kg. Height and weight were known for a subgroup of 54 patients. Sixty-five percent of those with a Body Mass Index (BMI) over 25 had eating binges, compared to 35% of those with a BMI under 25. Of those with BMI over 30 (*n* = 6, 11%), all had a pattern of varying weight and binge-eating.

2.14.3.2 Skipping Breakfast and Being Overweight

Children and adolescents who skip breakfast, the first meal of the day, are heavier than their peers who do eat breakfast. Research among Dutch families showed that one in seven families do not have breakfast; in Canada this is one in ten (Boere-Boonekamp et al., 2008; Dubois, Girard, Potvin Kent, Farmer, & Tatone-Tokuda, 2008; Mota et al., 2008). Compared to children who ate breakfast, those who did not appear to compensate by eating protein-rich lunches and more carbohydrates at the end of the afternoon. This led to a higher weight and BMI. Children who did eat breakfast also performed better at school (Berkey, Rockett, Gillman, Field, & Colditz, 2003). It is conceivable that when substituting for breakfast later in the day, there is no healthy meal, but rather snacks high in fat are eaten.

Adults with ADHD often skip breakfast and sometimes even lunch. It is conceivable that this increases appetite, as previous meals have been postponed or skipped. A pattern of postponing meals and forgetting to eat may be related to poor concentration and disorganization, but also to the disrupted biological clock, or circadian rhythm in ADHD (see Sect. 2.14.4). By shifting the biological clock earlier, mealtimes and sleep onset occur earlier, so in turn, other metabolic processes are better timed. After a three-week study of research in healthy volunteers, it was found that after a late evening meal, the glucose level does not drop sufficiently at night. This in turn creates a disturbed insulin response. Nocturnal eating and night-time activity are thus a risk factor for obesity and diabetes (Qin et al., 2003).

Obesity in ADHD can also occur as a result of increased appetite where there is comorbid seasonal affective disorder or winter depression (present in about 30%). Winter depression is also associated with a disturbance of the circadian rhythm (Lewy et al., 2006a). A correlation has been found between low mood, childhood ADHD symptoms, weight, and expression of the DRD4 gene, especially the 7-repeat allele, in a group of women with winter depression. These women tend to overeat during the winter months (Levitan et al., 2004). The DRD4 gene associated with

ADHD also appears to play a role in the common pattern of seasonal depression and obesity in this group. The DRD4 gene has been found more frequently in populations with alcohol/drug addiction, gambling, obesity, ADHD, and Tourette disorder (Blum et al., 1995).

As long as the reason for skipping breakfast in ADHD remains unknown, the simple advice to have breakfast is probably not enough. What is certain, however, is that those who succeed in having breakfast are more likely to control their weight. In addition, a side effect of treatment with stimulants may be that weight is better controlled, because of the known side effect of stimulants: loss of appetite.

The relationship between ADHD and obesity appears to be caused by skipping meals and poor meal planning, eating binges, sleep deprivation, and an increased prevalence of winter depression (which is accompanied by an increase in appetite).

2.14.3.3 ADHD in Obesity

Conversely, ADHD is found in 27% of severely overweight patients (BMI > 35) (Altfas, 2002; Cortese, Isnard, Frelut, Michel, & Quantin, 2007; Fleming, Levy, & Levitan, 2005). The risk of ADHD is greatly increased with the more severe forms of obesity: with a BMI > 40, the risk of ADHD is 42.6%. The exact correlation between the two is not yet clear and may be explained by abnormalities in dopamine and insulin receptor activity in the brain (Cortese, Konofal, Dalla Bernardina, Mouren, & Lecendreux, 2008). In ADHD a dopamine deficiency is assumed, which disrupts the dopamine reward system. This disruption of the dopamine system could also play a role in compulsive or addictive behavior such as binge-eating and obesity (Campbell & Eisenberg, 2007; Liu et al., 2008). The risk of ADHD is further increased by excessive daytime sleepiness in obese adolescents (Cortese et al., 2007, 2008). This may fit in with the previously mentioned hypothesis that a disturbance of the circadian rhythm affects several metabolic processes. Recent population studies have indeed shown that a short sleep duration and an irregular eating pattern in ADHD mediate the association with BMI (Vogel et al., 2015).

In families with a genetic cause for obesity (a mutation in the melanocortin-4 receptor (MC4R) (C271R)), the regulation of hunger and satiety is disturbed, leading to abnormal eating behavior. Homozygous twin patients had an 80% risk of ADHD, heterozygous patients 22%. Thus, genetically determined obesity also appears to be associated with ADHD (Agranat-Meged et al., 2008).

In prospective follow-up research among 12,500 schoolchildren, the mother's weight during pregnancy was associated with ADHD in the child. The following factors were controlled for: duration of pregnancy length, birth weight, weight gain and smoking during pregnancy, maternal age and education level, sex of the child, family structure, and country of origin. Women who were overweight before pregnancy and who gained a lot of weight during the pregnancy, were twice as likely to have a child with ADHD symptoms compared to women of normal weight (Rodriguez et al., 2008). These findings demonstrate the importance of weight management in the pregnant population, where there is an underlying increased genetic risk of the disorder.

The risk of ADHD is greatly increased with severe obesity and excessive daytime sleepiness. Excess weight gain during pregnancy also increases the risk of ADHD in the child. Problems with appetite, sleep, and weight in ADHD seem to be connected.

2.14.4 ADHD and Sleep Disorders

2.14.4.1 Sleeping Disorders in Children
A (subjective) questionnaire survey among parents of children with ADHD shows that these children often have difficulty falling asleep or do not feel like going to bed. They also experience difficulty getting up. Sleep is interrupted more often, sleep efficiency is decreased, which leads to drowsiness during the day. Objective research with the Multi Sleep Latency Test (MSLT), actigraphy, polysomnography, and measurements of Dim Light Melatonin Onset (DLMO) partly confirms the findings from questionnaire research. Children with ADHD are indeed more sleepy during the day than controls. Their sleep is more restless and agitated and they may also have Restless Legs Syndrome (RLS) or Periodic Limb Movement Disorder (PLMD) (Corkum, Tannock, Moldofsky, Hogg-Johnson, & Humphries, 2001; Cortese et al., 2005; Gaultney, Terrell, & Gingras, 2005; Konofal, Lecendreux, Bouvard, & Mouren-Simeoni, 2001; Lecendreux, Konofal, Bouvard, Falissard, & Mouren-Simeoni, 2000; Sadeh, Pergamin, & Bar-Haim, 2006). ADHD, RLS, and PLMD are associated with dopamine imbalance, and are treated with dopamine agonists. More research into overlap and differences between the three disorders is needed. It is possible that too low a level of ferritin, which has been demonstrated in children with ADHD, plays a role in the disturbing dopamine metabolism (Konofal, Lecendreux, Arnulf, & Mauren, 2004; Konofal et al., 2008; Oner, Dirik, Taner, Caykoylu, & Anlar, 2007). Furthermore, the onset of melatonin release in children with ADHD who fall asleep 45 minutes later than controls may be related to a delayed sleep phase due to circadian rhythm disruption (Van der Heijden et al., 2005; Van der Heijden, Smits, & Gunning, 2006). Treatment with melatonin brought forward the sleep phase in these children and extended the duration of sleep (Van der Heijden, Smits, Van Someren, Ridderinkhof, & Gunning, 2007). The genetic backgrounds of circadian rhythm disorders in ADHD are gradually becoming clearer (Coogan & McGowan, 2017).

2.14.4.2 Presentation Type and Sleeping Problems
Children with the inattentive presentation type of ADHD have fewer sleep problems than children with the combined presentation. Comorbid anxiety or depression are associated with more sleep problems, whereas comorbid oppositional defiant disorder is not. Daytime somnolence is most common with the inattentive presentation type, where sleep duration is also longer than normal (Mayes et al., 2008). A similar connection between ADHD and sleep problems was found among students. Those with the combined presentation type had shorter sleep duration, while the predominantly inattentive presentation type required more sleep (Gau et al., 2007). On the

other hand, impulsivity appears to occur more frequently in people with an evening chronotype, where there appears to be a connection between the delayed sleep phase and the hyperactive/impulsive type of ADHD (Caci et al., 2004, 2005; Wynchank et al., 2018). In adults, a possible link was found between the inattentive presentation type and longer sleep duration (van Veen et al., 2010).

2.14.4.3 Sleeping Disorders in Adults

Adults with ADHD have similar sleep problems as children. They report a lower quality of sleep associated with sleep problems, and fatigue when getting up (Schredl et al., 2007). Almost 80% of adults with ADHD go to bed late (between 1 and 3 am) and prefer to get up late as well. Problems with falling asleep occur when going to bed too early. Sleeping through the night is also difficult for them. Over 60% of ADHD adults experience daytime sleepiness. This drowsiness worsens concentration difficulties in ADHD. The majority have had these sleeping problems from childhood onwards (Bekker, Kooij, & Buitelaar, 2008; Dodson, 1999).

This sleeping pattern is typical of a late sleep phase, described in the DSM-5 as: "Circadian Rhythm Sleep Disorder, Delayed sleep phase." In research, "Dim Light Melatonin Onset," is late in ADHD. This measurement refers to the production of melatonin in the evening, under dimmed light conditions, which is a biomarker for late chronotype. Sleep phase is also delayed in ADHD compared to controls (Coogan & McGowan, 2017). The volume of the pineal gland, where melatonin is produced, is smaller in ADHD compared to controls, and this is correlated with both a late chronotype and the increasing severity of ADHD (Bumb et al., 2016).

People with this sleeping pattern are also called evening types. In the normal population, the evening type occurs at about 25%. Evening types have poorer health do night shift work and are also unemployed more often than morning people. Chronotype (being an evening or morning person) appears to be independent of gender, ethnicity, and socioeconomic status, but not of age (Paine, Gander, & Travier, 2006). Younger age (30–34 years) is more often associated with the evening type than older age (45–49 years).

A late sleep phase often results in a shortening of sleep duration, because of needing to get up early for work. In turn, short sleep duration appears to be associated with obesity in children and adults. Here, the relationship between sleep and weight gain emerges (Cappuccio et al., 2008). The first comparative study on the Dim Light Melatonin Onset (DLMO) of adults with ADHD, with and without insomnia, indicates a greatly delayed sleep phase due to a late onset of melatonin production in those with insomnia, results which are similar to those found in children (Van Veen et al., 2010). When using actigraphy to measure 24-hour muscular activity, this was found to be delayed in ADHD. In another study of twelve adults with ADHD versus controls, the late onset of melatonin release was replicated. The time of falling asleep and body temperature also shows a circadian rhythm. In this study, along with sleep onset time, both were delayed in ADHD (Bijlenga et al., 2013). As far as cortisol release is concerned, the studies are not unanimous (Coogan & McGowan, 2017).

In a comparative study of patients with ADHD, with obesity and controls, the ADHD group had shorter sleep duration on free days, later chronotype, more frequent indicators of delayed sleep phase, and an irregular eating pattern compared to the other groups (Vogel et al., 2015). The disturbance of the circadian rhythm proved to be a mediator between ADHD and obesity.

Treatment with a low dose of melatonin at the end of the afternoon and/or light therapy in the morning can be effective here (Lewy et al., 2006b; Pandi-Perumal, Srinivasan, Spence, & Cardinali, 2007). Initial experiences with melatonin in practice show positive effects, with earlier falling asleep and waking up times (Kooij, 2010).

Descriptions of nocturnal motor activity, as measured with actigraphy, vary in the adult literature. It has been shown that adults with ADHD, compared to controls, have more difficulty falling asleep, lower sleep efficiency, and interrupted sleep more often (Boonstra, Kooij, Oosterlaan, Sergeant, & Buitelaar, 2007; Kooij et al., 2001). In adults with Restless Legs Syndrome (RLS), as in children, ADHD is found more often than in controls (Wagner, Walters, & Fisher, 2004). Iron deficiency (and ferritin stores) may be an aetiological factor that links hypodopaminergic disorders such as ADHD, RLS, and Gilles de la Tourette syndrome (Cortese et al., 2008). Iron is needed for the metabolism of dopamine.

Adults with ADHD, especially those with obesity and cardiovascular disease, are more likely to suffer from respiratory problems that can lead to sleep apnea. Sleep apnea produces daytime sleepiness and cognitive problems (Gosselin et al., 2006; Mazza et al., 2005; Naseem, Chaudhary, & Collop, 2001; Yuen & Pelayo, 1999). The relationship between sleep apnea, obesity, and cardiovascular disease is also referred to as metabolic syndrome (Vgontzas, Bixler, & Chrousos, 2005).

RLS or PLMD, sleep apnea, late sleep, and daytime sleepiness are more common in children and adults with ADHD. These processes appear to occur via dopaminergic metabolic problems, which probably involve low ferritin and delayed melatonin release. All these sleep problems have interrupted sleep and shorter sleep duration in common.

Finally, excessive daytime sleepiness that can accompany ADHD may cause diagnostic confusion with narcolepsy or hypersomnia. A comparative study with questionnaires in a group of hypersomnia and/or narcolepsy patients and a group of ADHD patients indeed showed an overlap. Almost 20% of the hypersomnia group also met the ADHD criteria and 38% of the ADHD group was sleepy during the day (Oosterloo, Lammers, Overeem, De Noord, & Kooij, 2006). It seems appropriate to investigate both disorders in the case of such complaints.

In summary, nocturnal motor hyperactivity (RLS or PLMD), sleep apnea, late sleep, and daytime sleepiness are more common in children and adults with ADHD. The interrelationships between these phenomena seem to occur via dopaminergic pathways, in which low ferritin and late melatonin onset may play an aetiological role. All sleep problems share interruptions and short sleep duration.

2.14.4.4 Sleep Duration, Obesity, and Cancer

Short sleep duration is associated with obesity, diabetes, cardiovascular disease, and cancer (Cappuccio et al., 2008; Hill et al., 2015; Knutson & Van Cauter, 2008). Melatonin, the hormone that regulates our day and night rhythm, also has a protective effect against cancer. The total amount of melatonin produced at night could be related to the duration of sleep and thus the duration of melatonin production. Sleep duration in the general population has only decreased since the beginning of the last century (from 8–9 hours to 6–7 hours). A shorter sleep duration is associated with longer exposure to artificial light in the evening. This exposure to artificial light breaks down melatonin and is associated with a higher risk of cancer (Kayumov, Lowe, Rahman, Casper, & Shapiro, 2007). One hypothesis is that a lower melatonin level due to shorter sleep duration (and exposure to light) contributes to a higher risk of cancer in the long term. Evidence for this hypothesis comes from research in a large group of men in which a long sleep duration is associated with a lower incidence of prostate cancer (Kakizaki et al., 2008). Other indications come from the Nurses' Health Study, reported by the Health Council of the Netherlands in 2006 (Gezondheidsraad, 2006). In this study, years of nightshift work (especially if ≥30 years) and exposure to light were found to be associated with a lower melatonin level in morning urine and an increased incidence of breast cancer (Schernhammer & Hankinson, 2005; Schernhammer, Kroenke, Laden, & Hankinson, 2006).

In addition to this hypothesis, there are many other factors that increase the risk of breast cancer, such as heredity, frequent air travel, hormone therapy, alcohol abuse, obesity, and parity (Moser, Schaumberger, Schernhammer, & Stevens, 2006). However, research into risk factors for cancer is complex and no single factor can be identified as the most important. On the other hand, the clustering of cancer risk factors in ADHD patients (alcohol abuse, smoking, shorter sleep duration and obesity, possibly lower melatonin levels due to a late sleep phase, night work, and exposure to light) is a signal for further research. The anti-estrogenic and oncostatic properties of melatonin are increasingly substantiated in animal and in vitro research (Hill et al., 2013). Initial research into the anti-carcinogenic effect of melatonin on human cancer cells is ongoing (Bartsch et al., 2000; Panzer & Viljoen, 1997; Sabzichi et al., 2016). Much more research into these links is needed before definitive conclusions can be drawn.

2.14.5 ADHD and Mood

ADHD is often accompanied by shorter- or longer-term mood problems, mood swings, and mood disorders. Low mood can be linked to season (especially autumn and winter), menstrual status (premenstrual, postnatal, or perimenopausal), a reaction to a life circumstance or setback or have no clear cause. These comorbidities create a puzzling differential diagnosis. The following sections provide tools for the differential diagnosis of mood problems.

2.14.5.1   ADHD and Mood Swings

Almost all adults with ADHD exhibit a lifelong pattern of rapid irritability and frequent mood swings four to five times a day. Such a pattern has been found in studies in 90% of adults (Kooij et al., 2001). In the United States, the relationship between ADHD and mood swings has been noted. This has led to the Emotional Lability subscale in the Conners Adult ADHD Rating Scale (CAARS) (Conners et al., 1999). Mood swings are often reactive, when setbacks result from ADHD symptoms. For example, forgetting a key and being locked out. But even without a clear reason, rapid mood swings from cheerfulness to irritability are common. The so-called "short fuse" that characterizes many people with ADHD is one of the manifestations of mood lability. The following factors suggest that mood swings belong to the ADHD syndrome rather than a mood disorder in a narrower sense: high prevalence of mood swings in adults with ADHD (90%), chronic, persistent course (i.e., not episodic as in a mood disorder) and response to treatment with stimulants (Skirrow & Asherson, 2013). Mood lability, including irritability, usually decrease with stimulant treatment, as do the other ADHD symptoms. If this response is insufficient, an SSRI can be added.

Many women with ADHD suffer from a cyclical, violent, premenstrual worsening of mood swings that can include suicidality (Dorani, Bijlenga, & Kooij, 2017). Recent research indicates a significantly increased prevalence of premenstrual dysfunction in women with ADHD (46% versus 1–4% in controls) (Dorani et al., 2017, submitted; Dueñas et al., 2011). This may be due to increased sensitivity to reproductive hormone fluctuations that interact with dopamine function during the menstrual cycle.

Women with ADHD and PMDD also suffer from low mood during the rest of the cycle and may have a history of depression. Treatment with SSRIs throughout the cycle is usually effective (Shah et al., 2008). No research has yet been conducted into the treatment of this comorbidity in women with ADHD.

Daily mood swings in ADHD should be distinguished from a depressive episode with irritable mood, (rapid cycling) bipolar disorder, and borderline and antisocial personality disorder associated with emotional lability. There seems to be an overlap between ADHD and the diagnostic criteria of ultrarapid cycling bipolar disorder, cyclothymia, or the so-called cyclothymic temperament. There is currently much debate as to whether they are part of the bipolar spectrum or the temperament/personality spectrum (Angst, Gamma, Benazzi, Ajdacic, & Rossler, 2008; Bauer, Beaulieu, Dunner, Lafer, & Kupka, 2008; Phelps, Angst, Katzow, & Sadler, 2008).

Given that many mental health practitioners are unfamiliar with emotional lability in adult ADHD, a bipolar, or cluster B personality disorder is more likely to be considered as the cause of the mood swings. This lack of knowledge about ADHD in adults may manifest in (population) studies that use diagnostic instruments which do not (yet) include ADHD, such as the CIDI, the SCID, and the SCAN. Incidentally, the CIDI has a section on ADHD in adults (Fayyad et al., 2007).

The following criteria are used for the differential diagnosis:

1. Frequency of mood swings (four to five times a day in ADHD and cluster B personality disorders, lasting at least two to three days in a hypomanic episode)
2. Course (chronic in ADHD and cluster B personality disorders, episodic in bipolar disorder)
3. Age of onset (childhood in ADHD, usually later in bipolar and personality disorders)

In children with ADHD, irritable mood is often present, but this is usually associated with comorbid oppositional defiant disorder. The severity and duration of irritability are considered an indicator for the comorbid diagnosis, which can vary from ADHD (mood lability /short fuse), to depressive episode (severe/long-lasting irritability), to bipolar disorder (explosive/violent irritability) (Spencer, 2007).

It is necessary to obtain as much clarity as possible about the type of mood swings in the patient prior to treatment. Making a life-chart of the changing mood over time can help. A comorbid bipolar disorder or a depressive episode must first be treated prior to the treatment of ADHD. Chronic, rapid mood swings that occur four to five times a day do not need to be treated first and often diminish with stimulant treatment.

Ninety percent of adults with ADHD suffer from lifelong, rapidly changing moods (four to five times a day) and anger outbursts.

2.14.5.2   ADHD and Depression

Depression and dysthymia are common in adults with ADHD. It is conceivable that a prolonged pattern of failure will lead to loss of perspective and a gloomy outlook. However, having a reason for melancholy does not exclude the diagnosis of depression. If the low mood and anhedonia persist for more than two weeks and lead to functional limitations, the diagnosis of depression should be considered (APA, 2013). Recurrent depressive episodes occur in 55% of adults with ADHD in clinical populations (Amons et al., 2006; Kooij et al., 2004). Conversely, ADHD is found in approximately 20% of those with depression in both clinical and epidemiological studies (Alpert et al., 1996; Kessler, 2007).

In the NESDA population study among people with anxiety and depressive disorders, the prevalence of ADHD symptoms appears to increase with the severity and presence of the depression: 0.4% ADHD in controls, 5.7% in depression in remission, and 22.1% in a current depressive episode. The severity of ADHD further increased in those with more severe depression, chronic depression, and an earlier onset of depressive symptoms (Bron et al., 2016). This is an important finding for (clinicians treating) patients with depressive disorders, especially those with severe and chronic depression.

Research among young women with ADHD showed that they have a 2.5 times higher risk of depression compared to controls. Their depression started earlier, lasted more than twice as long, was associated with more severe dysfunction and more suicidality, needing admission more often than controls. Mood disorders also occurred more frequently in family members: depression in the parent(s) and mania in a sibling predicted depression in women with ADHD (Biederman et al., 2008).

Symptoms of ADHD and a depressive episode overlap in terms of concentration problems, sleep problems, possible psychomotor agitation or retardation, and fatigue or loss of energy. In ADHD however, these symptoms are present from childhood onwards, whereas in depression there is a symptom-free period before and after the episode. A depressed patient can distinguish between his/her normal self and the depressive episode; an ADHD patient has only a lifelong experience of symptoms. Both patterns can be distinguished in the combination of ADHD and depression.

2.14.5.3   ADHD and Winter Depression

The lifetime prevalence of depression in adults with ADHD is 55% in clinical trials (Amons et al., 2006). Of those with depression, 61% were found to show a seasonal pattern of mood disorder, also known as seasonal affective disorder (SAD) or winter depression. The incidence of winter depression in the total group of adults with ADHD was estimated at 27%. Women were more likely to have a seasonal pattern of mood disorder than men. This prevalence is comparable to the prevalence of 19% in the only other (Canadian) study on adults with ADHD and winter depression (Levitan, Jain, & Katzman, 1999). The prevalence of seasonal depression in the general population in the Netherlands is estimated at 3% (Mersch, Middendorp, Bouhuys, Beersma, & Van den Hoofdakker, 1999). Thus, winter depression is almost ten times more common in ADHD. Some patients are depressed all year round, with the atypical symptoms of winter depression being added in the winter (eating more, gaining weight, and needing more sleep). According to the Multidisciplinary Guideline on Depression, depression is treated with an SSRI; for winter depression, the first choice of treatment is light therapy (Multidisciplinary Guideline on Depression, 2013).

There is a link between the increased prevalence of seasonal depression and the late sleep phase in adults with ADHD. The late sleep phase in ADHD mediates the increased risk of seasonal depression (Wynchank et al., 2016). Both are related to a disturbance of the biological clock, or the melatonin rhythm (Lewy et al., 2006a). Interestingly, light therapy is effective for both winter depression and the late sleep phase, if administered at the right time (early in the morning).

Open-label research with light therapy also showed an effect on ADHD symptoms (Rybak, McNeely, Mackenzie, Jain, & Levitan, 2006, 2007). Controlled research is still lacking. It is not known exactly how light influences mood and sleep rhythm; however, melatonin production is interrupted under the influence of light received through the eyes, so that the body and brain "wake up" as a result.

Genetic variations for the photopigment melanopsin in the retina appear to be associated with winter depression, and with changes in the timing of sleep and activity in healthy controls. This study sheds new light on the retinohypothalamic compounds, where light from the environment captured by the retina is translated into signals to certain brain nuclei that regulate the circadian, neuroendocrine rhythm and behavior. The sensitivity of the retina is reduced during winter depression compared to controls, as shown by measurements of the pupil response to light. Remarkably, adults with ADHD report a hypersensitivity to light in 70%. Adults with ADHD therefore frequently wear sunglasses during the day, even when the sun is not shining brightly. This can further destabilize the circadian rhythm as it limits synchronization to light during the day (Kooij & Bijlenga, 2013). Further research into the functioning of the eye and pupil response to light is ongoing in ADHD.

Depressive episodes (lifetime) occur in 55% of adults with ADHD. Of these, 60% have a winter depression for which light therapy is the appropriate treatment. With light therapy in the morning, the day–night rhythm is also *reset*, which is important for the treatment of the late sleep phase in ADHD.

2.14.5.4 ADHD and Bipolar Disorder

Bipolar disorder occurs in 2–5% of adults (Merikangas et al., 2007). Bipolar disorder is more common in children with ADHD, i.e., 10–20% (Biederman et al., 2005; Hinshaw, Owens, Sami, & Fargeon, 2006). Adults with ADHD are also more likely to have bipolar disorder (in 10%) (Biederman et al., 1993, 2002). Conversely, 20–30% of bipolar II disorder patients also have ADHD (Sentissi et al., 2008; Viktorin et al., 2017).

The Juvenile Onset Bipolar Disorder (JOBD), with onset in childhood, occurs in 15% of those with bipolar disorder. This early onset of bipolar disorder makes differentiation from childhood-onset ADHD difficult. Moreover, JOBD is frequently associated with ADHD (up to 85%). This combination forms a more serious subgroup of bipolar disorder (Singh, DelBello, Kowatch, & Strakowski, 2006). ADHD and JOBD are more common in families, suggesting strong genetic predisposition (Faraone et al., 2003; Masi et al., 2006). Another combination that may predispose to bipolar disorder is ADHD comorbid with oppositional defiant disorder (ODD) or conduct disorder (CD) in childhood (Harpold et al., 2007).

Population studies in the United States show that ADHD is 6.2 times more likely to be associated with bipolar disorder I or II in adulthood (Kessler, 2007). ADHD and bipolar disorder thus occur relatively often together, which can complicate treatment. There is genetic overlap between ADHD and bipolar disorder. There are probably different genes implicated in early and later onset bipolar disorder (van Hulzen et al., 2017).

In summary, ADHD and bipolar disorder type II in particular, often occur simultaneously. The disorders are clinically distinguished by examining the symptoms, onset, and course of both disorders. There is an interrelationship between seasonal or winter depression, bipolar II disorder, and delayed sleep phase disorder (DSPD), and all occur to an increased extent in ADHD. Combination of a mood stabilizer with methylphenidate did not generate mania in a large Swedish study. However, mania was reported where methylphenidate was used as mono-treatment in patients with ADHD and bipolar disorder (Viktorin et al., 2017).

Differentiating between ADHD and Bipolar Disorder

ADHD and bipolar disorder can be distinguished on the basis of age of onset, course, and symptoms. ADHD begins in childhood, bipolar disorder usually in puberty. ADHD patients are chronically agitated, irritable, or hyperactive, while patients with bipolar disorder are episodically agitated (Leibenluft, Cohen, Gorrindo, Brook, & Pine, 2006). ADHD patients do not experience episodic sexual disinhibition, but they are "chronically in love." In bipolar disorder, there is increased libido and sexual acting out, but only during a (hypo)manic episode. People with ADHD generally have a negative self-image, while patients with bipolar disorder may be grandiose during a (hypo)manic episode. Furthermore, due to the heredity of both ADHD and bipolar disorder, the presence of either disorder in family members can be a diagnostic clue. Finally, there is the response to medication, which of course is not a diagnostic criterion, but can give an indication of whether the diagnosis is correct.

When ADHD and bipolar disorder coexist, more severe comorbidity is observed, including oppositional and antisocial behavior, anxiety, and alcohol abuse, compared with ADHD alone. In 88% of comorbid ADHD and bipolar disorder, type II bipolar disorder is present. Here, the severity of ADHD symptoms is greater than in ADHD alone. Functioning is worse, there are more depressive episodes, more suicide attempts, and aggression. There is a shorter duration of well-being between episodes of mood disorder. As a result, the mood disorder has a more chronic course. Due to the emotional lability seen in ADHD in combination with bipolar disorder, periods of euthymia are rare (Wilens et al., 2003). Where there is a chronic course, complex presentation, and poor response to treatment, a combination of ADHD and bipolar disorder (and/or other disorders) should be considered and investigated.

During treatment, different diagnostic problems can arise in patients with ADHD and a depressive episode: if after remission of the depression the patient becomes more active, this can resemble (hypo)manic behavior. To distinguish between bipolar disorder and ADHD, one should assess whether this is long-term behavior or whether it is an episode. The patient and his/her partner should assess the behavior. Evidence of excessive hyperactivity, may suggest a (hypo)manic episode.

ADHD and bipolar disorder often co-occur: about 20% of bipolar II patients have ADHD and 10% of adults with ADHD have bipolar disorder (almost always type II). This combination increases the risk of suicidality and chronicity.

Neuroimaging and Neuropsychology

In a first neuroimaging study of brain volume of adult patients with ADHD, bipolar disorder, both disorders, and normal controls, it was found that ADHD and bipolar disorder could be differentiated. In ADHD, the neocortex was smaller, especially the prefrontal cortex and anterior cingulate, as well as the cerebellum and gray matter. In bipolar patients, the thalamus was enlarged, and the left orbito-prefrontal volume decreased. In patients with ADHD and bipolar disorder, structural abnormalities characterizing both disorders were found. These results suggest that each disorder has its own typical pattern of brain volume changes (Biederman et al., 2008).

For a discussion of the overlap between ADHD and borderline personality disorder, see Sect. 2.14.8.

In a study of adolescents with bipolar disorder with ($n = 11$) and without ADHD ($n = 15$), an fMRI scan was performed during a Continuous Performance Test. Where ADHD was comorbid with bipolar disorder, there was less activation of the ventrolateral prefrontal and anterior cingulate cortex, and more activation of the posterior parietal cortex and mid-temporal gyrus (Adler et al., 2005). Both disorders could be differentiated in this study using neuropsychological testing. These research methods are not available in clinical practice, but they do indicate the presence of objective, structural differences between ADHD and bipolar disorder (Fig. 2.1).

Suicidality

The risk of suicidality in adolescents and adults with ADHD compared to controls appears to be particularly increased in the presence of hyperactivity/impulsivity, depression, dysthymia, and antisocial personality disorder (Barkley & Fischer, 2005; Semiz, Basoglu, Oner, & Munir, 2008). In adolescent studies, 36% of patients with ADHD before the age of eighteen had suicidal thoughts, versus 22% in the control group. For suicide attempts, these numbers were 16% versus 3%. After the age of eighteen, the difference in the prevalence of suicidal thoughts and attempts remained, although less pronounced (Barkley & Fischer, 2005). In a large English study of 7000 adults, ADHD was associated with double the risk of suicide (Stickley, Koyanagi, Ruchkin, & Kamio, 2016). In adolescent offenders, (comorbid) ADHD increased the risk of suicidal ideation and attempts, whereas alcohol and drug abuse further increased the risk (Ruchkin, Koposov, Koyanagi, & Stickley, 2016). Young women with ADHD also have an increased risk of self-harm and suicide attempts, especially in the presence of childhood and/or adulthood impulsivity (Swanson, Owens, & Hinshaw, 2014). Given the combination in

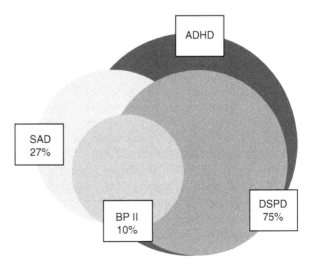

Fig. 2.1 Aggregate occurrence of ADHD with delayed sleep phase disorder (DSPD), (SAD), and bipolar II disorder (BP II)

ADHD of impulsivity, depression, and substance abuse, the increased risk of suicide is not surprising, but is often dangerously ignored in clinical practice (Furczyk & Thome, 2014).

2.14.6 ADHD and Anxiety

The lack of perspective in ADHD may lead to anxiety or panic, for example, when losing track of time or mislaying the keys for the umpteenth time. This panic clearly depends on the situation where there is chaos. Often these patients do not meet the criteria for panic disorder. The panic seems to be a consequence of the chaos. However, if there are physical symptoms of anxiety such as palpitations or hyperventilation, avoidance behaviors, or extreme anxiety, an anxiety disorder should be considered. Commonly comorbid with ADHD are anxiety disorder NOS, panic disorder, PTSD, (social) phobia, and generalized anxiety disorder.

2.14.6.1 ADHD, Fear of Failure, and Perfectionism

Patients with the predominantly inattentive presentation type (ADD) may have developed a compulsive coping style to compensate for their chaos and forgetfulness. This is appropriate and understandable, but in the long run, this coping style can become restrictive. The compulsive or perfectionistic style should be distinguished from obsessive–compulsive disorder (OCD). If for some reason the ritual cannot be performed and irritation results, this suggests AD(H)D; if anxiety or panic arises, OCD should be considered. Of course, the presence of both disorders should then be investigated.

Anxiety of failure is very common in AD(H)D and seems to be associated with a far-reaching history of failure. It is a real fear, which decreases when ADHD is treated, with the subsequent positive experiences in the areas of education, work, and relationships.

2.14.6.2 ADHD and Anxiety Disorders

In 25–63% of cases, adults with ADHD have one or more anxiety disorders (Biederman et al., 1993; Kooij et al., 2004). In American population studies, an anxiety disorder is found in 51% of those with ADHD, and in the Belgian population, the risk of anxiety disorders in ADHD is 7.5 times higher (De Ridder, Bruffearts, Danckaerts, Bonnewyn, & Demyttenaere, 2008; Kessler, 2007). Generalized anxiety disorder, panic disorder, PTSD, and social phobia predominate. Conversely, in population studies in the United States, ADHD is diagnosed in 17% of patients with anxiety disorders and in 20–33% of clinical anxiety disorder patient populations (Chao et al., 2008; Fones et al., 2000; Van Ameringen, 2008).

Anxiety disorders, especially when accompanied by physical anxiety symptoms, should always be treated prior to ADHD. Stimulants may cause tachycardia or palpitations as side effects, which people with (previous) anxiety complaints tolerate poorly. They may experience these symptoms as a return of an anxiety disorder; such an unpleasant experience that they refuse stimulant treatment again. To prevent this, the anxiety disorder should be diagnosed and treated first. Based on clinical experience, the anxiety disorder is best treated with an SSRI, which reduces the physical anxiety symptoms in a few weeks. After this, a stimulant can be added without increasing anxiety. It is unclear whether cognitive behavioral therapy successfully diminishes the anxiety-inducing side effects of stimulants. Some patients will need both treatments to control their anxiety.

Distinguishing between anxiety disorders and ADHD is not difficult when it comes to an episodic anxiety disorder. After all, it is possible to distinguish between these based on the course: chronic versus episodic. Differentiating between ADHD and generalized anxiety disorder is more challenging, as the former is chronic, with a young age of onset, and shares overlapping characteristics with ADHD (such as irritability, concentration problems, worrying). If anxiety symptoms are present, they should be identified so that they can be promptly treated. If chronic hyperactivity, attention problems, and impulsivity coexist, the comorbid diagnosis of ADHD should be considered.

Anxiety disorders and ADHD often occur together. This mainly concerns social phobia, generalized anxiety disorder, PTSD, and panic disorder.

2.14.6.3   ADHD and PTSD

Trauma and PTSD are common in ADHD. In childhood, both disorders are difficult to distinguish, as both can be accompanied by irritability and concentration problems. This problem occurs in sexually abused children who develop PTSD but who also have an increased risk of ADHD (Nickel et al., 2004; Weinstein, Staffelbach, & Biaggio, 2000). The presence of ADHD may increase vulnerability to traumatization. For example, inattention not only increases the risk of accidents, but can lead to high-risk situations. *Thrill seeking,* or looking for excitement and sensation, can further contribute to these risks. Furthermore, as parents of a child with ADHD have an increased risk of ADHD, they may be less able to provide structure and safety, so that the risk of family violence may increase. Research indeed indicates an increased risk of both perpetrator violence and repeat victimization in patients with ADHD (Henrichs & Bogaerts, 2012; Sugaya et al., 2012). Where ADHD and bipolar disorder are comorbid, the risk of victimization is even higher (Wozniak et al., 1999). In a comparative study of veterans with PTSD and veterans with panic disorder, ADHD was found more frequently in the PTSD group (36% versus 9% in childhood, and 28% versus 5% in adulthood) (Adler, Kunz, Chua, Rotrosen, & Resnick, 2004). In a meta-analysis, the relative risk of PTSD in ADHD was 2.9 and conversely, the relative risk of ADHD in PTSD was 1.7. Therefore, there appears to be a bidirectional association between ADHD and PTSD that requires further research. Cannabinoid receptor (CNR1) has recently been associated with an increased risk of ADHD and possibly also of PTSD (Lu et al., 2008).

Focussing on the increased risk of PTSD in ADHD: MRI scans investigated whether the "fear circuit" functions differently in untraumatized, medication-naïve young adults with ADHD versus controls. Here, learning and memory extinction tasks were performed (Spencer et al., 2017). A number of abnormalities were found in ADHD that resembled those found in PTSD. The emotional dysregulation in

ADHD may be responsible for this. In research among veterans with and without PTSD, ADHD symptoms appeared to increase the severity of PTSD; inattention especially played a role in this (Adams, Adams, Stauffacher, Mandel, & Wang, 2015). In a 10-year follow-up study in children, ADHD was an independent risk factor for the development of PTSD, as was smoking by the mother during pregnancy (Biederman et al., 2014). Problems with handling arousal in ADHD may play a role.

2.14.7   ADHD and Addiction

2.14.7.1   ADHD and Smoking

Adolescents with ADHD smoke twice as often as controls. It is assumed that the relative deficiency of dopamine in ADHD is compensated for by nicotine, a dopamine agonist. ADHD patients have good reason to smoke, because from an early age they notice the beneficial effects on their restlessness and concentration problems. Smoking can therefore be regarded as a form of self-medication in ADHD.

ADHD adolescents start smoking at a younger age and have more difficulty quitting. Treatment of ADHD seems to delay the early onset of smoking (Huizink, van Lier, & Crijnen, 2009). Smoking has been shown to be a risk factor for later alcohol and drug abuse (Wilens et al., 2007). In adolescents, a linear relationship has been found between the number of self-reported inattentive and hyperactive/impulsive symptoms and smoking. After checking for comorbidity, the risk of smoking increases with each ADHD symptom. In those who smoke, more ADHD symptoms are associated with an earlier onset of smoking, and with more smoking overall (Kollins et al., 2005).

Prospective mothers who smoke during pregnancy are more likely to have a child with ADHD, and there appears to be an interaction between exposure to smoking and certain genotypes in the child (DRD4, DAT1 440). These genotypes, when present and coupled with smoking exposure, increase the severity of ADHD (Linnet et al., 2003; Neuman et al., 2007). On the other hand, mothers who are smoke during pregnancy have an increased risk of having ADHD themselves, which also increases the genetic risk of ADHD in the child (Milberger, Biederman, Faraone, Guite, & Tsuang, 1997). There are indications that both factors, i.e., both heredity and exposure to nicotine in pregnancy, contribute to the risk of ADHD in the child.

In the acute phase of treatment, methylphenidate is associated with a dose-dependent increase in the number of cigarettes smoked (Rush et al., 2005). Some fear, therefore, that treatment with methylphenidate may induce nicotine addiction. In a first study, methylphenidate did not induce nicotine addiction, and was in fact associated with a later onset of nicotine use (Huss et al., 2008). Dutch research in ADHD adults showed different findings. Here, at baseline those with ADHD smoked twice as often as controls (50% versus 25%). However, after three months of treatment with methylphenidate, tobacco consumption increased by 1.3 cigarettes per day; that is 23 packets per year. Craving for nicotine increased by 20% after two weeks, and this stabilized at 29% after three months. In particular, light smokers (1–12 cigarettes per day) had an increased risk of tobacco consumption with methylphenidate treatment. This study should be repeated with objective measurements and a randomized design rather than using self-report. However, these findings suggest that smoking cessation should be attempted by all patients with ADHD who want to be treated with methylphenidate (Bron et al., 2013). This can be done with targeted counselling and by prescribing the dopaminergic antidepressant, bupropion hydrochloride (Upadhyaya, Brady, & Wang, 2004).

People with ADHD smoke twice as often, start earlier, smoke more, and have more trouble quitting than those without ADHD. The severity of ADHD predicts the number of cigarettes smoked per day. When treating with methylphenidate, prior smoking cessation should be considered because of a possible increase in tobacco consumption on this treatment.

2.14.7.2 ADHD and Addiction to Alcohol and Drugs

The risk of addiction to alcohol, cannabis, and a variety of other drugs is greatly increased in ADHD with odds ratios of 1.5 to 7.9, depending on the drug and the degree of dependence measured (Simon, Rolland, & Karila, 2015). Comorbidity with conduct disorder, antisocial personality disorder, eating disorder, bipolar disorder, early school leaving, and childhood neglect increase this risk (Kollins, 2008; Upadhyaya, 2008; Wilens et al., 2008). Adolescents with ADHD start abusing alcohol and drugs at a younger age. Around the age of 40 years, there is a second peak in substance abuse compared to controls (Wilens, Biederman, Mick, Faraone, & Spencer, 1997). Possibly this is related to giving up hope of improving the symptoms. Adults with ADHD do not use a particular drug, but all drugs (Carpentier, 2002). In addiction care, ADHD is found among hard and soft drug users and alcohol addicts. In psychiatry clinics, cannabis, and alcohol abuse are most common. All drugs affect the dopaminergic system, also known as the reward system. Neuroimaging in ADHD patients with a high risk for addiction shows an imbalance between an underactive inhibition control network and an overactive motivation reward network (Adisetiyo & Gray, 2017).

As with nicotine, patients with ADHD who abuse drugs appear to be self-medicating. Patients themselves report that on alcohol or drugs, they feel calm, relaxed, or clear-minded, and that they cannot sleep or function without drugs. Cannabis appears to improve the chronic delayed sleep phase in patients with ADHD (see Sect. 2.14.4.3), and cannabis abuse may be a persistent as a result. There is only one study in the literature showing that the level of melatonin increased significantly under the influence of cannabis (Lissoni et al., 1986). More research into the effects of cannabis and melatonin on sleep problems in ADHD is necessary.

Addiction has a negative effect on the course of ADHD and on quality of life. People with addictions often suffer from poor memory, making it extra difficult for them to recall the symptoms necessary to make the diagnosis. The memory problems are related to cognitive damage because of substance abuse. On the other hand, substance abuse can mimic the symptoms of ADHD, which can lead to overdiagnosis. If early-onset and lifelong course of ADHD symptoms are identified, alongside the onset, nature, and severity of substance use, patients with this comorbidity can receive appropriate treatment (Levin & Upadhyaya, 2007). Internationally, a conservative estimate of the prevalence of ADHD among alcohol and/or drug addicts is 20–40% (Van de Glind et al., 2004, 2013; Goossensen et al., 2006; Schubiner et al., 2000; Wilens, 2007; Wilens et al., 1994, 2007; Wood et al., 1983; Van Emmerik-van Oortmerssen et al., 2012).

With ADHD and addiction, the practitioner should be aware of an increased risk of other psychiatric disorders such as anxiety, depression, bipolar disorder, and personality disorders (Wilens et al., 2005). Addiction in patients with ADHD is more severe and chronic than without this disorder (Wilens, 2007).

Practitioners fear an increase in addictive behaviors when using stimulants in addicts with ADHD, so they are reluctant to prescribe the medication. While there are no indications that stimulant treatment of ADHD increases the risk of addiction, there is a greater risk of drug diversion: where stimulants are spread by patients and family members (Carpentier, 2007; Faraone & Upadhyaya, 2007; Wilens et al., 2003). The non-stimulant atomoxetine is recommended for substance disorder patients with ADHD, but it appears to be less effective than stimulants (Upadhyaya, 2008). Long-acting stimulants are less easy to abuse and are therefore preferred in patients with ADHD and (a history of) addiction (also see Sect. 4.19.6).

In positron emission tomography (PET) studies of adolescents with ADHD with and without addiction, methylphenidate blockade of the dopamine transporter (DAT) is similar. This overlap may shed light on the usefulness and role of stimulant use in addicts with ADHD. More neurobiological research is necessary (Szobot et al., 2008).

ADHD patients are addicted to alcohol and drugs more often than people without ADHD and they start earlier. Addicts with ADHD have more comorbidity and a worse prognosis than addicts without ADHD. Treatment with stimulants can prevent addiction in adolescents. Stimulants themselves are not addictive if long-acting preparations are used.

2.14.8 ADHD in Personality Disorders

ADHD and personality disorders overlap, and they can occur simultaneously, leading to diagnostic confusion. ADHD is a lifelong pattern from childhood with the typical characteristics of hyperactivity, impulsivity, and attention problems. Personality disorders are also defined by a chronic pattern of symptoms, which, may to a diagnosis in adolescence. Research into both diagnoses has increased in clinical studies. The combination of ADHD and personality disorder usually results in more comorbidity on axis I, particularly anxiety, depression, addiction, and sometimes criminality. Most of the research into ADHD and personality has addressed the cluster B personality disorders. Here, a high prevalence of ADHD has been shown, ranging from 33 to 65%. This raises the question of whether both disorders exist on a spectrum, or whether the diagnosis of ADHD was missed in the adult psychiatry setting, where clinicians diagnose personality disorders more readily than adult ADHD.

In German research among 118 women with borderline personality disorder, 41% had a history of ADHD in childhood, and 16% had concurrent ADHD. In this patient group, childhood ADHD was correlated with childhood emotional abuse, increased comorbidity on axis I and II, and more severe borderline symptoms (Philipsen et al., 2008). Similar results were found in Italian research (Fossati et al., 2002). In Dutch research in 103 borderline patients, ADHD was also found in 33% (Van Dijk et al., 2011). In the same study, the presence of hyperactivity did not distinguish between patients with borderline personality disorder and ADHD. Inattention was correlated with the cluster B personality traits risk *seeking* or novelty seeking. It is well known, that impulsivity is a core symptom of both disorders (Van Dijk et al., 2012). These data raise the question of whether ADHD and borderline personality do not have more in common than factors that separate them. Thinking about these two conditions existing on a dimensional spectrum may influence the differential diagnosis (see also Table 2.7).

In a Turkish study of 105 men with antisocial personality disorder (ASP) in detention, 65% were diagnosed with ADHD. Comorbidity with ADHD was associated with childhood neglect, severe and earlier onset of self-mutilation, suicide attempts, and psychopathy, than in those without ADHD (Semiz et al., 2008). These authors strongly recommend that all patients with borderline or antisocial personality disorder be specifically investigated for ADHD and, if necessary, treated for it.

Of the patients with cluster B personality disorders, 30–65% have a history of ADHD in childhood.

2.14.8.1   Cluster B Personality Disorders in ADHD

In a study of 53 adults with ADHD, a structured interview revealed a borderline or antisocial personality disorder in 6% (Kooij et al., 2006). Subclinical diagnoses of these personality disorders were made in 25%. Matching the data from follow-up studies in children, the development of cluster B characteristics was linked to a history of oppositional defiant disorder and/or aggressive behavior in childhood

Table 2.7 Differences and similarities between ADHD, bipolar disorder, and borderline personality disorder

Symptoms and course	ADHD	Bipolar	Borderline
Mood swings, irritable	X	X	X
Frequency of mood swings	4-5x per day	2–3 days	4-5x per day
Agitation, hyperactive	X	X	X
Impulsive	X	X	X
Attention issues	X	X	X
Increased associative thinking	X	X	–
Grandiosity	–	X	–
Sexual disinhibition	–	X	–
Onset in early childhood	X	+/–	–
Chronic/episodic course	Chronic	Episodic	Chronic
Family history	Positive for ADHD	Positive for bipolar disorder	–

(Biederman et al., 2008). Furthermore, in 90% of ADHD patients, the symptoms of "mood swings" and "inappropriate or excessive anger" overlapped in both ADHD and the borderline and antisocial personality. Impulsivity is the third overlapping symptom. Due to clinicians' unfamiliarity with the diagnosis of ADHD in adults, the presence of impulsivity, mood swings, and irritability can lead to the (mis)diagnosis of borderline or antisocial personality disorder, because these symptoms are common to both disorders Both diagnoses should be considered to improve the success of treatment. After all, if cluster B personality disorder symptoms that are so often treatment refractory are recognized as belonging to ADHD when making the diagnosis, this may open new treatment perspectives.

Follow-up studies of adolescents with ADHD have shown that the risk of developing personality disorder is increased: particularly borderline (odds ratio 13.16), antisocial (odds ratio 3.03), avoidant (odds ratio 9.77), and narcissistic personality disorder (odds ratio 8.69) (Miller et al., 2008).

Studies of Cloninger's personality dimensions of (Temperament and Character Inventory) in adults with ADHD have shown that the combined type of ADHD and hyperactivity/impulsivity are correlated with higher scores for novelty seeking and *persistence* and lower scores for *cooperativeness*, while the inattentive type of ADHD is more correlated with harm avoidance and self-directedness (Perroud et al., 2016; Salgado et al., 2009). More research into these clinically diverse ADHD presentations is necessary.

In comparative research, patients with the combination of ADHD and borderline personality disorder are more impulsive than patients with borderline personality disorder alone and controls. Patients with both disorders have more substance dependence and aggression than the other groups (Prada et al., 2014).

Initial open-label research indicates the effect of methylphenidate in the treatment of adolescents with borderline personality disorder and ADHD. In addition to the severity of ADHD symptoms, the severity of personality symptoms and aggressive behavior decreased with treatment (Golubchik et al., 2008). Controlled research into these effects is necessary.

ADHD increases the risk of (cluster B) personality disorders.

2.14.8.2   Differentiation of ADHD and Personality Disorders

Table 2.7 gives an overview of overlapping and distinguishing features of ADHD, cluster B personality disorders, and bipolar disorder.

In practice, ADHD is distinguished from other disorders on the basis of symptoms, course, and age of onset. This is complicated by research showing that ADHD and borderline personality disorder have more similarities than differences. The distinguishing features of hyperactivity and inattentiveness in ADHD are not as specific as previously thought. Dutch research shows that almost every borderline patient also has these symptoms, and impulsivity is central to both disorders (Van Dijk et al., 2011, 2012). Conversely, ADHD patients have mood swings and/or anger outbursts as often as borderline patients (4–5 times per day). Age of onset in ADHD does not appear to be consistently earlier than in borderline personality disorder. Longitudinal research points to a variant of ADHD with a later onset (after the twelfth year), the so-called "late-onset ADHD" (see also Sect. 1.3.2).

Personality disorders are diagnosed from adolescence onwards, so that age of onset is not a distinguishing feature unless the onset of ADHD is clearly in childhood. Cognitive problems are not unique to ADHD and may occur in borderline personality disorder too (Van Dijk et al., 2014). It, therefore, seems sensible to consider both diagnoses for any patient one suspects of having either ADHD or borderline personality disorder. Perhaps the borderline personality disorder should be seen as a more serious form of (or predisposition to) ADHD, precipitated by extra stressful environmental factors, such as sexual abuse and neglect (Ferrer et al., 2017). However, a large twin study from Sweden shows that abuse in childhood also predicts the persistence of ADHD into adulthood (Capusan et al., 2016).

Research into the antecedents of personality disorders also seems to provide indications of overlap and comorbidity. Personality disorders are preceded by behavioral disorders in childhood, including ADHD (Soderstrom, Nilsson, Sjodin, Carlstedt, & Forsman, 2005). A history of sexual abuse, violence, or neglect in childhood increases the likelihood of a cluster B personality disorder. It is important not to reject the diagnosis of ADHD too quickly because of a cluster B diagnosis: DHD does not rule out cluster B diagnosis. A history of neglect does not exclude ADHD (even in the family); both problems can reinforce each other, especially if there is also conduct disorder or personality *disorder in the* parents. A careful diagnosis ensures appropriate and effective treatment. Treatment of ADHD can have a rapid effect, and by reducing impulsive behavior and irritability, it can benefit the psychotherapeutic treatment for the personality disorder.

Overlapping features of ADHD and cluster B personality disorders are impulsivity, mood swings, and anger. Hyperactivity and inattention are also common in studies of borderline personality disorder The distinction with ADHD is therefore often unclear. Also, the earlier age of onset of ADHD does not always distinguish the two disorders due to the existence of a possible "late-onset ADHD."

2.14.8.3 Precursors to Cluster B Personality Disorders

A 10-year follow-up study of children with ADHD and comorbid behavioral disorders showed that the oppositional defiant disorder ODD persists in a minority. When these children were followed up at 4 and 10 years, childhood ODD was associated with depression and it increased the risk of Conduct Disorder (CD) and antisocial personality disorder (ASP). Have the diagnosis of CD alone also strongly increased the chance of developing ASP. CD also greatly increases the risk of substance abuse, bipolar disorder, and smoking (Biederman et al., 2008).

Research in adults with ADHD and CD in their history shows a similar pattern of comorbidity, particularly with cluster B personality disorders (Dowson, 2008). Therefore, ADHD is characteristically associated with behavioral disorders (ODD and CD) in adolescence, which increases the likelihood of cluster B personality disorders developing in adulthood.

2.14.8.4   ADHD and Sexual Abuse

It is conceivable that the presence of ADHD and behavioral problems that frequently coexist in the family can compound the risk of aggression and violence, including sexual violence. These behavioral disorders include impulsivity, sensation seeking, inattention, irritability, rebellious and aggressive behavior, and where bipolar disorder coexists, possibly sexual disinhibition. Such comorbidity leads to an explosive mixture. The hereditary nature of these disorders suggests that both perpetrator and victim may have characteristics that increase the risk of abuse. However, this is only a hypothesis that needs to be investigated further. Research has shown that children who have been sexually abused have a 14–46% risk of ADHD. Conduct Disorder (CD) is also more common in this group (McLeer, Callaghan, Henry, & Wallen, 1994; Merry & Andrews, 1994). Research among more than 14,000 adolescents shows that children with ADHD, inattentive presentation, have a 2.6 times higher risk of sexual abuse, and 2 times higher risk of physical neglect (Ouyang, Fang, Mercy, Perou, & Grosse, 2008). Sexual abuse was more common in a group of 144 girls with ADHD (14.3%) than in a matched control group (4.5%). In this study, sexual abuse was more common in the combined presentation method ADHD than in the inattentive presentation type (Briscoe-Smith & Hinshaw, 2006).

In another study among 104 children with ADHD and other behavioral disorders, children with ADHD were significantly more physically (96.2% versus 87.5%) and emotionally abused (46.2% versus 34.6%) compared to control children, but they were less physically and emotionally *neglected* than control children (5.8% versus 24.0%). However, there was no significant difference in witnessing family violence (56.7% versus 47.1%) or sexual abuse (5.8% versus 1.9%) (Sari Gokten, Saday Duman, Soylu, & Uzun, 2016). Female students with ADHD are more likely to be victims of sexual violence than controls (Snyder, 2015).

In the first study on sexual abuse in adults with ADHD compared to controls, a questionnaire on childhood trauma was used. Emotional neglect and abuse were more common in ADHD patients than in controls. Sexual abuse and physical neglect were more common among women than men with ADHD (23% versus 12.5%). Sexual abuse was associated with a later-onset of anxiety and depression. ADHD also proved to be a better predictor of severe psychosocial dysfunction in adulthood (Rucklidge, Brown, Crawford, & Kaplan, 2006). In Dutch research among 54 adults with ADHD, a history of childhood sexual abuse was found in 18.5% of the total group, and in 30% of the women. This number is comparable to previous research on ADHD and to the percentage of sexual abuse in other psychiatric disorders (Bryer, Nelson, Miller, & Krol, 1987; Kooij, 2002). Women with ADHD and a history of sexual abuse were more likely to have bulimia nervosa, lifelong aggressive behavior, less frequent gainful employment, and borderline personality disorder than women with ADHD without a history of abuse (Kooij et al., 2006). Thus, these two studies provide evidence for an increased frequency of sexual abuse in adults with ADHD, especially in women. It has long been recognized that a history of sexual abuse increases the risk of developing a borderline personality disorder (Zanarini et al., 1997; Zanarini, Frankenburg, Reich, Hennen, & Silk, 2005); such a history in adults with ADHD may help to establish comorbidity with a cluster B personality disorder.

Sexual abuse occurs in at least 14% of children with ADHD, and is reported by 18.5% of the total adult group, and in 30% of women with ADHD.

2.14.9   ADHD and Crime

Psychiatric disorders, including ADHD and behavioral disorders appear to be very common in offending adolescents and adults (Einat & Einat, 2008; Rasmussen, Almvik, & Levander, 2001; Vermeiren, De Clippele, & Deboutte, 2000; Vreugdenhil, Doreleijers, Vermeiren, Wouters, & Van den Brink, 2004). The prevalence of ADHD in adolescent and adult offenders with borderline or antisocial personality disorder is greatly increased: 40–70% have ADHD in addition to depression, anxiety disorders, and addiction (Andrade, Silva, & Assumpção Jr, 2004; Ginsberg, Hirvikoski, & Lindefors, 2010; Wetterborg, Långström, Andersson, & Enebrink, 2015). Conversely, children with ADHD who were followed up to the age of 31 years, were convicted for criminal activities in adulthood in almost half (47%) of the cases compared with controls in the general population. Half of these offenders with ADHD did not have antisocial personality disorder. Girls were also convicted more often (Dalsgaard, Mortensen, Frydenberg, & Thomsen, 2013).

Longitudinal studies of 15,000 children with ADHD also show significant associations with being arrested in adolescence and adulthood (RR: 2.2), convictions (RR: 3.3), and imprisonment (RR: 2.9). Children with ADHD are more likely to start antisocial behavior and have an increased risk of criminal recidivism. The most common criminal activities are theft, assaults, and drug- and weapon-related crimes (Mohr-Jensen, Amdisen, Jørgensen, & Arnfred, 2016).

Most research has been done on men, but female offenders who were investigated for ADHD had a *lifetime* ADHD diagnosis in 25% of cases, with 10% still meeting all criteria in adulthood. Women with ADHD had more comorbidity, were younger at the time of their conviction and received heavier sentences compared to women without this diagnosis (Rosler, Retz, Yaqoobi, Burg, & Retz-Junginger, 2008). Treatment of ADHD among offenders reduces ADHD symptoms, but also the risk of recidivism. This was found in three-year follow-up research and is clearly socially relevant (Ginsberg, Långström, Larsson, & Lindefors, 2015). A similar pattern emerged in longitudinal research among 25,000 people with ADHD in Sweden: during periods of medication use for ADHD, crime decreased by 30% and 40% (in men and women, respectively) (Lichtenstein et al., 2012). This is reason enough to track down and treat offenders with ADHD actively.

A 30-year prospective study of boys with ADHD and behavioral disorders compared to controls shows that hyperactivity is significantly more often associated with arrest, conviction, and imprisonment. Antisocial behavior in childhood, socioeconomic status, and IQ predicted adult criminality. Boys who had been intensively treated for ADHD for three years in childhood did no better than those who had been on medication alone. Hyperactivity without behavioral problems did not increase the risk of later crime (Satterfield et al., 2007). This study also shows that short-term treatment in childhood is insufficient to prevent such a course. In other prospective follow-up research on crime in boys with ADHD compared to controls, ADHD boys had been arrested (39% versus 20%), convicted (28% versus 11%) and imprisoned (9% versus 1%) significantly more often.

Conduct Disorder or antisocial behavior predicts an increased risk of crime, whether or not in combination with addiction. ADHD itself is not unequivocally associated with crime, but the associated behavioral disorder/ASP mediates the relationship with crime (Mannuzza, Klein, Bessler, Malloy, & LaPadula, 1998). Nevertheless, according to other research, boys with ADHD can develop criminality later in life without additional behavioral disorders. This, in turn, is linked to the development of ASP and to addiction during adolescence (Mannuzza, Klein, & Moulton 3rd., 2008). Hyperactivity and impulsivity predicted later criminal behavior, not inattentiveness (Babinski, Hartsough, & Lambert, 1999).

Hyperactivity in combination with behavioral disorders and addiction increases the risk of crime.

2.14.9.1 ADHD in Sex Offenders

ADHD is more common among sex offenders compared to controls (14% versus 8%). Research shows that 65% of sex offenders have a psychiatric disorder. Interestingly, those with ADHD begin with criminal activity 10 years earlier and are convicted more often (Blocher et al., 2001). In other studies of sex offenders with a variety of psychiatric disorders, only childhood ADHD is associated with paraphilia and socially deviant, aggressive forms of sexually impulsive behavior (Kafka & Prentky, 1998). In other studies, ADHD occurred in 43% of men with paraphilia. Conduct Disorder, mood disorders, and cocaine addiction were comorbid disorders (Kafka & Hennen, 2002). When ADHD is comorbid with other psychiatric disorders, it appears to add to the severity of the sexual offense. ADHD appears to be a risk factor for the severity of sexual offense in convicted men with comorbidity. Little is known about how this group responds to treatment. One study examined 26 men with ADHD, mood disorders, paraphilia, and related disorders who had not responded adequately to treatment with either a stimulant or an SSRI. Here, an SSRI or a stimulant (respectively) was added to the treatment regimen. Outcome measures were the severity of ADHD, mood disorder and paraphilia symptoms. Addition of the SSRI was significantly associated with reduced paraphilia-related behavior. Addition of the stimulant was associated with improvement in symptoms of paraphilia, mood, and ADHD (Kafka & Hennen, 2000). In general, it is advised to treat comorbid psychiatric disorders with a wide spectrum of pharmacological agents, but data on this is still limited (Kafka, 2012).

2.14.10 ADHD and Autism Spectrum Disorder

ADHD is not the only child psychiatric or developmental disorder that continues into adulthood; this is also true for behavioral disorders (called personality disorders in adulthood) and autism spectrum disorder (ASD). In the DSM-5 the distinction between different forms of autism has been abandoned (for example, PDD-NOS and Asperger syndrome). All forms now fall under autism spectrum disorder.

Autism is a complex neurobiological developmental disorder with lifelong consequences. Heredity and environmental factors contribute to the risk, but the exact etiology is still unknown. The current prevalence is estimated to be at least 1.5% in the Western world, with an increased prevalence in those with normal IQ. Population research has identified advanced parental age, preterm birth, a short time between pregnancies, and possibly prenatal exposure to air pollution, as risk factors. More research is needed on the contribution of nutrition, metabolic conditions, and the endocrine system (Lyall et al., 2017).

Autism is a multifactorial hereditary disorder that is associated with lack of empathy, reduced reciprocity in social communication, strangeness or eccentricity, difficulty integrating information, social withdrawal, repetitive stereotypical movements or behaviors, perseverance, rigidity, difficulty in tolerating change and rapidly becoming over stimulated. Two-thirds of those with an autistic disorder are mentally retarded (Van Berckelaer-Onnes, 2004). Scientific interest in autism where IQ is normal or high is fairly recent. English population studies estimate the prevalence of autism in children (and adults) at over 1%; previous estimates were lower. A distinction has been made between defining autistic spectrum disorders strictly (prevalence 0.4%) and slightly more broadly (0.8%). It is unclear whether the increase in prevalence is related to better recognition, broader diagnostic criteria, or an increase in incidence. Despite the uncertainty, children and adults with social communication and interaction problems deserve attention and care (Baird et al., 2006).

The recognition of autism spectrum disorders in psychiatry leaves much to be desired; it should be included in psychiatric training. Diagnostic instruments include: the Autism Diagnostic Observation Schedule (ADOS), the Autism Diagnostic Interview-Revised (ADI-R), and the Diagnostic Interview for Social and Communicative Disorders (DISCO) (Kan, Buitelaar, & van der Gaag, 2008). The comorbidity in autism spectrum disorders is diverse, but schizophrenia or other psychotic disorders predominate (Mouridsen, Rich, & Isager, 2008).

2.14.10.1 Overlap and Differences between ADHD and ASS

Autism spectrum disorders are often associated with ADHD symptoms. In the general population, twin studies of children show significant correlations (0.54) between those with symptoms of ADHD and autism, both where parents and teachers respond to questionnaires about phenotype, but also in terms of genetics. There is also substantial overlap between the two disorders: 41% of children with autism spectrum disorders also have ADHD symptoms, and 22% of those with ADHD also meet the diagnosis of autism spectrum disorder. These findings suggest a common genetic influence in both disorders (Ronald et al., 2008). Other twin studies in the general population examined the occurrence of autistic features in children with and without ADHD. Children with the inattentive and combined presentation of ADHD had significantly more autistic characteristics than children without ADHD (Reiersen, Constantino, Volk, & Todd, 2007). Owing to a lower cut-off point for girls than boys, more girls reached the threshold for ASD diagnosis than boys. The number of positive symptoms was lower for girls because they generally have better social skills than boys. In studies of children with ADHD, their siblings, and controls, more autism symptoms were found in children with ADHD, (especially combined presentation type), and in boys in general. Symptoms of autism were found to be familial and occurred more often when two children in a family had ADHD. Regarding the correlation between ADHD and autism in boys: 56% could be attributed to common genetic influences in the family (Mulligan et al., 2009). However, this correlation was not found in ADHD girls with symptoms of autism. Furthermore, in girls, it was striking that higher autism scores were associated with ADHD and other comorbidities: For example, children with ADHD and high autism scores had more oppositional defiant disorder (ODD), conduct disorder (CD), movement disorders (clumsiness), and language development problems, similar to Gillberg's concept "Deficits in Attention, Motor control and Perception" (DAMP) (Gillberg, 2003).

In a Swedish birth cohort of almost two million adults, associations between ASD and ADHD were found within individuals and families. People with ASD had a 22 times higher risk of ADHD compared to people without autism. This was especially the case in high-functioning ASD. Family members of people with ASD also had an increased risk of ADHD (in monozygotic twins seventeen times, in dizygotic twins and siblings four times) (Ghirardi et al., 2017). This pattern indicates genetic overlap between the two disorders. In DSM-5, unlike in DSM-IV, both ADHD and ASD can be diagnosed in the same patient.

When making a differential diagnosis, it can be difficult to distinguish ASD from the social awkwardness due to inattention and impulsivity so common in ADHD. Also, where ADHD is comorbid with social anxiety, social phobia, or obsessive-compulsive disorder (OCD) the picture becomes more complicated. ASD can be distinguished clinically from social anxiety or OCD as those with primary anxiety disorders are not aloof or eccentric. Rather, they avoid social situations or performs ritualistic actions out of fear.

In ASD, social avoidance is present because of a lack of social-emotional reciprocity and deficits in non-verbal communicative behaviors used for social interaction. As a result, relationships are poorly developed, maintained, and understood.

In contrast, in OCD and social anxiety disorder, social interaction is avoided to lessen anxiety caused by performance and relationships. Both social anxiety disorder and OCD respond to treatment, unlike ASD. Hence careful diagnostic assessment is imperative (Cath, Ran, Smit, Van Balkom, & Comijs, 2008). Patients with inattentive presentation (or ADD) often suffer from anxiety and depression, which impacts their social competence. Social awkwardness as a result of ADD lowness, should be distinguished from eccentricity or not knowing what is expected in a social context. Diagnostic instruments for anxiety, depression, and autism spectrum disorders can be helpful in unravelling this diagnostic tangle. Where there is doubt as to the diagnosis of ASD is present in addition to ADD, (and possibly anxiety or depression), one should first treat the anxiety or depression, then the ADD and finally, reassess the likelihood of ASD being present.

ADHD and autism spectrum disorders both have a strong genetic background and often occur together in the same family. The two disorders appear to exist on a continuum: there is no strict separation, rather, a dimension.

2.14.11   ADHD and Tourette's and Other Tic Disorders

Tourette's and Persistent vocal or motor tic disorders start in childhood, are familial and are accompanied by repetitive movements such as blinking, facial twitching, or movements of the neck (motor tics). Vocal tics include growling, sniffing, or other sounds. The blurting out of foul language as originally described by Tourette is quite rare. In studies of children with tics, 39% also had ADHD and 40% had obsessive-compulsive symptoms or OCD. Twenty percent had both ADHD and OCD. In patients with Tourette's, ADHD was present in 25–80%; the combination of OCD and Tourette's was even more common. This argues in favor of a common basis for all forms of tic disorders and for genetic links with ADHD (Fernandez-Alvarez, 2002). Conversely, tics occur in 50% of children with ADHD (Knell & Comings, 1993). Tic disorders usually decrease in severity with age, and at the age of eighteen, half are free of tics. In adults, tics persist for about 20%, but they are often less severe than in children (Leckman, Bloch, Scahill, & King, 2006). As a result, tics rarely pose a major problem in the treatment of adults with ADHD. However, adults who had tics in childhood may have children with the same condition. Sometimes adults who used to have tics will stutter; this appears to be a remnant of the tic disorder, which can suddenly disappear with stimulant treatment. In one-third of children with tics, these increase during treatment with stimulants, but in the majority, the tics decrease or the severity remains the same. Hence the clinician is advised to use stimulants where ADHD and tics coexist, recording the frequency and severity of the tics (Gadow & Sverd, 2006; Palumbo, Spencer, Lynch, Co-Chien, & Faraone, 2004; Poncin, Sukhodolsky, McGuire, & Scahill, 2007). A study of the effectiveness of methylphenidate in adults with ADHD and tics was conducted (Spencer, Coffey, & Biederman, 1997, published in Weiss, Hechtman, & Weiss, 1999). Eleven percent of over 300 adults with ADHD had tics. These were almost all male, and for 90%, the tics had started in childhood but later than the ADHD. Those with tics also had OCD more often. Treatment with methylphenidate in the past had no influence on the occurrence of tics, their age of onset or severity. A review published in 2006 came to the same conclusion (Cooke & So, 2016).

Tic disorders are more common in children than in adults with ADHD. For the majority, treatment with stimulants has no adverse effects on the tics.

2.14.12   ADHD and Dyslexia

Dyslexia or reading disorder occurs in 3–4% of the population and is often associated with ADHD. Dyslexia is a disorder of reading or spelling, or both. Trouble with the sounding out of written language reflects a technical problem, not a disorder of comprehension. This slows the pace of reading. However, the technical problem can also adversely affect understanding of the text. Dyslexia is persistent and improves only with remedial teaching not with extra reading exercises. The treatment of dyslexia consists of specific training in sound-sign coupling and learning to compensate using strategies and computer-based tools.

Remediating reading problems in dyslexia may fail if there is also an attention deficit, and more serious reading problems may arise. Treatment of the attention deficit with stimulants can thus improve the treatment response in dyslexia (Wasserstein & Denckla, 2009). Research among severely dyslexic students shows that they have attention problems more often than controls, as well as in half of the cases, anxiety, depression, and behavioral problems (Knivsberg & Andreassen, 2008).

The diagnostic tools for dyslexia and learning disabilities are much less developed in adults than in children, although this area is improving (Nichols, McLeod, Holder, & McLeod, 2009). Initial research into biomarkers for ADD, ADHD, and dyslexia, using neuroimaging, magnetic encephalography, and psycho-acoustics was able to distinguish the three groups from controls with great precision (89–98%). This relates to the neuro-audit system. If replicated, this study could lead to a diagnostic test distinguishing these conditions based on brain functions (Serrallach et al., 2016).

Dyslexia is often hereditary and occurs in families. There is a history of a late start with reading, slow, inaccurate, and effortful reading which persists once the skill has been mastered. There may be spelling errors or difficulty with written expression (e.g., problems with grammar, punctuation, or organization). Even when the text is checked, errors are often missed. In addition to computer spell checks, various specific programs have been developed to remediate dyslexia.

In ADHD, attention deficit leads to learning difficulties because of lack of focus, persevering with certain tasks (causing dislike and avoidance of homework). These, coupled with poor working memory ultimately lead to underperformance. Of children and adults with ADHD, 60% have (had) learning problems, and 30% have not progressed academically. Thus, there are clear differences between the symptoms of ADHD and dyslexia; not infrequently both occur in one person, which exacerbates the learning problems and underperformance.

2.14.13   ADHD and Psychosis

The combination of ADHD and psychosis was long considered a rarity. The two disorders have opposing neurotransmitter aetiologies: reduced or increased dopamine metabolism. The totally different clinical pictures made it seem unlikely that they could coexist. However, research shows that 5% of all ADHD patients have psychotic episodes (Stahlberg, Soderstrom, Rastam, & Gillberg, 2004), and conversely that schizophrenia is preceded by ADHD symptoms in childhood in 17% of cases (Peralta, Campos, De Jalon, & Cuesta, 2010). A follow-up of 208 children with ADHD to age 31 years showed that 3.8% developed schizophrenia, a relative risk of 4.3 (Maibing et al., 2015). Common genetic and neurobiological vulnerability, in addition to interaction with environmental factors, may predispose to the co-occurrence of will underlie these increased prevalences of ADHD and psychosis (Pallanti & Salerno, 2015).

In longitudinal cohort research among 5500 children, the presence of underlying psychiatric disorders predicted the onset of psychotic *experiences* at the age of 12 years and psychotic *disorders* at the age of 18 years (odds ratios 1.7 and 2.3, respectively). In particular, the combined presentation of ADHD at age seven was strongly associated with psychotic experiences at the age of 12 years (odds ratio 3.3) (Hennig et al., 2017). In the same study, where the number of children had increased to 8000 children, it was found that children with ADHD at the age of 7 years were more bullied at the age of 10 years (odds ratio 3.6). Children involved in bullying had more psychotic experiences, and bullying proved to be an important mediator in the relationship between ADHD and psychosis, contributing 41–50% to the effect. Traumatic experiences before the age of eleven were also associated with psychosis later, but this was not a mediating factor (Hennig et al., 2017). All in all, comorbid ADHD and psychosis or schizophrenia are not rare. It is time to pay attention to this group of, particularly afflicted patients.

2.14.13.1 Differential Diagnosis

Psychotic symptoms occur in schizophrenia but also in bipolar disorder, personality disorders and depression, and should be differentiated. In patients presenting with the negative symptoms of schizophrenia (without a history of florid psychosis), the inattentive presentation of ADHD, or ADD, should also be considered. These patients are severely impaired due to their inattention, memory problems, lack of overview, planning, slowness, and indecisiveness. This clinical picture may resemble the negative symptoms of schizophrenia. For successful treatment, careful differential diagnostic examination is recommended in these patients. For treatment of ADHD in psychosis, see Sect. 4.19.4.

Diagnostic Instruments

3

3.1   Ultrashort Screening list for ADHD in Adults

General practitioners and other care providers who wish to examine a patient briefly and specifically for the core symptoms of ADHD can use an ultrashort screening instrument consisting of four questions: three questions about the core symptoms of ADHD and one question about their lifelong course.

This ultrashort screening list (see section "Ultrashort Screening List for ADHD in Adults" in Appendix) has not been validated in research. However, it is consistent with the DSM-5 requirements for the diagnosis of ADHD and covers the three core symptoms, namely restlessness or hyperactivity, impulsivity, and concentration or attention problems. A symptom cannot be transient, it should have been present consistently. If this is so, it should be lifelong, from childhood (before the twelfth year). These four questions identify all three presentation types of ADHD. This questionnaire shows that the core of ADHD is not so much the presence of one or more symptoms, but rather its chronicity (usually lifelong).

If one or more core symptoms have been present for life and the patient experiences distress as a result, the more extensive self-report questionnaire on attention problems and hyperactivity can be completed (see Sect. 3.2). For further diagnostics, the semi-structured Diagnostic Interview for ADHD in adults can be used (DIVA-5, based on the DSM-5 criteria, 2017).

3.2   Self-Report questionnaire on Attention Problems and Hyperactivity for Adulthood and Childhood

The *self-report questionnaire on attention problems and hyperactivity* (see section "Self-report Questionnaire on Attention Problems and Hyperactivity for Adulthood and Childhood" in Appendix) is based on the DSM-5 criteria for ADHD. It questions 23 items twice, once for childhood and once for adulthood.

© The Author(s), under exclusive license to Springer Nature   85
Switzerland AG 2022
J. J. S. Kooij, *Adult ADHD*, https://doi.org/10.1007/978-3-030-82812-7_3

There are eighteen DSM-5 criteria, nine for attention deficit or inattention, and nine for hyperactivity/impulsivity. The 23 items derived from the 18 criteria, where five complex items are reformulated in two single statements, making a total of 23 items. On the score sheet, these are later reduced to the original 18 criteria (Kooij et al., 2005). The cut-off point for the diagnosis in childhood is six of the nine criteria; in adulthood the cut-off point is five of the nine criteria. Self-reporting may introduce underreporting, so the advice is to consider further diagnostic testing for ADHD where there are 4 or more criteria in both childhood and adulthood.

In the diagnostic examination, the final number of criteria is determined by the researcher on the basis of a semi-structured interview, such as the DIVA. The self-report questionnaire on attention problems and hyperactivity has been examined in both epidemiological and clinical research (Kooij et al., 2004, 2005).

3.3   Diagnostic Interview for ADHD (DIVA-5) in Adults

The Diagnostic Interview for ADHD (DIVA-5) *in adults* is based on the DSM-5 criteria and is the first semi-structured Dutch interview for ADHD in adults (Kooij and Francken 2007a, b, c). In order to facilitate the assessment of the presence or absence of each criterion in childhood as well as in adulthood, concrete examples are given for both stages of life. In five areas of daily life, practical examples of dysfunction caused by the symptoms are given. The DIVA interview occurs when possible in the presence of the partner and family members in order to assess direct and collateral history simultaneously. The DIVA takes one to one and a half hours.

DIVA-5 only investigates ADHD. Each diagnostic examination should also check for the comorbid disorders that are frequently present. These include anxiety, sleep, mood, autism spectrum, personality disorders, and addiction. To this end, instruments and guidelines for the diagnosis of other psychiatric disorders may be used.

The DIVA has been translated into many languages and can be downloaded for a minimal charge from www.divacenter.eu. DIVA 2.0, the predecessor of DIVA-5, was based on the DSM-IV criteria and has been validated in Spanish and Swedish research (Pettersson et al. 2017; Ramos-Quiroga et al. 2019a, b).

Treatment

4

The treatment of an adult with ADHD consists of:

- Psycho-education
- Medication
- Contact with other people with ADHD (see Chap. 5)
- Coaching/cognitive therapy (see Chap. 5)
- Psychotherapy (see Chap. 5)

4.1 The Attitude of the Therapist

ADHD patients have a great need for a structured treatment program. For example, the therapist will rapidly notice that asking open questions is counterproductive. The patient is unable to answer them in a targeted manner. Poor concentration probably makes it more difficult to answer open-ended questions. It is, therefore, better to ask more specific, concrete questions. When treating a patient with ADHD, the therapist should provide the necessary structure, such as clear agreements about time, the subjects to be discussed and any subsequent assignments. The therapy session itself also needs to be structured, otherwise, there is a good chance that the discussion will digress and essential issues will not be covered. Effective treatment of patients with ADHD is described by Nadeau as follows (1999):

- Practice-oriented: Practical learning to deal with daily recurring problems.
- *Goal oriented:* Focusing on specific goals instead of going from one topic to another at random.
- Directive: The therapist gives guidelines, practical advice, and proposes concrete interventions.
- *Solution focused: The* goal is to achieve the desired result, taking feelings into account.
- Educational: The patient's understanding of ADHD and its consequences is increased during treatment.

© The Author(s), under exclusive license to Springer Nature Switzerland AG 2022

J. J. S. Kooij, *Adult ADHD*, https://doi.org/10.1007/978-3-030-82812-7_4

- Supportive: The therapist's attitude toward the patient is understanding and encouraging.
- Linking insight to action: Insight into symptoms or problems is always linked to specific solution-oriented actions.

4.2   Psycho-Education

Treatment for ADHD always begins with psycho-education. When information is transferred to the patient, he/she understands the process that is beginning, what the diagnosis and treatment are so that expectations are realistic. Patients have a great need for knowledge about the diagnosis and treatment; where it is lacking, it is a great loss (Matheson et al., 2013). Psycho-education is described in detail in articles and handbooks on the treatment of ADHD in adults (Barkley & Murphy, 2006; Murphy, 1995; Nadeau, 1994, 1999; Quinn & Nadeau, 2004; Safren et al., 2006a, 2006b; Triolo, 1999).

Psycho-education enables the patient to make the best choices independently and from a well-informed perspective. In this sense, psycho-education *empowers the* patient. Armed with this information, the newly diagnosed patient is more resilient when asked about the diagnosis and proposed treatment. Certainly, the newly diagnosed adult is often faced with a lack of understanding about this "trendy diagnosis" and treatment with stimulants. In practice, psycho-education appears to be an indispensable part of treatment of adult ADHD.

Adults diagnosed with ADHD have an almost inexhaustible need for information; they are curious and enterprising, which may make them request information more than other patients. They ask many incisive questions and exchange all kinds of experiences and information on the Internet. Not infrequently, they have downloaded information and completed questionnaires from the Internet. They may take these along to the intake interview.

Patients with ADHD require ongoing psycho-education from the practitioner(s). This is necessary for the acceptance of the diagnosis(es) so informed choices can be made for treatment. Information about the consequences of ADHD so that choices improve in education, the workplace, and in relationships.

Partners and parents of patients with ADHD also need information and the opportunity to exchange experiences. The family and/or partner should be involved from the start of the diagnostic process and, if desired, during treatment. The partner is present when psycho-education is given about the diagnosis(s) and the treatment plan. In addition, groups have been developed for partners and parents, in which they can tell their side of the story undisturbed, get information, and exchange tips. Often, the partner becomes so involved in (the prevention of) failures in the patient's life that there is little time or space left for his or her own agenda. If this balance is restored, patient and partner can often renegotiate their position in the relationship.

Sometimes the diagnosis evokes a strong emotional response or resistance in family members, which may interfere with treatment. ADHD symptoms may be identified in themselves or even rejected. Both of these situations may make the patient feel vulnerable and hinder acceptance of the diagnosis. Psycho-education focuses on discussing these processes and their effects on the patient. Family members are invited to receive the same psycho-education as the patient. This prevents the uncomfortable situation of a patient having to explain the disorder to the family or having to account for the difficulties experienced.

4.2.1 Online Psycho-Education

An interactive form of information is provided via the Internet through peer-to-peer contact on websites and forums. Here information and experiences are exchanged. Through websites and social media, the latest news from science is rapidly made accessible to the public. Of course, there is also a lot of chaff mixed in with the wheat. For reliable information sources, please refer to the sites listed at the back of the book.

Apps that support patients and/or therapists are a new development in the field. They give information, coaching and tips, monitor symptoms, and prevent relapse.

4.2.1.1 Digital Medicine: Super Brains App for ADHD

Psychiatric interventions should be cheaper, better, and at the same time serve more people. The e-health platforms that have been developed so far are too slow, boring, and user-unfriendly. E-health is usually conceived by health care providers and therefore does not fully meet the needs of the patient/consumer. Super Brains changes this: this app is an initiative of Rutger den Hollander, himself an ADHD patient and director of a Tech company. He created the app in collaboration with the following contributors: the author of this book, the Parnassia group, PsyQ, Lucertis Den Haag, the patient association Impuls, parents' association, Balans and the Dutch ADHD Network.

It is an app for ADHD patients of all ages, but also for family, practitioners, employers, and teachers. The name Super Brains refers to the qualities and talents of people with ADHD that are stimulated with the app. But it is also a reference to how the daily support, tips, and reminders reduce the burden of ADHD. Super Brains can be used by people with ADHD who may not yet have embarked on treatment, by therapists and patients during treatment, and after discharge from a treatment program, to prevent relapse. Super Brains, therefore, supports treatment strategies, and prevents relapse.

Super Brains is an example of "Digital Medicine," where the patient can collaborate with the specialist via a mobile phone and consult them at all times. The app contains:

- Tips on how to deal with poor planning, chaos, forgetfulness, irritability, agitation, relationship problems etc.
- More than 150 lifestyle habits to adopt or lose (e.g., adequate sleep, exercise, morning and evening routines, developing hobbies, and healthy eating.).
- The option to schedule tasks directly in the electronic calendar with reminders.

- A reward system with points that give access to new activities and games that help improve working memory.
- Access to games (gamification).
- Individualized profiles for each user with a photo or avatar.
- Points that are visible in each profile are visible to others so they can also monitor one's progress. These points give access to new activities and games.
- Interactive communities with chat rooms for children and adults with ADHD, partners and family members, practitioners, employers, and teachers.
- A buddy system where answering questions or helping others earns points.
- Information about ADHD and concomitant disorders.
- Treatment advice.
- Digital coaching and cognitive therapy through weekly animated videos with Dr. Brains, an avatar who gives personal feedback.
- Live video chats with the practitioner.

The app works by providing visual information and short texts. The content is based on the latest scientific knowledge. As a result of continuous feedback from users and the website "analytics," improvements are constantly being implemented.

Clinicians also have their own profile with a photo or avatar, and a "Virtual Practice" in which the progress of their patients is monitored (medication adherence or other treatment goals). This provides the practitioner with a rapid overview of how patients are doing. There is a community of practitioners to ask each other questions and exchange knowledge, where they can anonymously compare the progress of their own patients with that of colleagues. Clinicians who have more experience in handling ADHD help others more often, have more access to games and have more successfully treated patients. They will receive more points, which are visible in their profile, and have more access to games. Again, the game element introduces an element of competition.

Through the "ADHD University" component of the app, diagnostic tools and experiences are shared. Clinicians can follow "e-journeys," which refers to online training by the so-called Dr. Brains. In this way, patients and practitioners receive the same information about ADHD and the treatment, which unifies the process. The progress of Super Brains can be followed via www.superbrains.nl. Super Brains has been available since 2018 via Google Play and the App Store. The costs of Super Brains for patient and practitioner have been kept as low as possible and maybe reimbursed by health insurers.

4.2.2   Psycho-Education During Treatment

In general, it seems best to vary and repeat psycho-education at different times. Psycho-education by the practitioner can be offered individually, in groups, and through Super Brains. Psycho-education during group treatment and in Super Brains has the important advantage that not only the practitioner is informed, but that fellow patients can share their experiences directly with each other.

Patients themselves are involved in psycho-education: for example, experienced patients can share their experiences with the diagnosis and treatment with fellow ADHD adults who are about to start treatment (Schuijers & Kooij, 2007). This form of information was developed at the request of experienced patients who wanted to share their knowledge with newcomers. They indicated that when they first sought help, they would have liked to have had support and feedback from an adult with ADHD who had already been through the process. In the project "ADHD patients for each other," experienced patients were specially selected for this informative task and trained by a counsellor. The results of this sharing initiative are very positive for both clinicians and those newly diagnosed. Common questions about the use of medication and acceptance of the diagnosis are addressed in a more direct way than during standard psycho-education sessions. The experiential aspect plays an important role: someone with personal experience is far more convincing than an expert. This can save time during treatment, so that patients are motivated to use medication and do not need convincing.

During intake, the initial questions are answered and leaflets from the patient organization may be distributed to family members and patients. They also receive information about the treatment program and medication, as well as a list of useful websites and books. During the interview, the patient and family discuss the following: the diagnosis(es), severity, impact on functioning to date, heredity and biological background of ADHD, sequence of treatment steps for the comorbid disorders, the effectiveness and side effects of medication, the importance of coaching for the practical problems of ADHD, learning skills, prognosis, and the duration of treatment. Rules for cancelling appointments, the costs and consequences of not showing up for appointments are also discussed. By educating the patient and family about the characteristics, causes, and brain function in ADHD, blame and prejudice are diminished. The focus is taken off an alleged faulty upbringing and blame is not attributed of the fact that the patient does not function properly. This is of great importance, because every family has its own explanations for the patient's difficult life; often all parties feel powerless and the relationships are burdened with the question of guilt. The explanation is that ADHD is a neurobiological disorder, usually hereditary, usually has an exculpatory effect. This explanation creates room for the family members to redefine relationships, which benefits the patient and the treatment process. After all, a patient without family or network support is vulnerable, even if the treatment is effective. Psycho-education is best provided verbally and in writing. After the emotional upheaval of the intake consultation, it is helpful to refer to the information later, on a website or in a leaflet.

During treatment, psycho-education will continue to play an important role for any subject the patient or practitioner raises. In general, patients with poor concentration can absorb less information. The practitioner should take this into account by using short sentences and closed questions as much as possible. It helps if information is unambiguous and repeated, and both oral and written. Once pharmacological treatment begins and there is a positive treatment response, the patient's ability to process information improves considerably.

At the end of treatment, psycho-education focuses on how to deal with medication after discharge, how long to continue with medication, what to do in the event of an increase in symptoms or relapse and how to re-enter a treatment program, if necessary. Usually, the advice is to continue effective medication at the same dosage after discharge. This applies to both antidepressants and treatment for ADHD. Patients are advised to apply the tools and interventions that they acquired during treatment in the case of emerging complaints. With the Super Brains app, new goals can be formulated after discharge, for example, maintaining routines and adhering to and medication.

4.3 Important Points for the Practitioner

Acceptance of the diagnosis is a recurring theme for many patients and the practitioner must always be aware of this struggle. The significance of the diagnosis and the proposed treatment should be examined in each patient. Relief, grief, or anger are all possible emotional responses on receiving the diagnosis. The consequences of diagnosis differ depending on how the patient views the past. It may provide relief and a good explanation for years of problems, or the diagnosis may confirm the patient's self-construed poor self-esteem and weakness ("someone with ADHD is a loser"). The attitude toward medication can also vary greatly, from "medication is poison, I don't take it" to "if it can help me function better, let me start today rather than tomorrow." Daily intake of medication, especially short-acting medication, reminds some patients that they need medication in order to function. This may be interpreted as a reminder of their vulnerability and can reduce adherence. For this reason (amongst others) long-acting medication is preferable.

4.3.1 Possible Answers to FAQs in Psycho-Education

4.3.1.1 What Is the Impact of Untreated ADHD?

The impact of untreated ADHD is considerable; in addition to the persistence of concentration problems, hyperactivity, and impulsivity, the patient also has to deal with the consequences of the disorder: underperformance in education and work, lower income, changing jobs and partners, (car) accidents, teenage pregnancies, early onset of substance abuse and the risk of addiction, low self-esteem and insecurity, chronic fatigue and sleep problems. Psycho-education extends to the clinical picture of ADHD, the consequences of the disorder and the frequent comorbidity. It reduces stigmatization and provides an explanation for the effort it has taken to function, that he/she is "not lazy, stupid or crazy" (Kelly et al., 2006). On the other hand, it becomes clear that ADHD is not about minor problems. On average, adult patients with ADHD have sought help for 12.5 years without being diagnosed. The additional diagnoses such as anxiety, depression, and addiction may have been diagnosed and treated, but insufficiently (Kooij et al., 2001). Epidemiological research has shown that untreated ADHD can contribute to the chronicity of comorbid disorders (Fayyad et al., 2007; Kessler et al., 2006).

4.3.1.2 Is ADHD a Fashionable Diagnosis?

Perceiving ADHD as a "trendy diagnosis" may confuse the newly diagnosed patient. Psycho-education then focuses on distinguishing between fact and fiction. The fact that ADHD has been increasingly diagnosed in recent years, does not mean that it is suddenly more common, but that it is being better recognized by professionals. The clinical picture of ADHD was described in 1937 by Dr. Bradley, who noted that hyperactive children were calmed by amphetamine. In the 1960s, symptoms now associated with ADHD were referred to as "Minimal Brain Damage" and then the disorder was also treated with stimulants. Scientific research over the past 45 years has provided a solid, objective basis for diagnosis and improved treatment. Now that science has shown the genetic basis for ADHD and that it continues into adulthood, adults are also eligible for treatment. The term "trendy diagnosis" suggests that ADHD is a temporary hype. The well-documented scientific history of ADHD contradicts this. Perhaps every new development in psychiatry deserves some limelight for a while, to get the necessary attention. Ultimately, clinicians will become aware of the validity of the diagnosis and the effectiveness and safety of treatment (compare ADHD to the discussion about the wave of depression diagnoses some time ago). It takes time before the diagnosis is accepted as a "standard" disorder amongst others. Further research into ADHD will lead to refined diagnostics, different classification of symptoms, further elucidate the biological parameters, and possibly provide biomarkers as diagnostic tests. However, the clinical picture of ADHD has long been recognized and will not disappear.

4.3.1.3 Does ADHD Only Occur in the Western World?

One often wonders whether ADHD is only diagnosed in the West. This does not appear to be the case: ADHD is not a Western invention, but occurs in population studies of children and adults all over the world (Faraone et al., 2003; Fayyad et al., 2007; Kessler et al., 2006).

4.3.1.4 Is ADHD Outgrown? And If So, in Whom?

The question of whether ADHD disappears deserves a clear answer. After all, until 1990, the notion that ADHD was outgrown prevailed. ADHD continues to cause complaints and dysfunction in many adults who had it as children. Those who "grow out of it" tend to have high intelligence, little comorbidity, and a safe, supportive childhood (Biederman, Faraone, Milberger, Curtis, et al., 1996, Biederman, Faraone, Milberger, Guite, et al., 1996). Longitudinal population studies show that childhood-onset ADHD diminishes fairly often in adulthood, and that there is another variant of ADHD with late-onset, which has similar symptoms and dysfunction in adulthood. All this can change the diagnosis of ADHD (see also Sect. 1.3.2).

4.3.1.5 What Does ADHD Medication do to the Brain?

The pharmacological effect of stimulants is briefly explained on the basis of an illustration (see Fig. 4.1). ADHD probably involves a shortage of dopamine (DA) and to a lesser extent, norepinephrine (NA), in the synapse. These substances are important for inhibiting behavior. This applies to inhibiting movement

Fig. 4.1 Dopamine production, release,
and reuptake in synapses

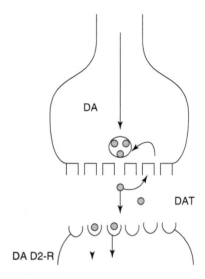

(hyperactivity), impulsivity (impatience), distractability (inattention), and emotions (mood swings and anger). ADHD is therefore also called a disorder of the braking mechanism, and the stimulants methylphenidate (MPH) or dextroamphetamine are the "brake fluid" (Fig. 4.1). The hypothesis is that dopamine (DA) is produced in the synapse, but that it is rapidly reabsorbed into the cell via the dopamine transporter (DAT) (genetic control). This creates a net shortage of the neurotransmitter available to enable stimulus transfer to the receptor (Da D2-R). The first drug choice for ADHD, methylphenidate, inhibits the reuptake of dopamine (and norepinephrine), resulting in more dopamine available to act as an inhibitory neurotransmitter. The other stimulant, dextroamphetamine, stimulates the release of dopamine and thus has a different mode of action. As a result, where there is non-response to methylphenidate, dextroamphetamine may be effective. If necessary, both can be tried successively.

The mechanism of atomoxetine, a non-stimulant, is similar to that of methylphenidate, although atomoxetine inhibits the reuptake of norepinephrine, not dopamine.

4.4   Medication

4.4.1   Introduction

Adults with ADHD usually have a long history of underperformance and failure. The diagnosis is usually made around the age of 30 years. This is preceded on average by 12.5 years of seeking help (Kooij et al., 2001), without receiving a diagnosis or treatment. Comorbid disorders, may have been inadequately treated, leading to chronicity of symptoms. After such a delay in diagnosis, intervention should be optimal. Stimulants are the most effective and safest treatment for ADHD. Medication should be started immediately after psycho-education. Stimulants are effective in

50–70% of children and adults with ADHD, as long as they are taken (Faraone & Biederman, 2002; Faraone et al., 2002; Kooij et al., 2004; Spencer et al., 2005). If doses are skipped or if medication is discontinued, the symptoms return. The first and commonest question about treatment is: "Can't it be done without medication?" The answer is "Not really." In other words, so far no other modality has a comparable effect on the concentration problems, restlessness, irritability, and emotional lability of ADHD. But this does not mean that medication is the only treatment. Coaching and/or cognitive behavioral therapy provide a practical approach to planning and organization. These interventions can be supported by the Super Brains app. Medication should be the first step in treatment, because experience has shown that without it, coaching is unsuccessful because of inattention, forgetting appointments, and defaulting from therapy. After three months, once the novelty of the diagnosis has worn off, a patient who is not on medication may be unable to implement the necessary changes, or simply will no longer show up at appointments. Many people with ADHD recognize this pattern of dropping out. The attentional problems of ADHD, therefore, hamper the treatment itself. That is why it is advisable to start with medication.

ADHD is also called an inhibition disorder or a disorder of the brake. There is no braking of inattention, so concentration is diminished. Similarly, motor actions and emotional responses are not inhibited, leading to hyperactivity, impulsivity, and mood swings. The brake function is driven by the neurotransmitters dopamine and norepinephrine, which appear to be diminished in ADHD. The stimulant medications are dopamine and norepinephrine agonists, which increase these neurotransmitters in the synapse, and thus activate the brain's braking function. The stimulating effect on the inhibition makes it clear that stimulants actually calm patients. The calming effects of amphetamine-like substances on hyperactive children have been known since 1937 (Sandberg, 2002). Stimulants are now among the best-researched drugs in medicine, precisely because they are amphetamine-like substances that were initially only prescribed to children for whom all the necessary checks and balances were required.

By activating the brake as described, stimulants promote mood stability, calm, peace, a better overview, and clearer thinking.

In adults, all medication is prescribed *off-label, with the* exception of atomoxetine, which is registered for children and adults with ADHD. Methylphenidate is registered in The Netherlands for children with ADHD, but not for adults. This is different in many countries, including the United States.

All medications for ADHD, except one of the long acting methylphenidate brands and atomoxetine, are prescribed *off-label* to adults in the Netherlands.

Research shows that when taken as prescribed, stimulants are effective, safe, and not addictive in children, adolescents, and adults. If the medication is taken haphazardly (the dose is forgotten or taken late), the effect will not be felt, or unpleasant effects may occur (see Sect. 4.9.4.3). This is particularly a problem with short-acting stimulants such as Ritalin and dextroamphetamine, which should be taken every two to four hours to prevent premature effects and rebound. Adults who are active for 16 hours per day should take short-acting medication six to eight times daily, on time. Practice has shown that no ADHD patient is able to do this in the long term because of the nature of the disorder itself: forgetfulness is a core problem of ADHD. In adult patients, the long-acting forms of methylphenidate are not reimbursed and short-acting stimulants may cause side effects or require multiple doses. This means that the available treatments leave much to be desired. Poor adherence to medication also affects psychological treatment. As a result, treatment as a whole becomes unnecessarily inefficient, lengthy, and costly.

4.4.2 Stimulants and Addiction Risk

In most countries, stimulants are scheduled medications because they contain amphetamine-like substances. National legislation controls the prescriptions at pharmacy and practitioner levels to prevent potential abuse. However, the prescribed stimulants are less potent than amphetamines available on the street, and are therefore less likely to cause dependence. If stimulants are taken as prescribed, addictive effects are usually not observed. Psychiatric patients do not find methylphenidate habit forming. On the contrary, the clinician often needs to motivate them to continue taking the medication rather being concerned about them taking too much. Short-acting stimulants in particular can be taken intravenously or intranasally in order to get a kick. When administered via these routes, addictive effects similar to those of cocaine may occur (Volkow et al., 1995). The speed of administration determines whether a euphoric effect occurs. If patients abuse their prescription medication, short-acting stimulants should be stopped. Abuse is rare in psychiatric patients, but occurs more often in (ex-)addicts. For this reason, they are better treated with long-acting stimulants or with atomoxetine.

Abuse or misuse of stimulant medication during treatment may produce the following symptoms: the patient does not recover as expected, the patient misses appointments, and/or looses prescriptions several times (losing a script once is possible, especially in chaotic people with ADHD). All these findings necessitate a discussion about the correct dosing, efficacy, possible side effects, and abuse of the medication. If a patient feels that he or she is being taken seriously by the practitioner, these questions are likely to be answered honestly. Taking a patient seriously means: the practitioner is responsible for prescribing the correct dosage, timing doses appropriately, and addressing any adverse side effects. For example, if the medication effect is too short, there will be no effect in the evening, and a craving for drugs results. The practitioner should then be willing to add an evening dose. Underdosing is a reason for patients to relapse into drug abuse.

Long-acting medication has been specially developed to improve compliance, efficacy, and to reduce the risk of misuse: the methylphenidate is encased in a hard capsule and dissolved in gel form (Oros-methylphenidate or Concerta) or in an easy-to-open capsule with granules containing both short- and long-acting methylphenidate (Equasym and Medikinet). In the long-acting form of dextroamphetamine, the active substance is linked to L-lysine, from which it cannot be detached (Faraone, 2008). This makes intravenous or intranasal administration more difficult.

It is conceivable that patients with comorbid depressive disorder might be in need of the mood-enhancing effects of a stimulant. Treating depression first with an SSRI (see Sect. 4.20.3) addresses this problem.

However, there are increasing concerns about the spread and misuse of stimulants by young adults and students in the United States (Faraone & Upadhyaya, 2007). The medication is used by those wishing to memorize exam material in a short period of time. Research into this group shows that they report poorer concentration, are less motivated during cognitive tests and have worse study habits compared to controls (Ilieva & Farah, 2013). This raises the possibility that they are undiagnosed and untreated patients with ADHD, or family members of treated patients. They may have easy access to the medication and experience enhanced attention and concentration when taking it. There is little research on the effects of stimulants in normal controls, but available research in children with and without ADHD indicates that stimulants produce similar effects (Rapoport & Inoff-Germain, 2002). However, those with **no** concentration problems experience little benefit from medication and, above all, are bothered by the side effects.

4.4.3 Improvement of Cognitive Functioning

Healthy people without ADHD are increasingly coming into contact with ADHD patients who are taking stimulants, so the medication can be diverted for a once-off trial in a person without ADHD. But there are also indications that the use of other cognitive-enhancing drugs is increasing. In addition to coffee, tea, and nicotine, these include cholinesterase inhibitors (treatment for Alzheimer's dementia), ecstasy, methamphetamine, modafinil, and stimulants (Franke et al., 2014; Sahakian & Morein-Zamir 2015). Users will perceive a small improvement in cognition, but the side effects and drug interactions are a cause for concern. A systematic review of fourteen studies in adolescents aged 12–25 years showed that modafinil improves reaction time, logical reasoning, and problem solving. Methylphenidate improved performance in new tasks, tasks requiring attention, and reduced planning delays in more complex tasks. Amphetamine improved the consolidation of information, resulting in better recall, but more research with comparable methods and outcome measures is needed (Bagot & Kaminer, 2014).

4.4.4 Effect of Stimulants on Addiction

There is little evidence of stimulant abuse by patients with ADHD, and no link has been found between treatment with stimulants and the later development of substance abuse. On the contrary, stimulant treatment has been shown to reduce the risk of substance abuse in ADHD adolescents to that of their peers (Faraone & Upadhyaya, 2007). Short-acting stimulants have the highest risk of abuse whereas long-acting stimulants are designed to prevent abuse. The uptake of the medication in the brain with oral ingestion of stimulants is slow and provides effective treatment without producing euphoric effects. Even when confirmed cocaine addicts were given oral methylphenidate, no craving developed unless the medication was accompanied by a conditioned stimulus (pictures or videos of cocaine abuse) (Volkow et al., 2008). In general, long-acting stimulants are preferable because they are less likely to be abused. They are more effective because repeated dosing is not necessary and they are less likely to be forgotten (Faraone & Upadhyaya, 2007). In addiction care, certain risk groups may benefit from non-stimulants such as atomoxetine. In a recent review, the treatment of ADHD with stimulants appears to be effective in addicts. It is important to assess and monitor the potential risks of stimulant use in this population (Kollins et al., 2008).

Innovative research is needed to clarify in the long term, which treatment is suitable for which patient group. Treatment with stimulants and cognitive therapy can have a positive influence on substance abuse, as well as on ADHD. This was demonstrated among cocaine users (Levin et al., 2015). In all cases, management should be adapted to fit the person with individual-level tailoring ("precision medicine") approaches (Luo & Levin, 2017).

Treatment with stimulants reduces the risk of addiction. Long-acting stimulants are preferred because of the better compliance and lower risk of abuse.

4.4.5   Functioning of Stimulants in the Brain

After dopamine is secreted into the synaptic cleft for excitatory neurotransmission, the dopamine transporter removes it and pumps it back into the presynaptic neuron (Fig. 4.1). The density of the dopamine transporter is increased in ADHD compared to controls. It seems plausible that in ADHD patients, dopamine is removed from the synapse too quickly, even before adequate neurotransmission has taken place (Krause et al., 2003). Imaging studies show that methylphenidate blocks dopamine transport, inhibiting reuptake, and increasing the amount of dopamine available for neurotransmission (Dresel et al., 2000; Volkow et al., 2002). Addicts have reduced dopamine in various brain areas, including the striatum, which may explain why they seek to supplement this deficiency (Volkow et al., 2004). In ADHD, a dopamine deficiency is believed to exist in the frontal cortex and striatum, areas responsible for attention and impulse control. Stimulant treatment increases the quantity of dopamine (and to a lesser extent, norepinephrine) available in these areas and improves inattention and impulse dyscontrol (Solanto et al., 2001). Dextroamphetamine increases the release of dopamine, with a similar effect on the improvement of ADHD symptoms. Because dextroamphetamine has a different mechanism of action in the brain, it is worth trying dextroamphetamine if methylphenidate is not effective. In children with ADHD, the total response rate for methylphenidate and dextroamphetamine was 90% (Elia et al., 1991). This response rate is so high that treatment with stimulants is very similar to supplementing a deficiency, as is the case with providing insulin in type 1 diabetes.

Methylphenidate inhibits dopamine reuptake. Dextroamphetamine increases the release of dopamine.

4.4.6 Order of Treating Comorbid Disorders

Three-quarters of adults with ADHD have one or more co-existing psychiatric disorders, such as anxiety, depression, bipolar II disorder, sleep disturbance, or addiction. These disorders should be treated, preferably prior to the treatment of ADHD. Generally, the most severe or disabling disorder is treated first. After all, ADHD is chronic, and rarely a reason for acute distress. An underlying anxiety disorder, depression, or addiction also masks the efficacy of ADHD medication. Side effects from stimulants can also be counterproductive: an anxious patient experiences the accelerated heartbeat that occurs as a result of treatment as a return of panic, and will immediately stop the medication. Clinical experience shows that after treating the anxiety with a modern antidepressant (SSRI), the stimulant-provoked tachycardia is no longer experienced as anxiety. A depressed patient may not be able to recognize the improvement caused by the stimulant due to a negative outlook, and an addicted patient using alcohol or drugs, increases the risk of side effects, making it impossible to assess the effect. Depression is therefore first treated with an antidepressant and alcohol and drugs are reduced as much as possible before starting stimulants.

ADHD patients tend to default treatment if there is no rapid improvement in symptoms. For this reason, it is preferable to treat comorbid anxiety and depression with an SSRI and not psychotherapy (where treatment duration is 12–16 weeks). After four to six weeks of treatment with an SSRI, when the depression/anxiety symptoms have subsided, stimulant medication can be started. Clinical experience shows that long-term psychotherapy for comorbid disorders is not completed if the ADHD remains untreated.

Bipolar disorder is treated with a mood stabilizer, after which a stimulant can be added. Where a severe sleep disorder prevents patients from attending appointments during the day because they are asleep, the sleep disorder should also be treated first. The combination of medicines (e.g., SSRI + long-acting methylphenidate + melatonin) provides the quickest reduction in symptoms. In the case of additional personality disorders, it is advisable to treat the ADHD first (and any other axis I comorbidity), and then to start psychotherapy for the personality disorder. Once the impulsivity, inattention, and irritability associated with ADHD have decreased, treatment of the personality disorder has a greater chance of success.

When treating comorbid disorders, the most serious disorder takes precedence. Anxiety and depressive disorders are treated first and substance abuse is first stopped or reduced as much as possible; only then is methylphenidate added.

4.4.7 Medication Available (in The Netherlands)

There are different types of medications for ADHD: stimulants and non-stimulants, registered and non-registered medications, and those registered for children, or for both children and adults with ADHD (see Table 4.3). There are three types of stimulants: methylphenidate, (lis) dextroamphetamine, and dexmethylphenidate. Brand names of long-acting methylphenidate are: Concerta, Equasym XL, Medikinet CR, and the non-label methylphenidate Retard Sandoz or Mylan. Short-acting methylphenidate is called Ritalin or Medikinet. Dextroamphetamine exists in a registered short-acting form (Amfexa or Tentin 5 mg), an unregistered short-acting form (dextroamphetamine), and as unregistered long-acting form (dextroamphetamine Retard and Elvanse (though the latter is registered for children and adolescents). According to the Dutch guideline for adult ADHD, the British NICE guideline, and the guideline of the British Association of Psychopharmacology (BAP) (De Crescenzo et al., 2017), stimulants (methylphenidate and dextroamphetamine) are first choice drugs because of the highest effect size, i.e., the highest chance of effect (NVvP, 2015; De Crescenzo et al., 2017). The next choice is atomoxetine (Strattera), and then long-acting bupropion (Wellbutrin) (see also Table 4.1).

Modiodal has been registered for narcolepsy or sleeping sickness, and was also effective for ADHD in five studies in children and adolescents (Wang et al., 2017). However, a controlled study in adult ADHD was negative (Arnold et al., 2014). Long-acting guanfacine (Intuniv), an alpha-2-adrenergic agonist is registered for children and adolescents with ADHD for whom stimulants are inappropriate or ineffective. This drug has been little studied in adults. Initial studies with guanfacine in adults, comparing guanfacine plus stimulant with stimulant plus placebo, showed no added value of guanfacine (Butterfield et al., 2016). A small randomized adult study comparing short-acting guanfacine with dexamphetamine showed similar efficacy and minor side effects (Taylor & Russo 2001). Guanfacine is currently prescribed off-label to adults, especially those with cardiovascular risks (e.g., hypertension) and tic disorders, but more research is needed. Long- and short-acting clonidine is registered in the United States for ADHD children aged six to seventeen years, but not in Europe. Clonidine is an alpha-2-adrenergic agonist, used as an antihypertensive drug with strong sedative properties. There are no double-blind studies of its use in ADHD adults (Kooij et al., 2001). The sedation is a limiting factor for its use in adults, as this causes further reduction in concentration, as well as potentially dangerous rebound hypertension if a dose is missed.

Table 4.1 Choice of medication order for ADHD in the Netherlands, based on effectiveness and side effects

Medication	Effectiveness	Side effects
1. Stimulants (methylphenidate, dexmethylphenidate, and D-dexamphetamine)	+++	Headaches, dry mouth, loss of appetite, anxiety, palpitations, sleep problems
2. Atomoxetine	++	Loss of appetite, abdominal pain, nausea, flu-like symptoms, skin rash, accelerated heartbeat, drowsiness, sexual side effects, possible increase in suicidal thoughts
3. Long-acting Bupropion	+	Dry mouth, drowsiness, at higher doses increase the risk of seizures
4. Guanfacine XR	+/−	Hypotension, drowsiness, sedation, bradycardia, weight gain, headache, abdominal pain, increased heart rate, and blood pressure

Long-acting medication is generally preferred for adult ADHD because it needs to be taken less often and is therefore less often forgotten. This improves effectiveness, reduces rebound symptoms, and provides better cover when driving a vehicle. Long-acting medication is a safer choice for ADHD with comorbid addiction.

4.4.7.1 Registered Medications Versus Off-label Use

The branded drugs Ritalin, Medikinet CR, Equasym XL, Concerta, Strattera, and Intuniv are registered in the Netherlands for children and adolescents with ADHD. In the United States and many other countries most are also registered for adults. In our country, Strattera and Medikinet are the only drugs registered for ADHD in children and adults. Non-registered drugs are prescribed "off-label" if the drugs are proven effective and safe in controlled trials in the relevant age group.

4.4.7.2 Dosage

Adults with ADHD use different doses of long-acting stimulants. The best dose is the lowest dose that produces an optimal effect and with minimal side effects. This varies from person to person. The dosage level is likely to depend on the genetically determined sensitivity to the substance. The cost of treatment with long-acting medication varies depending on the dose.

4.4.8   Medication Available in the United States

In the United States, all of the drugs listed in Table 4.1 are available, plus a range of different types of stimulants with different duration of action. For example, there are long-acting forms of Ritalin (Ritalin Long Acting and Ritalin Slow Release), which last eight and six hours, respectively. There are short- and long-acting forms of a d-isomer of methylphenidate (Focalin), with duration of action of three to four and eight to ten hours, respectively (Spencer et al., 2007). Finally, there is the methylphenidate patch (Daytrana TM) with an duration of action of twelve hours (Findling et al., 2008; Pierce et al., 2008). The long-acting amphetamine preparations consist of a combination of different amphetamines (Adderall and Adderall XR), which are effective for four to six and ten to twelve hours, respectively (Weisler et al., 2006). Dexedrine spansule contains long-acting dexamphetamine (six to eight hours) (Pelham et al., 1990). The latest dexamphetamine, (Vyvanse), has a twelve to fourteen hours duration of action. Abuse is prevented as an L-lysine molecule is linked to dexamphetamine (Blick & Keating, 2007; Faraone, 2008). The non-stimulants include short- and long-acting guanfacine, an alpha-adrenergic agonist related to clonidine (Biederman et al., 2006, Biederman et al., 2008; Taylor & Russo, 2001). Guanfacine is thought to have less serious side effects than clonidine (although fatigue and drowsiness are most common).

4.4.9   Drugs in the Pipeline

Nicotinergic drugs, including a patch, are still under investigation and appear to be effective for ADHD (ABT-418, ABT-089) (Poltavski & Petros, 2006; Wilens & Decker, 2007; Wilens et al., 2006). Finally, a combination of amphetamines, with a 16-h duration of action seems promising: the so-called triple-bead mixed amphetamine salts (SPD-465). This should last for the entire adult working day.

4.5   Dealing with Alcohol and Cannabis USE Before and During Treatment with Medication

Prior to starting stimulant medication, alcohol, and drug abuse must be stopped. The patient's motivation for quitting is usually increased when they are told that their need for these drugs will decrease, once the stimulants are taken. Firstly, the number of alcoholic drinks, joints, or other drugs used per day should be recorded, giving an impression of the severity of substance use. Depending on this, an individually tailored program can be created for phasing out and stopping the substance. Sometimes this requires specialized help within the addiction care setting **before and during treatment**. Preferably, the patient should be clean before starting the medication. Sometimes it is not possible to phase out completely before starting the treatment. In this case, in consultation with the patient, drug use can be stopped while the medication is being built up. This often works better when the symptoms of ADHD have decreased as a result of the medication.

Patients and practitioners often ask how to deal with moderate alcohol and cannabis use during the treatment of ADHD with methylphenidate or dextroamphetamine. Abuse of alcohol or cannabis should be stopped prior to starting medication so that the impact of treatment can be properly assessed. Another reason is that the side effects of alcohol and stimulants can potentiate each other. Furthermore, heavy alcohol consumption is depressogenic. If ADHD patients before and during treatment use excessive drugs and alcohol, they should refrain from using these altogether. After all, one should question their appropriateness of treatment if they cannot stop their addiction. Those who can are able to use in a moderate way, should be permitted to have a drink once in a while. No research has been done into the effects of moderate alcohol consumption on stimulants. In practice, the following rule of thumb is applied: no alcohol during the week, and on the weekend or at a party, a maximum of two glasses a day. If alcohol is stopped during the week, this indicates more control and restricted consumption; at weekends or at parties moderate alcohol use is tolerated. In this way, the patient does not have to go through life as a total abstainer.

Cannabis is often **before and during treatment** used to combat symptoms of ADHD such as restlessness and sleep problems. Cannabis increases the concentration problems of ADHD and therefore negates the beneficial effects of stimulants on concentration. It is also difficult to assess the effects of stimulants in the presence of cannabis. For the common sleep problems associated with ADHD, melatonin is the treatment of choice, although more research into this is necessary (see Sect. 4.20.2). Experience shows that addiction to cannabis can be very persistent. It is difficult for patients to cut down on their habitual use of one joint a day, which is usually taken at bedtime. Nevertheless, ADHD medication is incompletely effective as long as cannabis use continues. Treatment often stagnates because patients miss appointments, and cannot maintain their attention during conversations and therapy.

If the stimulants are effective, abstinence tends to be successful. Therefore, patients are not required to be completely abstinent before starting the medication, but are required to reduce to a pre-agreed maximum **before and during treatment** number of drinks or joints, and to stop completely or use in moderation during stimulant treatment.

Rules of thumb for the amount of alcohol and cannabis when using stimulants: no alcohol during the week, and a maximum of two glasses a day at the weekend or at a party. Minimize cannabis to one joint per night and if possible, replace it with melatonin where there are sleeping problems.

4.6   Contraindications to Stimulant Use

Contraindications for stimulants are pregnancy, current psychosis, and congenital dysrhythmia.

Pregnant women are currently discouraged from using stimulants because there is as yet insufficient data on the consequences for the child. Initial data on exposure to methylphenidate in the first trimester of pregnancy in 180 women showed four children with abnormalities, slightly less than the number naturally occurring in pregnancy (Dideriksen et al., 2013). This is a reassuring first finding, but to ensure the safety of methylphenidate use in the first trimester, data from 1000 pregnancies are required according to EMA (European Medicine Agency) guidelines. So, more research and follow-up after exposure to methylphenidate in pregnancy are needed.

A Danish population study of all pregnancies ($n = 989,932$) between 1997 and 2008 reports that 0.02% of the women ($n = 186$) used methylphenidate or atomoxetine during pregnancy because of ADHD. They were compared with pregnant women with ADHD ($n = 275$) without medication use, and a control group. Medication use in pregnancy was associated with spontaneous abortion, but the diagnosis of ADHD without medication use also showed this association. Apgar scores <10 at birth were more common among women with ADHD who used medication during pregnancy than among women who did not use medication during pregnancy (Bro et al., 2015).

The use of dexamphetamine preparations in pregnancy appears to be on the increase in the United States, without clear knowledge of the effects. Research into this is recommended (Louik et al., 2015).

Therefore, the advice for the time being is to be cautious: the medication should be stopped as soon as an early pregnancy test is positive (or the period is one week overdue). The fetus will then have been exposed to the medication in utero for a maximum of two weeks. The risk of this must be weighed up by the patient and partner together with the doctor. The following risks should also be taken into consideration: if medication is stopped before conception, the woman will have a longer time off treatment. This may also be associated with higher risk of relapse into drug abuse.

Too little is known about breastfeeding and methylphenidate. Methylphenidate is secreted in small amounts in breast milk. The advice is to be cautious, unless the condition of the mother requires treatment with methylphenidate. In that case, it is best to prescribe short-acting methylphenidate, so that breastfeeding can take place after a dose has been metabolized, in order to minimize the risk of exposure. Children breastfed by mothers taking methylphenidate should be monitored for irritability, sleep problems, and insufficient weight gain. In the limited case studies available, no short-term side effects have been observed so far (Marchese et al., 2015). After childbirth and breastfeeding, methylphenidate can be resumed.

Fortunately, certain modern antidepressants can now be continued during pregnancy, so that the expectant mother does not relapse. Patients with psychosis should always be treated with an antipsychotic first. Stimulants can exacerbate or precipitate psychosis in predisposed people. In these cases, stimulants are not recommended. Patients with schizophrenia are better advised to try other non-stimulant medication, although it appears from case reports that stimulants are effective in patients with ADHD and psychosis (Blom & Kooij, 2012) if they are protected with an antipsychotic (see also Sect. 4.20.4).

An exception can be made for those diagnosed with schizophrenia who have never had florid symptoms, but only negative symptoms. This clinical presentation may resemble the inattentive presentation of ADHD. If the diagnosis of ADHD is confirmed, treatment for ADHD can be initiated under proper supervision and control.

Patients with drug-induced psychosis or a history of psychotic episodes with mental retardation have an increased risk of relapse with psychosis with stimulants. In these patients, antipsychotic before starting a stimulant will provide protection. They can also be treated with atomoxetine or other non-stimulant medication. Patients treated with an antipsychotic where the psychosis is in remission, may be treated with a stimulant under supervision. However, no systematic research has been done in this group with this combination of drugs. Bipolar patients are first treated with a mood stabilizer, after which stimulant medication can be added. Initial clinical experience with this combination is favorable (see Sect. 4.20.3). Patients with a cluster B personality disorder with associated (micro)psychotic or paranoid episodes may benefit from a low dose of an antipsychotic, to which a stimulant may be added. Although this remains to be confirmed by research, clinical experience suggests that the antipsychotic effect is not reversed by the use of stimulants, and both drugs appear to be predictably effective in these patients.

In the case of congenital dysrhythmia (e.g., velocardiofacial syndrome, Marfan syndrome, Wolff-Parkinson-White syndrome), patients are discouraged from using stimulants, where the associated tachycardia can aggravate the arrhythmia. In such cases, consultation with the cardiologist is essential. If an arrhythmia is suspected, an ECG and, if necessary, further cardiac examination is advised. Before starting stimulants, the doctor should always inquire about arrhythmia and measure blood pressure and pulse. Sudden death is increased in children with congenital heart defects. Children with these heart defects who also have ADHD may run an additional risk when treated with stimulants if the heart defect goes unrecognized. However, in a study comparing ADHD children with congenital heart defects who were treated with ADHD medication and those who were not, no difference was found in the number of deaths. It could not be demonstrated that stimulant medication contributed to mortality (Conway et al., 2008; Wilens et al., 2006; Winterstein et al., 2007). More information on this subject can be found via **www.fda.gov** and www.aacap.org. During the course of life, most heart abnormalities become known, which means that adults are probably less at risk than children, some of whom were not yet diagnosed when they started treatment for ADHD. Incidentally, adults or children whose arrhythmias are treated can take stimulants with the consent and supervision of the specialist.

4.6.1   Relative Contraindications

Epilepsy, hyperthyroidism, hypertension, glaucoma, arrhythmia, and anxiety disorders are relative contraindications for the use of stimulants. The reasons for this are that stimulants:

- Lower the insulin threshold.
- Exacerbate the pre-existing tachycardia in hyperthyroidism.
- Can increase (but also decrease) the blood pressure.
- Can increase eyeball pressure.
- Can worsen arrhythmias.
- Exacerbate fear or panic in sensitive individuals by acceleration of the heartbeat.

Therefore, these conditions are always checked before starting with stimulants and further investigated if required. These conditions must be treated and controlled before methylphenidate can be added. Existing tics may worsen with methylphenidate, but the majority do not (Gadow et al., 1999). It is useful to monitor the severity of any tics prior to and during treatment. Stuttering can be regarded as a form of tic disorder and, like tics, sometimes improves with methylphenidate.

4.7   Measures Prior to and During the Use of Medication

The patient first receives extensive psycho-education about the effect, side effects, and duration of action of the medication. The severity of the ADHD symptoms and the adverse effects can be charted using the Symptom and Adverse Drug Reaction List (see see section "List of Symptoms and Side Effects of ADHD" in Appendix) or only the severity of the ADHD symptoms with the total score of the ADHD Rating Scale (see Sect. 4.8.2 and section "ADHD Rating Scale, Self-Report" in Appendix). It is also possible to use a list of measurable target symptoms, drawn up specifically for the individual patient, where one expects to see improvement (see

Sect. 4.8.3). It is important that the patient does not underreport the severity of the symptoms prior to treatment, so that any decrease in the severity of the symptoms over time accurately reflects improvement. ADHD patients may present with the paradox of being more aware of the severity of their symptoms **after** effective treatment. As a result, they sometimes score higher after treatment than before. It is therefore up to the practitioner to ensure that the baseline severity scores are accurately filled in.

(Relative) contraindications are discussed with the patient as described above. Blood pressure, pulse, and weight are routinely measured, and then repeated after several weeks of medication use. Where indicated, laboratory, ECG, or EEG investigations are performed, with or without referral to a specialist.

4.8   Instruments for Drug Treatment

4.8.1   Symptom and Side Effects List

This list (see Annex 2.1) contains a number of ADHD symptoms, such as restlessness, concentration problems, and a number of side effects of methylphenidate. Symptoms and adverse reactions are recorded daily for one week prior to the start of use of methylphenidate. The severity of symptoms and side effects ranges from 0 (absent) to 3 (severe/frequent burden). During the use of the medication, the patient continues to fill in the list until the therapeutic effect and the side effects are sufficiently clear to both patient and clinician. These lists can be discussed at the next appointment, two weeks later. Alternatively, the ADHD Rating Scale can be used to evaluate the effect of treatment (see section "ADHD Rating Scale, Self-Report" in Appendix).

4.8.2   ADHD Rating Scale

The ADHD Rating Scale is based on the DSM criteria for ADHD and consists of the same 23 items as the self-report questionnaire for attention problems and hyperactivity. The difference when this rating scale is used during treatment is that the subscores of attention deficit and of hyperactivity/impulsivity are not ascertained to make a diagnosis, but rather, the total score of the current symptoms is used to evaluate treatment response. To calculate the total score of the original eighteen DSM criteria, all the items that form a criterion are added up. Once all items are answered, the total score is calculated. Of the items 1+3, 2+4, 8+9, 10+11, 12+13, per pair the highest score is taken. Where a patient scored 1 on item ten and 3 on item eleven, the relevant score is 3 (the higher of the two).

The list is completed prior to and during treatment with medication. The aim is to achieve at least a 30% reduction in the total score of ADHD symptoms with treatment. This measure for improvement results from research on treatment response, which examined the reduction of symptoms with the same questionnaire (Kooij et al., 2004; Spencer et al., 2005). Therapeutic effect can be expected within a few weeks after starting the correct dose of a stimulant; in the case of atomoxetine, the effect occurs four to six weeks after the highest dose was initiated.

4.8.3 Example of an Individual Target Symptom List

For patients who have difficulty filling in long questionnaires at home or reflecting on changes in symptom severity over time, it may be helpful to take a different route; in this way treatment efficacy can still be objectively assessed. For example, in consultation with the patient, the clinician identifies three objectives for treatment, or three symptoms that should reduce in severity with treatment (see Table 4.2).

It is important that a goal is quantified, preferably in minutes, or in number of times a week. In this way, reduction in the severity of the complaints can be measured and checked during the next consultation. The advantage of this method is that the therapeutic goals are chosen by the patient, and that he or she feels involved in the evaluation process.

4.8.4 QbTest

The effect of medication can be also be measured objectively by using the QbTest, a continuous performance test (CPT) that also measures hyperactivity with an infrared camera. A baseline QbTest is done before starting medication and repeated after reaching an effective dose. The test measures executive functions, which is a slight deviation from the clinically observable symptoms of ADHD. Nevertheless, patient and practitioner can document visible differences before and after medication. This guides the decisions on what constitutes an optimal dosage. Nonresponse is also immediately apparent from the QbTest. Differences between various ADHD medications can also be objectified by using the QbTest (see also Sect. 1.1.9).

Table 4.2 Example of an individual target symptom list

Target	Frequency now	Frequency after treatment
1. Be able to read for longer periods of time without being distracted	3 minutes	
2. Being less irritable in the family	Quarreling 4 times a week	
3. Less effort with tidying up	1× per month, with reluctance and requires a lot of effort	

4.9   Prescribing Methylphenidate to Adults

In general, the stimulants methylphenidate and dexamphetamine are the first choice for treatment. In many countries, there are three brands of methylphenidate available, three of which are long-acting: Concerta, Equasym XL, and Medikinet CR (see Table 4.3). The short-acting form of methylphenidate is best known as Ritalin, but short-acting Medikinet is also available (see Tables 4.3 and 4.4). There is a right-turning enantiomer of methylphenidate: dexmethylphenidate, in short- and long-acting forms.

When choosing a methylphenidate preparation, the aim is to provide the patient with a stable blood level of the drug for the duration of the adult day (from 8 a.m. to midnight, sixteen hours). None of the available medications have an adequate duration of action for adults, so different preparations can be combined. The duration of action of the same medication may vary from patient to patient. Therefore a treatment regime should be tailor-made to suit the individual patient.

In practice, Concerta, the longest-acting methylphenidate, appears to work seven to ten hours in adults, rather than twelve. Therefore, after taking the first dose at 8 a.m., patients should take another dose at 3 p.m., so that the effect is maintained until bedtime. *The second dose of stimulant can also be of Equasym or Medikinet, if Concerta has worn off by 5 p.m.* The optimal combination, therefore, depends on how long each form of methylphenidate is active in the individual patient. In adults, immediate release Ritalin only works for two to four hours per dosage, so patients had to dose six to eight times a day until late at night to achieve adequate control of symptoms. Patients with ADHD tend to be forgetful with erratic compliance, so treatments with Ritalin often failed in the past. With long-acting methylphenidate, the maximum number of times a day that medication has to be taken is two, which significantly improves therapy compliance. Long-acting medication is the first choice for ADHD because of better compliance (Swanson & Hechtman, 2005), a lower chance of abuse and greater safety in traffic (Connor & Steingard, 2004; Cox et al., 2004a; Faraone & Upadhyaya, 2007; Ramos-Quiroga et al., 2008).

A disadvantage of dosing long-acting stimulants twice a day is that the final total dose is higher. No data from scientific research are yet available on the impact of a higher daily dosage. The highest dose in controlled studies in adults is Concerta 72 mg/day, which was also reported to be the most effective dose compared to lower doses (Medori et al., 2008). Clinical experience with twice-daily long-acting methylphenidate dosing is favorable, with the optimal dose being determined on the basis of effect and side effects, such as blood pressure, pulse, and weight. An optimal dose is a dose with maximum efficacy and minimal side effects. Where

Table 4.3 ADHD medication, dose per tablet, duration of operation and dosages per day

Short-acting ADHD medication	Dose per tablet	Duration of operation	Dosages per day
Ritalin	10 mg (methylphenidate)	2–4 h	4–8
Medikinet	5, 10, 20 mg (methylphenidate)	2–4 h	4–8
Amfexa or Tentin	5 mg (dexamphetamine)	5–6 h	2–3
Long-acting ADHD medication			
Equasym XL	10, 20, 30, 40, 50 mg (methylphenidate)	6–8 h	2–3
Medikinet CR	5, 10, 20, 30, 40, 50, 60 mg (methylphenidate)	6–8 h	2–3
Concerta	18, 27, 35, 54 mg (methylphenidate)	8–10 h	1–2
Generic Methylphenidate Retard	18, 36, 54 mg	6 h	1–2
Strattera	10, 18, 25, 40, 60, 80, 100 mg (atomoxetine)	24 h	1
Intuniv	1, 2, 3, 4 mg (guanfacine)	24 h	1
Focalin (dexmethylphenidate XR)	5–40 mg	12 h	1
Long-acting medication registered for other indications			
Wellbutrin (long-acting bupropion)® for depression and smoking cessation	150, 300 mg	24 h	1
Modiodal (modafinil)® for narcolepsy	100 mg	24 h	1

Table 4.4 Starting dose, maintenance dose, and provisional maximum dose per stimulant

Stimulants	Starting dose	Common maintenance dose	Provisional maximum dose
Concerta (C)	18–36 mg	72 + 36 mg	150 mg/day
Methylphenidate Retard Sandoz	18–36 mg	72 + 36 mg	150 mg/day
Focalin (dexmethylphenidate)	10 mg	10 – 40 mg	40 mg/day
Equasym XL (E)	30 mg	C 72 + E 20 or 30 mg or E 2× 30 mg + C 36 mg	150 mg/day
Medikinet CR (M)	30 mg	C 72 + M 20 or 30 mg or M 2× 30 mg + C 36 mg	150 mg/day
Ritalin	4× 10 mg	6–8× 10 mg or 4× 15 mg and 2× 10 mg or 4× 20 mg and 2× 10 mg	150 mg/day
Amfexa or Tentin	1× 5 mg	2× 5–10 mg	20 mg/day

methylphenidate with a longer duration of action is used, the time of onset and the desired bedtime should also be taken into account.

4.9.1   Wearing off of Methylphenidate in the Evening and Its Effect on Sleep

When various long-acting methylphenidate preparations are combined, the duration of action is longer and rebound effect occurs later. Rebound is characterized by a temporary increase in restlessness, amongst other things), which is now closer to the desired moment of falling asleep. Rebound symptoms that occur around bedtime may delay sleep onset. To prevent rebound and promote sleep, a sufficient blood level of methylphenidate should be present until 11 p.m. The presence of methylphenidate facilitates the "winding down" that is necessary to fall asleep. If the long-acting preparation has worn off by evening, then 5–10 mg of Ritalin can achieve the desired effect. If the patient cannot fall asleep on methylphenidate, the rebound symptoms should be timed to take place a few hours earlier in the evening. Knowledge of the timing of the medication is, therefore, necessary to prevent patients from falling asleep too late or suffering from sleep-onset insomnia.

Animal studies show that methylphenidate delays the biological clock, even days after use (Coogan et al., 2017). This may exacerbate a delayed sleep phase, which is already present in the majority of patients with ADHD. More research is needed into these effects and how to overcome them, with well-timed melatonin treatment (see also Sect. 4.20).

However, a bigger problem than the medication and its metabolism are the chronic sleep problems that occur from childhood in most adults with ADHD. There are many indications that these sleep problems are related to a problem of the biological clock causing a chronically delayed sleep phase. Melatonin appears to be a promising treatment for this (Bekker et al., 2008; Smits et al., 2001; Van der Heijden et al., 2005, 2007; Van Veen et al., 2010) (see Sects. 2.14.4 and 4.20).

4.9.2   Short- and Long-term Effectiveness

Stimulants are among the best researched drugs; and most of the research has been done on their effectiveness and safety in children. Effectiveness is high, with response rates around 70–80%. This is much higher than for other medications. Various meta-analyses report on the short-term (six months) effectiveness of stimulants and atomoxetine in adults with ADHD. The mean differences between medication and placebo range from 0.4 to 0.7, with stimulants being more effective than atomoxetine. Short- and long-acting methylphenidate are effective for the core symptoms of ADHD, and improve executive functioning by inhibiting impulsiveness, improving working memory, and sustaining attention. The dexamphetamine preparations (dextroamphetamine, mixed amphetamine salts, lisdexamphetamine) are even more effective than methylphenidate, with effect sizes of 0.73–0.97 versus 0.51 (Faraone & Glatt 2010; Castells et al., 2011; Fridman et al., 2015; Maneeton et al., 2014; De Crescenzo et al., 2017).

In terms of long-term outcomes, a one-year study comparing methylphenidate to placebo plus group therapy, showed that methylphenidate was significantly better than placebo (Philipsen et al., 2015). The longest duration of a placebo-controlled study for both methylphenidate and atomoxetine was six months. There are also eleven open-label, follow-up studies, the longest with atomoxetine (three years). All of these support the benefits of drug treatment (Fredriksen et al., 2013). The evidence for bupropion, buspirone, aripiprazole, magnesium, and reboxetine is limited by small study populations and methodological limitations, as reported in systematic reviews (De Crescenzo et al., 2017).

Effects of stimulants can be measured by scores on cognitive performance, learning tasks, and even IQ scores (Berman et al., 1999; Gimpel et al., 2005). Other studies have used the QbTest (see also Sect. 4.8.4) with clinical variables such as symptom lists or observations of behavior (Kooij et al., 2004; Spencer et al., 2005). Imaging research using PET scans that show the effects of stimulants on the dopamine transporter (Volkow et al., 2002).

Stimulants improve the driving behavior of adults with ADHD, both in a driving simulator and on the road (compared to placebo) (Barkley et al., 2005; Verster et al., 2008; Gobbo and Louzã 2014). Stimulants also improve certain measures of executive functioning (sustained attention and verbal learning) in adults with ADHD, compared to those not on medication (Biederman et al., 2008). In follow-up studies, stimulants reduce the risk of recidivism in prisoners and criminals with ADHD (Lichtenstein et al., 2012; Ginsberg et al., 2015). Treatment with stimulants for ADHD also reduced the risk of depression in a large Swedish cohort study (Chang et al., 2016).

In children, it has been found that the total response rate of 90% is reached when methylphenidate or dextroamphetamine are used successively (Elia et al., 1991).

The effects of stimulants in healthy individuals are increasingly being investigated, especially in relation to the off-label use of stimulants as cognitive enhancers (see Sect. 4.9.2.1). The effects of stimulants on behavior in children both with and without ADHD are similar (Rapoport and Inoff-Germain 2002). This means that attention and impulse control improve to a similar extent in both groups. It is the existing brain function that determines whether this is an added value or not. It is unclear whether an improvement is relevant where the symptom previously posed no problem. Improved concentration seems to add value most where people experience problems in this area. Those without complaints will mainly experience the side effects of the medication.

4.9.2.1 Improvement of Cognitive Functioning in Healthy People

Users of stimulants that had not been prescribed for them were compared to controls in terms of attention: both objectively measured tasks and their subjective experience of their attention. Self-reported study habits and motivation during tasks requiring attention were also compared. The results indicate that users of non-prescribed stimulants have relatively more underlying attention problems. This emerged in the self-reported attention tasks and less clearly in the objective measures. Users also had lower motivation during cognitive testing and suboptimal study habits (Ilieva et al., 2019). These results point in the direction of more attention problems among students who use stimulants, possibly reflecting a form of self-medication.

Students appear to use different substances to promote concentration and improve their results. These substances vary from coffee and energy drinks to stimulants, modafinil, and glutamate stimulants (ampakin). Stimulants improve cognitive performance in children and adults with ADHD. In healthy controls, spatial working memory tasks also improve on stimulants. Of note, these tasks involve an area of the frontal cortex that is sensitive to damage (Elliott et al., 1997).

It is estimated that 5–10% of high school students and 5–35% of university students abuse stimulants (Clemow & Walker 2014). This occurs mainly in students and men with ADHD symptoms and anxiety complaints (Gudmundsdottir et al., 2016). Research among students aged 18–25 years with a high risk for eating disorders showed that more severe eating problems, binges, vomiting, depression, anxiety, and stress were associated with the abuse of stimulants. Targeted screening could be conducted in this population (Gibbs et al., 2016). Clinicians treating these patients should be alerted to the possibility of underlying ADHD, because the risk of ADHD is particularly increased in binge-eating, bulimia, as well as in obesity (see also Sect. 2.14.3.1).

In a systematic review of the literature on the effects of cognitive-enhancing drugs in adolescents aged twelve to fifteen, modafinil was found to improve reaction time, logical reasoning, and problem solving. Methylphenidate improved performance in new and attention-related tasks and reduced planning latency in more complex tasks. Amphetamine improved the consolidation of information, leading to better recall of information from memory (Bagot & Kaminer, 2014). Whether the use of stimulants in healthy brains causes any damage is unknown. There is a possible danger of excessively high doses with consequences for brain plasticity. More research into the effects of stimulants on healthy individuals is needed (Urban & Gao, 2014).

4.9.3   Differences Between Methylphenidate Preparations

The different methylphenidates do not vary in terms of the pharmacological constituent, but rather in terms of the amount of methylphenidate present, and the proportion of immediate and delayed release present. For example, Concerta contains 22% immediate release methylphenidate and 78% delayed release methylphenidate. With Equasym XL the ratio is 30:70, with Medikinet CR 50:50 (for available doses per stimulant, see Table 4.3). This ratio makes it possible to determine the quantity of fast release methylphenidate that is needed to get off to a good start in the morning.

If Concerta is the drug of choice because of its longer duration of action, but the amount of immediate release is insufficient for an efficient start to the morning, a tablet of Ritalin 10 mg may be added to the dose of Concerta.

Concerta's mechanism of action is independent of food intake. Equasym should be taken *before* breakfast while Medikinet should be taken *during or after* breakfast. Deviations from this dosing can adversely affect the mechanism of release. This can become a problem when combining the different methylphenidates, because the second dose may not be taken at mealtime. Patients should therefore be instructed to eat as much as possible *before taking* Equasym and *after* taking Medikinet if they want to benefit from the longest possible duration of action.

Another difference between the preparations is that in Concerta, the immediate release methylphenidate forms a layer on the outside of the capsule, and the delayed release methylphenidate is dissolved in gel form inside the capsule. Through osmotic pressure, the long-acting methylphenidate is released through a small laser-drilled hole in the capsule. If the capsule were to be opened, the contents could not easily be snorted or injected. Equasym XL and Medikinet CR capsules, on the other hand, can be opened and contain granules of both short- and long-acting methylphenidate. These granules can be sprinkled over custard or applesauce and ingested as required. This route of administration may be an advantage for those who have difficulty swallowing capsules or tablets. The granules are also designed to prevent abuse.

4.9.4 Adjusting to the Correct Dosage

4.9.4.1 Adjusting to Long-acting Methylphenidate

Concerta is the methylphenidate preparation with the longest duration of action. The starting dose is 36 mg, at a regular time in the morning, taken with breakfast. Patients who are sensitive to side effects can start with 18 mg. The dose is increased after one week, taking effect, duration of action, and side effects into account. For example, 36 mg daily is increased to 54 mg in the morning. The duration of the effect should be noted, and if necessary, a second dose (of 36 mg) can be added half an hour before that time. Some adults respond directly to a low dose, others only notice the effect at higher doses. If there is a need for additional immediate release methylphenidate at the first dosing, then Equasym XL 30 mg or Medikinet CR 30 mg can be added to the Concerta 36 mg. One week later, the effect, duration of action, and side effects can be evaluated. Blood pressure, pulse, and weight should be measured. The compliance to medication and timing of intake should be checked. Wherever possible, the optimal maintenance dosage and timing of dosages should be determined and continued. A stable patient is initially assessed every one to three months, then every six months. During this initial phase, coaching should be initiated with a psychologist or other practitioner. (For more information about ADHD, organizational training, support, and advice, see Chap. 5).

On average, adults take two times 36 mg Concerta as a morning dose (72 mg in total). This corresponds to approximately 60 mg Ritalin. If the medication effect is over by the afternoon, 36 mg can be added at 3 pm (this is half of the morning dose). The total dose per day is 108 mg. This dosage schedule is common. The second dose becomes inactive around 10 p.m. If the duration of action of the first dose of Concerta lasts until 5 p.m., an additional dose of Equasym XL or Medikinet CR of 20 or 30 mg taken at that time will provide symptom control until bedtime. Some adults may require higher doses, for example, two times 54 mg Concerta in the morning and once 36 mg in the afternoon (total 144 mg). In children, the maximum dose of short-acting methylphenidate is 60 mg per day. Maximum doses in adults are unknown as they have not been studied. However, both in the United States and in Europe, these doses and combinations are customary in the clinical treatment of adults with ADHD (Sadock et al., 2009). The aim is to achieve stability during the sixteen-hour day. The total dose of a stimulant per day can vary greatly from person to person, and is determined not so much by body weight as by polymorphisms of certain genes that determine susceptibility to the substance (Kooij et al., 2008; Mick et al., 2008). In clinical practice, these polymorphisms cannot be determined, and much remains unclear about their meaning. In the future, researchers hope to be able to use pharmacogenetics to determine a personal medication profile. This will increases the chance of optimal effectiveness and minimal side effects from medication (Stein & McGough, 2008). A maximum dose of 1 mg/kg per day was advised until recently, but this dose is inadequate to maintain stable blood levels until the evening. Until more information is available from research, a maximum daily dose of 150 mg methylphenidate per day is advised. The effect and side effects of the treatment regimen should be assessed for each individual patient, while monitoring blood pressure, pulse, and weight.

The individual dose of methylphenidate depends not so much on weight, but on the genetic susceptibility to the substance.

4.9.4.2 Short-Acting Methylphenidate: Disadvantages

Short-acting methylphenidate is an inferior agent for most patients with ADHD. This is due to its short duration of action. Parents and teachers of children with ADHD have to supervise the intake of the medication three times a day. For adults, dosing frequency increases to six to eight times a day, and they have no external prompts in place. A study of seventy patients shows that patients on short-acting methylphenidate improve after switching to long-acting medication (Ramos-Quiroga et al., 2008). As both drugs contain the same active ingredient, this outcome suggests that the short-acting preparation was taken erratically. Patients who struggle with adherence end up needing a longer treatment period because they remain symptomatic, forget their appointments and the treatment stagnates. Research shows that poorer compliance is associated with non-response to the medication (Kooij et al., 2004).

If treatment objectives are not met and attention and concentration remain poor, psychotherapy is less effective. Many patients may previously have received extended treatment in the mental health services for disorders comorbid with ADHD, such as addiction, anxiety, and depression. If the underlying ADHD were to be left untreated, these disorders would not improve. Better cost-effectiveness results when long-term medication is reimbursed by medical insurance companies, because the use of frequently dosed short-acting stimulants have increase costs in the long-term where treatment is ineffective (Faber et al., 2008).

Treatment with short-acting methylphenidate is ineffective because it necessitates frequent, regular daily dosing. This is unattainable for many chaotic patients with ADHD.

4.9.4.3 Prescribing Short-acting Methylphenidate

If it is not possible to prescribe long-acting methylphenidate due to the cost, availability, or lack of reimbursement, short-acting methylphenidate (Ritalin) can be prescribed four to eight times daily, with an alarm to remind of the dosing time. Initially, one tablet of Ritalin 10 mg, is prescribed to be taken four times a day at 8:00, 12:00, 16:00, and 20:00. Depending on the duration of action of a single dose, one week after starting, the times are adjusted to prevent an annoying rebound (a temporary increase in the severity of ADHD symptoms, such as restlessness, irritability, and poor concentration). Most patients should be dosed every three hours. This translates into five doses between 8 a.m. and 8 p.m. To achieve focus in the evening and to avoid rebound-related irritability during the evening, when patients are with family or their partner, the sixth dose should follow at 8 p.m. By 11 p.m., there is no more active drug in the system. The amount of methylphenidate used can be increased to one and a half to two tablets if necessary. However, in the evening, one tablet is given per dose. Common dosage regimens of Ritalin are: six times 10 mg or four times 15 mg and twice 10 mg or four times 20 mg and twice 10 mg.

Some patients notice an annoying increase in ADHD symptoms and inactivity of the drug after just two hours. These individuals should take one tablet eight times a day (every two hours). This regime turns out to be unfeasible, as patients complain that they are constantly taking medication. These complicated treatment regimens emphasize that the first choice in adults is clearly long-acting medication. Some parents, friends, or employers are willing to pay for long-acting medication once the contrast between (frequently missed) short- and (more stable) long-acting medication is observed. Cessation of cannabis or cigarette smoking can save money to pay for long-acting medication.

To prevent forgetting of doses and experiencing rebound effects, the patient should use a timer or alarm, preferably set on a mobile phone (which is usually not forgotten). The mobile phone should have the possibility of several alarm times, preventing the need to reset the alarm and to compensate for memory lapses.

4.9.5   Maintenance Treatment with Stimulants

After the adjustment phase, the optimized dosage and administration schedule is maintained during the treatment. Where patients are referred to a general practitioner for follow-up, the same dosage should be continuously increasing, decreasing doses, or changing medication is unsettling. Some patients begin to lose trust in the therapeutic process. The clinician may also lose faith, and the chance of non-response increases. The doctor should remain in control and be aware that the effectiveness of the medication decreases with each phase of the protocol; they are not equivalent options. Therefore, the gold standard is to prescribe the first-choice medication, with an active approach to managing side effects and comorbidity.

Many patients ask how long they should continue with the medication and what the long-term effects of the medication might be. Usually, when stimulants and other ADHD medications are discontinued, the symptoms return. This is immediately noticeable when a single dose is forgotten. Nevertheless, patients regularly want to re-experience life without medication. Patients may report ongoing benefits of stimulants even after these are discontinued. This may be possible, but experience suggests that symptoms recur whether or not they are noticed by the patient. Often, people around the patient notice a relapse before the patient does. Such a relapse may be unacceptable to family members, a spouse, or an employer. Suddenly, dismissal or divorce threatens the patient. The risks and consequences of relapse should be discussed. Some patients struggle to accept the diagnosis and the need for long-term medication, which reminds them of the disorder on a daily basis. It can help to discuss other chronic conditions (asthma, diabetes) where patients cannot function without medication. Metaphors can also help put the problem into perspective. For example, the management of ADHD can be compared to top-level athletics. Top athletes can run with rubber boots (without medication), or wear advanced running shoes (use medication). Discussions with a therapist or within a support group about accepting the diagnosis can also provide the necessary support and recognition (Schuijers & Kooij, 2007).

Regarding the long-term effects of stimulants, it is reassuring to note that they have been used clinically in children and adolescents since 1960, and in adults since 1990. So far, no serious risks of prolonged use have come to light. The only effect in children, attributed in part to stimulant use, is a slight decrease in the expected height and weight achieved (1 cm and 1.2 kg/year) (Swanson et al., 2008). Although these effects decrease with time and some data suggest that the final adult growth parameters are not affected, more research is needed to clarify the effects of continuous treatment from childhood to adulthood. Doctors are advised to continue to monitor the height of children, although the difference in height has shown no clinical consequences as yet (Faraone et al., 2008).

The longest placebo-controlled study for both methylphenidate and atomoxetine lasted six months. In addition, there are eleven open-label follow-up studies, the longest with atomoxetine (three years), all of which support the benefits of drug treatment (Fredriksen et al., 2013).

The best dosage and administration schedule of the medication is continued as the maintenance dose.

4.9.5.1 What Is (non-)response?

In short-term studies, the response rates to stimulants are unusually high, certainly compared to other psychotropics. Therefore, before determining that methylphenidate is ineffective, the following parameters should be carefully considered:

1. Is the dose high enough? Does the duration of action extend until bedtime?
2. Has the medication trial been sufficiently long (a few weeks at optimal dosage)?
3. Is the patient compliant with therapy? Is a timer or alarm being used? Is the patient adhering to the agreed dosage times? Is rebound between doses occurring because "the drug is worse than the ailment"?
4. Is there unknown comorbidity interfering with effectiveness? Think of a subclinical anxiety disorder that becomes only manifests with methylphenidate treatment. Tachycardia as a side effect is experienced as panic, which makes it impossible to evaluate the benefit of methylphenidate on ADHD symptoms. The anxiety disorder should first be treated with an SSRI, after which methylphenidate can be added. A comorbid depression has a similar effect: the effect of methylphenidate is not observed because the gloomy mood interprets everything as negative. Again, starting an SSRI is the quickest route to improving the mood disorder. An underlying addiction can also undermine the effect of treatment with a stimulant. All these possibilities should be investigated in case of non-response.
5. When patients complain that the stimulant no longer works (after a good initial response), check that they are taking the medication properly, at the correct dose.

Typical effects of methylphenidate are experienced as: inner peace, a sense of control and less impulsivity, less irritability and mood swings, better concentration, gaining an enhanced general grasp of a situation, and less reluctance to tidy up. Tidying up is really something people with ADHD dislike, so improvement in this regard is a clear indication of the effect of the medication for patients. The practitioner notices the effect of the medication because the consultation runs more smoothly and in an orderly fashion. The patient is more present, summarizes better, interrupts less, and answers more to the point. So now the consultation can be completed on time. Patients sometimes report that tasks that used to take hours are now completed rapidly. This saves a lot of valuable energy that can be spent on other things, more tasks are completed in less time, and the patient is more productive.

Important tools in the evaluation of response are those that measure the decrease in severity of ADHD symptoms. If the total score on the Symptom and Side Effect List, the ADHD Rating Scale or the Individual Target Symptom List decreases, there is a response (see see section "List of Symptoms and Side Effects of ADHD, ADHD Rating Scale, Self-Report, Individual Target Symptom List" in Appendices). The level of response is monitored after the dose has been optimized, side effects reduced or controlled and any manifest comorbidity treated. The aim is to achieve at least a 30% reduction in the severity of ADHD symptoms. Depending on effect, side effects, therapy compliance, and comorbidity, a good effect can be achieved within a few weeks but sometimes takes up to a year.

Evaluating responses is not always simple in practice. Patients with ADHD are not used to reflecting on their behavior, let alone observing precise differences in symptoms over time. They tend to focus more on their surroundings than on their own inner world. A partner is usually more likely to see that the patient is now calmer. A typical comment that patients make in the first week after starting medication is: I do not notice anything, except ... (side effects). When questioned further, it turns out that he or she is a bit calmer and organized, but because on a starting dose the differences are subtle, the patient does not immediately recognize the effect. Patients struggle to identify improvements in an abstract domain such as cognitive functioning, where there has formerly only been chaos. It is important to explain to patients individually what the desired effect is in their case, so that they can identify and recognize it. A thorough description of side effects and other symptoms experienced is also necessary. Helping patients distinguish between side effects and other ailments, such as the flu, is useful for further motivation and compliance.

There is a clear need for an objective cognitive test, such as the QbTest to determine the response to medication, the domains (of ADHD) in which the response occurs, and the effect of different doses of medication. Much research is being conducted into the applications of this test (Bijlenga et al., 2015).

Non-response occurs in 20–30% of patients treated with methylphenidate. Typical for non-response is that the patient says s/he feels like a "zombie," i.e., drowsy and slow. This is an undesirable effect. Such reactions must be distinguished from the symptoms of comorbid depression and from the effects of overdose of the stimulant. Where the stimulant dose is too high, the patient may feel inhibited, lose initiative, which is also described as "becoming a coach potato." The solution is then not to stop the stimulant, but to reduce the dose. If there is a comorbid depression, this should of course be treated. One determines non-response only if the patient has been treated adequately (high enough dose, sufficient duration of treatment, reverse side effects, exclude comorbidity, and ascertain good therapy compliance) and there is no discernible improvement. In that case, methylphenidate is stopped; this can be done overnight. Gradual dose reduction is not necessary because of the short half-life.

The development of tolerance to a stimulant is rare, i.e., after an initially good response the effect decreases or disappears dramatically. Decreasing effect is common at the beginning of treatment if the dose is inadequate and needs to be optimized; this is not tolerance. Loss of effect is something else, this can also be objectified with the objective QbTest. Patients feel desperate because they have experienced the benefits of treatment, but this is now taken away from them again. The only known solution is to temporarily stop the stimulant and resume it after a few days. Sometimes it appears that a comorbid depression or anxiety disorder has obscured the effect of the ADHD medication. After treatment of the comorbidity, the effect then returns.

Response to methylphenidate occurs in 50–70% of adults with ADHD. The total response to stimulants (methylphenidate and dextroamphetamine, tried consecutively) is 90% in children.Response is defined as a minimum of 30% decrease in the severity of ADHD symptoms as measured by questionnaires.

4.9.6   Side Effects

The most common side effects of stimulants are: loss of appetite and weight, initially, a headache and tachycardia. Less frequent side effects are dry mouth and difficulty falling asleep. Blood pressure can rise, but also fall. The safety of stimulants when used by adults is an important topic that has been well researched: there is little or no evidence of serious cardiovascular side effects, including no serious QT length abnormalities. In the available literature, the increase in blood pressure is limited to ≤7 mmHg on average and the increase in heart rate to ≤10/min on average (Martinez-Raga et al., 2017). In some cases, greater changes occur that may have clinical consequences. In these cases, the medication is adjusted in consultation with the cardiologist or general practitioner. More research into the possible cumulative long-term effects of stimulation use is needed (Hammerness et al., 2015).

In rare cases, stimulants can help to relieve psychosis in sensitive individuals. In principle, a previous psychosis is a contraindication to the use of stimulants, so one checks for the symptoms in advance. However, there are some reports of favorable responses where an antipsychotic is used concurrently with stimulants in (previously) psychotic patients with ADHD, see Sect. 4.20.4. If a psychosis occurs while treating with stimulants, the drug is immediately discontinued and the psychosis is treated. The same applies to (hypo)mania in the case of bipolar disorder. Symptoms of bipolar disorder should be investigated before starting treatment, and, if present, treated. If (hypo)mania develops spontaneously with stimulant treatment, stop the stimulant and start a mood stabilizer. Thereafter, the stimulant may be restarted with the protection of the mood stabilizer (see Sect. 4.20.3).

On average, weight loss of 1–2 kg occurs during the first few weeks (Kooij et al., 2004), after which weight usually stabilizes. Patients who have a low weight, to begin with may find it difficult to maintain their weight with stimulants. Their weight should therefore be well monitored, they are advised to eat three times a day, preferably at set times, even where there is a lack of appetite. They can be referred to a dietician if necessary. If they are underweight, treatment should be discontinued until the weight is back to a previously agreed-upon level. With time and perseverance, most patients manage to maintain their weight. For most patients, losing a few pounds is an advantage. However, excessive weight loss requires following a specific nutritional diet. Ironically, adherence to a diet is facilitated by stimulant use.

The headache is usually temporary. Due to a decrease in appetite, many patients forget to drink, which can cause the headache. By warning patients about this, this side effect can be prevented.

Tachycardia refers to an acceleration of the heartbeat by an average of 4–7 beats per minute (Wilens et al., 2005b). This permanent side effect is associated with amphetamine-like substances. Most patients experience no discomfort as a result. Those who do may have underlying anxiety complaints; they experience the acceleration of the heartbeat as a signal that the anxiety or panic is returning. Treatment with an SSRI, and then reintroduction of the stimulant, appears to overcome this phenomenon. Cognitive therapy may have some effect on the perception of the accelerated heartbeat. Patients who feel agitated by the rapid heartbeat, but who have **no** anxiety symptoms, can achieve symptom reduction with the addition of 10–40 mg propranolol per day (Wilens et al., 1995).

Dry mouth can increase the risk of caries, especially if other medications are used that produce this side effect. Frequent tooth brushing and possible use of a mouth gel can reduce the symptoms. For problems falling asleep with methylphenidate, see Sect. 4.8.1. Occasionally, a patient reports that visual accommodation has decreased since use of the stimulant. This is a recognized but rare side effect.

The most annoying side effect, however, is the rebound that occurs when methylphenidate has been metabolized. Rebound is associated with a temporary increase (for several hours) in ADHD symptoms, i.e., restlessness, irritability, concentration problems, and forgetfulness ("cotton wool in the head"), irritability, mood swings, and an increase in impulsivity. In addition, symptoms such as sweating, palpitations, and gastrointestinal complaints may occur. It is clear that rebound must be prevented as much as possible. This can be achieved by limiting the frequency of dosing to a maximum of twice a day. For this, long-acting medication is necessary. To prevent forgetting or delaying a dose, it is necessary that the patient uses an alarm or timer. With short-acting Ritalin, doses are needed six to eight times a day (and each dose can be forgotten), so that patients are often less stable than before treatment. Short-acting methylphenidate is therefore not suitable for adults where the predominant problems are chaos and forgetfulness. Even though ADHD children have support from parents and teachers in taking their medication, long-acting medication is often preferable. ADHD patients need stability and this cannot be achieved with fluctuating onset and offset of immediate release medication.

Adults need six to eight doses a day of short-acting methylphenidate. Each dose is easily forgotten, making them less stable than before treatment. Short-acting methylphenidate is not suitable for adults with ADHD whose main problem is chaos and forgetfulness.

4.9.7   Overdosage

With overdosing, overstimulation of the nervous system may produce: vomiting, agitation, trembling, exaggerated reflexes, muscle contraction, convulsions (possibly followed by coma), feelings of euphoria, confusion, hallucinations, sweating, flushing, headache, high fever, tachycardia, irregular heartbeat, high blood pressure, pupillary dilation, and dehydration of the mucous membranes.

4.9.8   Dexmethylphenidate

Dexmethylphenidate consists exclusively of the d-methylphenidate enantiomer. Methylphenidate consists of 50% l-methylphenidate (l stands for "levo," left) and 50% d-methylphenidate (d stands for "dextro," right). Another possible name would be: left- and right-oriented methylphenidate (d,l-methylphenidate). In the United

States, it is registered for ADHD under the names Focalin (XR) and Attenade. It is possible that dexmethylphenidate is stronger than d,l-methylphenidate, that patients experience fewer side effects and that its duration of action is longer, but this has not yet been properly investigated (Weiss et al., 2004). Clinical experience in 79 adults with ADHD treated with dexmethylphenidate at PsyQ in The Hague used a starting dose of 10 mg in the morning, which was increased in response to effect and side effects. The average daily dose ranged from 10 to 40 mg, an average of 20 mg per day. Most patients needed only one dose per day. Half reported a ten-hour duration of action. Side effects were similar to those known with stimulants: weight loss (−3 kg), increase in systolic blood pressure (+4 mm Hg) and increase in heart rate (+7/minute) (internal publication PsyQ). The study could not determine whether the side effects were milder than with the other stimulants.

4.9.9   Treatment of Physical Conditions During Stimulant Use

Before starting with a stimulant, raised blood pressure should be treated. Stimulants can increase or decrease blood pressure. Hypertension that develops just after starting a stimulant should also be treated. This may occur where there is a family history of hypertension. If the stimulant is effective, it should be continued while the blood pressure is controlled. Patients who are normotensive before the start of the medication should have their blood pressure checked a few times during the dose escalation stage, then once the dose is established, at least once or twice a year (Wilens et al., 2005). Hypertensive patients should be checked more often and referred to a general practitioner or specialist for treatment. Beta-blockers for the treatment of hypertension, such as metoprolol, can precipitate depression in sensitive individuals and should be avoided in such cases.

A similar approach applies to glaucoma. Stimulants can increase eyeball pressure. If diagnosed, glaucoma should first be treated and then stimulants can be prescribed while ocular pressure is monitored by an optician and/or ophthalmologist.

Hyperthyroidism should also be treated first because of tachycardia, which is enhanced by the use of stimulants. After treatment, a stimulant can be added.

In the case of cardiovascular complaints, a specialist referral may be necessary. In the case of arrhythmias, acute myocardial infarction and objective tachycardia, the stimulant should be stopped immediately. Where there is doubt, a consultation with the cardiologist should follow. Stimulants lead to an increase in the heart rate, but unlike tricyclic antidepressants, have no effect on cardiac conduction. Experience has shown that cardiologists are more concerned with the cardiac problems associated with tricyclics than with the effects of stimulants.

Children with epilepsy are 2.5 times more likely to have ADHD (Hesdorffer et al., 2004). In adults with epilepsy, the prevalence of psychopathology, including ADHD symptoms, is increased (Loughman et al., 2017). Epilepsy should be treated first because stimulants are believed to lower the seizure threshold. In children, treatment with a stimulant under cover of an anticonvulsant has been shown to be safe and effective. This should be carried out in consultation with the neurologist (Gross-Tsur et al., 1997, 2017; Gucuyener et al., 2003; Van der Feltz-Cornelis & Aldenkamp, 2006). A history of epilepsy is the reason for caution, even in the absence of recent complaints and no current use of an anticonvulsant. Consultation with the neurologist and an EEG, prior to the start of the stimulant, seems to be the safest way.

4.10   Dextroamphetamine

Dextroamphetamine shares first place with methylphenidate in the treatment of ADHD according to the Dutch Guideline on adult ADHD (NVvP, 2015). Differences between methylphenidate and dextroamphetamine are: mechanism of action, duration of action, and dosage used.

1. The mechanism of action of both stimulants differs due to a different site of action in the brain: dextroamphetamine increases more the release of dopamine and norepinephrine in the synapse, whereas methylphenidate more inhibits their reuptake. This explains why it makes sense to try dextroamphetamine in patients who are non-responders to methylphenidate.
2. Short-acting dextroamphetamine works longer than short-acting methylphenidate, for about four to five hours. Dextroamphetamine is therefore dosed three to four times a day, every four to five hours.
3. Dextroamphetamine is twice as strong as methylphenidate, so the dose is about half that of methylphenidate.

Effects, side effects, and (relative) contraindications of dexamphetamines are similar to those of methylphenidate (see Sect. 4.8), although the side effects appear to be milder. The pharmacokinetics of dextroamphetamine and short-acting methylphenidate appears to differ. In the United States, there are various long-acting dextroamphetamine preparations including the Dexedrine spansule (duration of action six to eight hours), a mixed amphetamine preparation (Adderall XR, mixed amphetamine salts, ten to twelve hours), and Vyvanse, lisdexamphetamine (combination of L-lysine and D-amphetamine, twelve to fourteen hours).

Lisdexamphetamine is a long-acting stimulant registered for adults with ADHD in the United States, England, Sweden, and Denmark. It consists of lysine plus dextroamphetamine, making it an inactive prodrug. This combination reduces the risk of abuse because after oral administration, the conversion of lisdexamphetamine to d-amphetamine is thought to occur gradually, resulting in a prolonged pharmacokinetic profile with a low peak but sustained plasma amphetamine concentrations. This prolonged profile is considered to be associated with slower effects on dopamine release, lower euphoric effects, and a possibly lower risk of misuse. After oral administration, lisdexamphetamine disintegrates and is absorbed only after passage through the stomach. It is significantly more effective than placebo for ADHD symptoms, general functioning, executive functions, and quality of life. Both first time stimulant users and non-responders to methylphenidate respond equally well. Research demonstrates a well-tolerated side-effect profile. Comparative studies with methylphenidate and atomoxetine are lacking (Frampton, 2016). In adults, lisdexamphetamine achieved the highest effect size of 1.07, compared to atomoxetine and methylphenidate (systematic review, Fridman et al., 2015). Lisdexamphetamine is also effective in reducing binge eating (McElroy et al., 2015).

4.10.1 Starting Dextroamphetamine

The starting dose of short-acting generic dextroamphetamine is 5 mg three times per day, one tablet every five hours (8 a.m., 1 p.m., and 6 p.m.). The drug works within thirty minutes. After one week, drug effects and side effects can be evaluated. The duration of action is determined. If the medication is inactive under five hours, dosing is then every four hours (8.00, 12.00, 16.00, and 20.00). The dose is increased to one and a half or two tablets of 5 mg at a time based on response and side effects. In order to keep to the correct dosing schedule and to avoid forgetting a dose, a timer or alarm, preferably on a mobile phone, is necessary. A common dose of dextroamphetamine is 5 to 10 mg three to four times a day, in total ranging from 15 to 40 mg per day. The maximum dose is not known, but the highest common doses of generic dextroamphetamine are around 80 mg per day. The starting dose of generic long-acting dextroamphetamine Retard is 10 mg, and the average duration of action is eight hours. Many patients can take a once daily dose. The dose per day ranges from 20 to 40 mg once to twice daily. The dose is determined on the basis of response, side effects, duration of action, required total duration of action per day, while blood pressure, pulse, and weight are monitored. The maintenance dosage is the optimal dosage with the corresponding administration times. Amfexa or Tentin seems to work a bit longer (6 hrs) and is dosed lower, 1–2× daily.

4.11 Pregnancy, Lactation, and the Stimulants

Methylphenidate is increasingly used by adults, about half of whom are women. Patients who wish to have children are advised to use the ADHD medication until an early pregnancy test is positive. See also Sect. 4.5 on stimulant use during pregnancy and lactation.

Women who take methylphenidate on prescription and want to become pregnant are advised to stop the medication as soon as the pregnancy test is positive.

An early pregnancy test seems advisable because the exposure to methylphenidate will be at most one to two weeks, an acceptable risk. The disadvantage of stopping stimulants earlier is that where it takes a long time to fall pregnant, the use of effective medication is delayed for too long.

The question of which alternatives can be offered during pregnancy is not easy to answer. In general, it is preferable to use substances where there is research data. Some tricyclic antidepressants, fluoxetine, and an increasing number of other serotonin reuptake inhibitors are considered safe in pregnancy, so comorbid disorders can be treated during pregnancy. This often makes a considerable difference to the severity of the symptoms, compared to the situation prior to diagnosis and treatment. Explaining and considering the best options with the patient and her partner is helps to determine the best treatment plan during pregnancy. For example, temporarily working fewer hours, asking for help from family or friends, can make a big difference to the symptom severity. After pregnancy, the patient can restart methylphenidate, as soon as any period of breastfeeding has ended.

4.12   Driving While Using Stimulants

Every country may have its own rules and regulations regarding driving in case of ADHD and/or its treatment. In the Netherlands, new and young drivers (18–23 years of age) with ADHD must undergo a once-off medical examination before obtaining a driving license on the basis of the self-filled Instruction Manual. During this examination, information should be given about the reduced driving ability in ADHD, the increased risk of accidents and the positive effect of ADHD medication on driving ability. It is also strongly recommended not to use alcohol and/or drugs while driving, as this increases the risk of accidents. Where adults have experienced multiple traffic violations and/or car accidents, ADHD should be excluded by a competent physician. If ADHD is diagnosed, medical treatment is recommended to prevent a recurrence. See also Sect. 2.7.1.

Current research indicates that stimulant use improves driving ability in people with ADHD.

4.13   Travelling Abroad

Using ADHD medications abroad is not everywhere allowed. For travel to Asia or other areas where stimulants might be considered illegal drugs, the patient should always contact the relevant embassy in advance. In this way the patient prepare for the measures to be taken. Also, in high-risk cases, the decision can be made to make a trip to another country or to temporarily discontinue the medication, although this may induce an undesirable return of the symptoms during the trip.

4.14   Atomoxetine

Atomoxetine (Strattera) is registered for children and adolescents with ADHD, and also for adults since 2014. Atomoxetine is a so-called noradrenergic reuptake inhibitor preventing the reuptake of norepinephrine (not dopamine) in the synapse. Atomoxetine is therefore not a stimulant and is not a scheduled medication. The advantage is that there is no risk of abuse, which can be especially important drug-dependent patients with ADHD (Jasinski et al., 2008). Atomoxetine has a lower effect size than the stimulants (0.6), but the advantage is that it only needs to be taken once a day because it works for 24 hours (Faraone et al., 2005a).

In controlled trials, the effect of atomoxetine was maintained for six months in adults (Adler et al., 2009). Furthermore, atomoxetine improved functioning (Adler et al., 2009), response inhibition, and performance on the Stroop test in ADHD adults with ADHD (Chamberlain et al., 2007; Faraone et al., 2005b). Emotional dysregulation, which is also frequent in ADHD, also improved (Reimherr et al., 2005). Atomoxetine was not effective in relieving depression in ADHD adolescents (Bangs et al., 2007).

Atomoxetine is prescribed for non-response to methylphenidate and dextroamphetamine, where there are contraindications to using stimulants (e.g., psychosis) or where there is comorbid addiction or social anxiety disorder (Adler et al., 2009; Rostain, 2008; Wilens et al., 2008). Patients with recently remitted alcohol addiction and ADHD showed improvement in the ADHD symptoms, but not clearly on drinking behavior (Wilens et al., 2008). In a meta-analysis of 13 RCTs in adults, atomoxetine was more effective than placebo (effect size 0.45), for both inattention and hyperactivity/impulsivity (Ravishankar et al., 2016).

A meta-analysis of studies comparing the effectiveness and safety of atomoxetine with a stimulant confirms the first choice of stimulants in the treatment of ADHD (Gibson et al., 2006). Comparative research in a small group of patients on the effectiveness of a stimulant (mixed amphetamine salts) and atomoxetine on driving ability in a driving simulator shows that the stimulant is much more effective (Kay et al., 2009). Open-label response prevention research suggested that non-responders to methylphenidate also did not respond to atomoxetine (Buitelaar et al., 2004). Crossover studies in more than 500 children comparing oros-methylphenidate to atomoxetine contradict this: oros-methylphenidate was more effective than atomoxetine, but those who did not respond to oros-methylphenidate did respond to atomoxetine in 43% of the cases. Conversely, those who did not respond to atomoxetine had a good response to oros-methylphenidate in 42% of past cases (Newcorn et al., 2008). Thus, there appears to be a different sensitivity to both drugs in patients with ADHD.

Clinical experience in combining stimulants and atomoxetine was first reported by Wilens during the congress of the American Association of Psychiatrists (APA) in 2007. He described adding a stimulant where there was a partial response to atomoxetine. This raised the question of whether stimulants alone would not have had the same effect in this group.

Atomoxetine is a noradrenergic reuptake inhibitor and not a stimulant; it works for 24 hours, but it is less effective than stimulants.

4.14.1   Starting Atomoxetine

A contraindication for atomoxetine is glaucoma. Prescribers should also note the following warnings: caution with hypertension, tachycardia, cerebrovascular and cardiovascular disease, and predisposition to hypotension. In case of jaundice or laboratory indications for liver damage, treatment should be permanently discontinued. Where concurrently administered medications are CYP 2D6 inhibitors, drug–drug interactions between atomoxetine and other medications may occur. Patients with a mutation in CYP 2D6 may be slow metabolizers of atomoxetine.

This occurs in 7% of the white population. For these people, one-third of the usual dosage may suffice. If the habitual dosage of atomoxetine is prescribed in slow metabolizers, additional side effects may result. When using atomoxetine, concomitant use of MAOIs is contraindicated up to two weeks after discontinuation.

The starting dose of atomoxetine for adults is 40 mg. After one to two weeks, the dose is increased to 80–120 mg per day (Simpson & Plosker, 2004). The posology of atomoxetine is 10, 18, 25, 40, 60, 80, and 100 mg, so the dose can be titrated if necessary. In contrast to the stimulants, the therapeutic effect of atomoxetine is achieved after six weeks. This must be explained to patients well in advance, otherwise, they may default treatment prematurely. With treatment, blood pressure and pulse may increase slightly and are checked before and during treatment.

The side effects of atomoxetine are: loss of appetite, abdominal pain, nausea, weight loss, flu-like symptoms, skin rash, an accelerated heartbeat, fatigue, drowsiness, and sexual side effects. Fewer sleep problems occur with atomoxetine than with methylphenidate (Sangal et al., 2006). Increase in liver enzymes occurred at 0.5% and was reversible in all cases (Bangs et al., 2008). In a meta-analysis of studies with atomoxetine in children, the frequency of suicidal thoughts was 0.37% (5 of 1357 patients treated), versus 0% (0 of 851 patients) in the placebo group. Thus, although suicidal thoughts are rare, the difference was significant. The frequency of suicidal thoughts when using atomoxetine or methylphenidate was not different (Bangs et al., 2008). The FDA decided to issue a warning (www.fda.gov). More research is needed to clarify the risk of suicidal thoughts in patients with ADHD treated with atomoxetine. However, practitioners of patients with ADHD should always be mindful of suicidality in their patients, either through the combination of ADHD with comorbid depression or bipolar disorder, or as an undesirable side effect of medication.

Overdose with atomoxetine in children leads to tachycardia, vomiting, and cognitive disorders (Lovecchio & Kashani, 2006). There is as yet little clinical experience with atomoxetine in adults, which is related, among other things, to the effectiveness of the stimulants and to the high cost of atomoxetine, which is often not reimbursed by medical insurance.

In the case of non-response or partial response to atomoxetine, it is advisable to check for possible underlying comorbidities, such as addiction, anxiety, depression, bipolar disorder, or a disordered late sleep phase. If found, these should be treated. If response does not improve, atomoxetine can be discontinued immediately and without problems. No withdrawal or rebound symptoms have been observed on discontinuation.

4.15   Guanfacine XR

Guanfacine, an α2A receptor agonist, increases noradrenergic neurotransmission in the brain. The long-acting form, Guanfacine XR, has been registered for children and adolescents with ADHD as stimulants are ineffective or not well tolerated, but it can also be added to a stimulant (Posey & McDougle 2007; Huss et al., 2016). A controlled study in adults did not demonstrate a difference in effect between 1 and 6 mg Guanfacine XR and placebo (Butterfield et al., 2016). Guanfacine stimulates the postsynaptic α2A receptors in the prefrontal cortex, and was originally known as a blood pressure-lowering agent. Side effects include: dry mouth, drowsiness, dizziness, headache, and constipation. Combined treatment of Guanfacine XR with lisdexamphetamine showed no clinically significant interactions in healthy controls (Roesch et al., 2013), but the added value of the combination seems limited (Taylor & Russo 2001).

4.16 Long-Acting Bupropion

Bupropion has been on the market for years. Initially, it was available as a short-acting form prescribed three times daily. Later, a prolonged release and twice daily form were developed (Zyban). Now, an extended release form exists with once daily intake. Long-acting bupropion (Wellbutrin XR) is registered for depression and smoking cessation. It inhibits reuptake of both norepinephrine and dopamine, and has been shown in controlled trials to be effective for ADHD in children and adults at doses of 300 to 450 mg per day (Solhkhah et al., 2005; Wilens et al., 2001, 2005a; Maneeton et al., 2011). Wellbutrin XR is not registered for ADHD and is therefore prescribed off-label. The drug has a half-life of twenty hours, which means that a once-daily dosage is sufficient. There are bupropion XR tablets of 150 mg and 300 mg. The dose for ADHD can be increased from 150 to 300, possibly up to 450 mg, with a week between steps. The effect occurs two weeks after the highest dose. In patients with impaired liver or kidney function, a lower dose should be maintained. Blood pressure is monitored prior to and during treatment with bupropion.

The side effects of bupropion are: headache, dry mouth, nausea, insomnia, constipation, rash, dizziness, tinnitus, visual disturbances, and high blood pressure. The risk of epileptic seizures is significantly increased with short-acting bupropion at doses above 300 mg. With long-acting Wellbutrin XR up to 300 mg, the risk of seizures is 1 in 1000. Above 400 mg the chance is 4 in 1000. In controlled trials, effective treatment of ADHD sometimes requires doses higher than 300 mg, up to 450 mg. Patients should be informed about the risk of seizures, and patients with epilepsy (in their history) are only prescribed the drug with the permission of their neurologist. Contraindications also exist for patients with alcohol or benzodiazepine addiction, diabetes, or drug use that may further lower the seizure threshold in interaction with bupropion. Concomitant use of MAO inhibitors is contraindicated up to two weeks after discontinuation. If a seizure occurs while on bupropion, the drug should be permanently discontinued.

Overdose results in drowsiness, loss of consciousness, and/or changes in the electrocardiogram (ECG), such as conduction disorders, arrhythmias, and tachycardia. In such cases, hospitalization is advised. Most patients recover without consequences.

Long-acting bupropion is a moderate inhibitor of CYP 2D6. When drugs metabolized by CYP2D6 are used in combination with atomoxetine, blood levels may rise. These include the drugs venlafaxine, tricyclic antidepressants (nortriptyline, imipramine, desipramine), citalopram (although it is not metabolized by CYP 2D6), risperidone, and beta-blockers. The dose of the antidepressants may be reduced in line with blood levels. When combined with carbamazepine and valproate, bupropion levels may decrease. When atomoxetine is combined with alcohol, patients may experience reduced tolerance to alcohol. A combination with a nicotine patch can increase blood pressure.

Long-acting bupropion is prescribed if the stimulants and atomoxetine are poorly tolerated or ineffective. For patients with ADHD and comorbid depression, who want to stop smoking, bupropion seems to be the ideal drug. However, both ADHD and depression should be treated first in order to maximize the chance of response. Extended release bupropion is an advantage in forgetful ADHD patients. In open studies, bupropion is also less likely than SSRIs to cause sexual side effects and maniform disinhibition (Wilens et al., 2003). Clinical experience generally indicates a good response to long-acting bupropion with relatively few side effects, although it is clearly less effective than the stimulants. The drug can be discontinued without withdrawal problems, but a phase-out period can be considered.

4.17   Other Antidepressants: Tricyclic Antidepressants, Venlafaxine, Duloxetine, and Reboxetine

Tricyclic antidepressants are somewhat effective in the treatment of ADHD in children and adolescents, but this has never been convincingly demonstrated in adults (Otasowie et al., 2014; Prince et al., 2000). In view of their cardiovascular and cognitive side effects, and toxicity in case of overdose, they are not an optimal treatment alternative.

Reboxetine, a noradrenergic reuptake inhibitor, was more effective than placebo in three RCTs in adults, but more research is needed before definitive conclusions can be drawn (Ghanizadeh, 2015).

Serotonin and noradrenaline reuptake inhibitors (SSRIs and SNRIs) show mixed results: venlafaxine was not more effective than placebo in a controlled study (Amiri et al., 2012), whereas duloxetine was (Bilodeau et al., 2014).

4.18   Modiodal

Modiodal (modafinil) is registered for narcolepsy, but not for ADHD. It improves alertness during the day. The precise mechanism of action of modiodal is still unclear; it binds to alpha-adrenergic receptors and affects the catecholamine, serotonin, glutamate, gamma amino-butyric acid, orexin, and histamine systems in the brain (Minzenberg & Carter, 2008).

In controlled trials of children and adolescents, modiodal at doses of 170–425 mg per day has been shown to be effective for symptoms of ADHD (Amiri et al., 2008; Biederman & Pliszka, 2008; Kumar, 2008). In a 9-week, placebo-controlled trial of modiodal in 330 adults, the drug was not superior to placebo, although a wide range of doses ranging from 255 to 510 mg/day was used (Arnold et al., 2014).

4.19   Drug Treatment of ADHD in the Elderly

In the elderly with ADHD, the clinician should be extra alerted to the possibility of medical comorbidities, other medications use and possible drug interactions. Differences in drug metabolism are important to consider for all medications in the elderly. Therefore, when prescribing, one should always start with a low dose, e.g., Oros-methylphenidate 18 mg daily, or short-acting methylphenidate 5 mg twice daily. Then, in response to the effect and side effects, the dose can be carefully increased to the optimal strength.

Both methylphenidate and dexamphetamine have clear, dose-related cardiovascular effects. By causing vasoconstriction and increasing peripheral resistance, an increase in heart rate and tidal volume may occur. As a result, blood pressure may increase. Prescribers should monitor cardiovascular status and condition prior to treatment with medication, and any cardiovascular side effects (palpitations, tachycardia, and dyspnoea) should be monitored before and during treatment. If the side effects are troublesome, the choice of drug, dosage, and treatment of the side effect should be reconsidered (NVvP, 2015).

It has been recognized that in adults, stimulants lead to a slight increase in blood pressure (1–5 mmHg on average) and pulse rate (4–10 beats/minute). These changes are almost always clinically insignificant. On ECG, there is no evidence of significant QT-interval prolongation with stimulants. Overall, long-term studies show that the cardiovascular risk for adults is limited. However, a review of three adult studies indicated that in two, stimulant use was associated with poorer cardiovascular outcomes (TIA, cardiac arrhythmias) (Westover & Halm 2012; Schelleman et al., 2012). Limitations of these studies included selection bias and failure to control confounders properly. Despite their limitations, these studies suggest that prior to treatment with stimulants in the elderly, the risk factors for cardiovascular disease should be identified. If necessary, they should be treated in consultation with a cardiologist. The side effects of stimulants, namely increased blood pressure and pulse rate, may exacerbate existing cardiac problems in the elderly. This should be taken into account when prescribing stimulants in this population. Table 4.5 presents a checklist of cardiovascular risk factors that can be used prior to drug treatment in patients aged 50 years and older.

4.19.1 Methylphenidate

No randomized controlled trials (RCTs) on the effectiveness of methylphenidate on the core symptoms of ADHD have been conducted in the elderly. However, case

Table 4.5   Screening cardiovascular risk factors in patients ≥50 years of age

In patients ≥50 years of age:
1. Cardiac complaints in the past six months (dyspnoea on exertion, chest pain, or pain between the shoulder blades, fatigue, arrhythmias, nocturnal dyspnoea, nocturia >1×, peripheral oedema)
2. Cardiac history, high cholesterol, high blood pressure, diabetes, medication for these disorders
3. Family history of cardiac or cerebrovascular problems including CVAs, heart attacks, or cardiac death
4. Physical examination: Pulse frequency, blood pressure, weight, edema
5. ECG
Where limited cognitive disorder is suspected and/or age ≥65 perform:
Laboratory studies: Full blood count, electrolytes, kidney and liver functions, vitamins B1, B6, B12, D, folic acid, fasting glucose, TSH, creatinine, CRP.
Check-ups after starting medication, at every medication increase, and at stabilization, every six months check:
Heart rate Blood pressure Pulse Weight Other checks where indicated:

studies describe a beneficial effect of medication. For example, a 67-year-old woman with ADD was prescribed 10 mg of methylphenidate three times a day (Da Silva & Louza, 2008). After the second week, she and her family reported significant progress in her concentration and improved functioning in daily activities. Biederman describes a similar situation where a 55-year-old man diagnosed with ADHD was also prescribed 10 mg methylphenidate three times a day and indicated that the medication "worked immediately," helped him focus and complete tasks (Biederman, 1998). One pilot study on drug treatment of the elderly with ADHD was conducted in Israel among eleven elderly people with ADHD (aged 56 to 70 years) (Manor et al., 2011). Each elderly person was prescribed methylphenidate, but the dosage, frequency of administration, and duration of action of the drug differed. Three persons received methylphenidate three times a day (25 mg or 30 mg), five received methylphenidate twice a day (22.5–35 mg), two received delayed-release methylphenidate (60 mg) and one was prescribed OROS methylphenidate, 108 mg/day. While two of the eleven participants discontinued their medication due to a lack of improvement, the others experienced an improvement in attention and impulsivity. This study shows that elderly people with ADHD may need a daily dose that is similar to that of younger adults with ADHD. Although RCTs are needed to investigate the effectiveness and safety of methylphenidate in the elderly, these first pilot studies show that methylphenidate can also have a positive effect on their ADHD symptoms. A naturalistic follow-up study among 113 older patients with ADHD showed that, after careful cardiovascular monitoring before and during stimulant treatment, there was a similar response and side effects as in younger adults (Michielsen et al., 2020).

4.19.2 Methylphenidate in the Elderly with Depression and Dementia

Although treatment with methylphenidate has not yet been studied in the elderly with ADHD, methylphenidate has been used and researched in the elderly with depression and dementia. This research can provide general information about the effects and safety of methylphenidate in the elderly.

Various case reports describe the successful treatment with stimulants of therapy-resistant depression in the elderly. Stimulants were even given to patients with serious physical conditions and to patients after heart surgery (Katon & Raskind, 1980; Kaufmann et al., 1984; Fisch, 1985). A rapid improvement in mood without serious side effects was reported.

In a double-blind controlled study, methylphenidate was added to the treatment with citalopram in 143 elderly with depression (Lavretsky et al., 2015). Doses of citalopram ranged from 20 to 60 mg/day, and methylphenidate ranged from 5 to 40 mg/day. The improvement in mood was faster and better in the group using the combination treatment compared to the groups using one of the two drugs. There were no differences in the number of side effects, degree of drop-out, and reasons for drop-out between those who took only citalopram, only methylphenidate, or both drugs. However, there was a significant increase in heart rate in the methylphenidate-only group and in the methylphenidate + citalopram group, but not in the citalopram-only group. The greatest increase in heart rate occurred in the methylphenidate + citalopram group. The results of this study should be interpreted with caution. The US Food and Drug Administration recommends a maximum dosage of citalopram of 20 mg per day in the elderly because of possible cardiac side effects. This study shows that it is worth considering treating an elderly person with ADHD *and* depressive disorder with methylphenidate, in addition to citalopram. This is on condition that the clinician thoroughly evaluates the cardiac status and somatic comorbidity, and monitors cardiac parameters before and during treatment.

A review of treatment with methylphenidate in patients with dementia concludes that methylphenidate can be applied for apathy in this group (Dolder et al., 2010). Psychostimulants were not effective for behavioral problems or cognitive symptoms in dementia. An RCT in sixty patients treated with methylphenidate for apathy in Alzheimer's disease showed a significant improvement in apathy and a trend for improvement in overall cognition, with minimal side effects. Two out of sixty patients had serious side effects such as delusions, agitation, anger, irritability, and sleep problems (Rosenberg et al., 2013). It is not known whether treatment with stimulants in the elderly with ADHD and limited cognitive decline or dementia has benefits for one or both disorders. This needs to be investigated.

4.20   Combining Stimulants with Treatment for Comorbidity

4.20.1 Combining Stimulants with Antidepressants

Where they coexist with ADHD, severe anxiety disorders, dysthymia, and depressive episodes should be treated first. First choice medications are SSRIs and tricyclic antidepressants (TCAs) (Multidisciplinary guideline on depression, 2013). Anxiety and mood disorders can present more acutely and severely than the more chronic ADHD. Depression is known for suicidality, and a potentially lethal course. Where comorbid depression remains untreated, few positive effects can be gained from treating ADHD. For these reasons, patients should always be questioned about depressive symptoms. If the diagnosis of dysthymia or depression is met, treat it first. The effectiveness of the antidepressant can usually be determined after four to five weeks, and the dose is increased if necessary. After the depression has subsided, methylphenidate for ADHD can be added to the drug treatment. When using a TCA, determine its blood level as this can increase when interacting with methylphenidate (Weiss & Sutureman, 1993).

Although the above order probably applies to the more severe forms of depression, this does not seem to apply in all cases. Depression may need to be treated prior to ADHD only where it is severe. In other cases, ADHD can be treated first, with good results. In a large national longitudinal study conducted over a year, almost 2000 patients with ADHD and depression were compared to the same number of patients with depression alone. The group with ADHD and depression were significantly more likely to be resistant to two or more different antidepressant treatments of adequate dosage and duration compared with patients with depression alone (odds ratio 2.32). Where the ADHD had been treated, the risk of therapy resistance to antidepressants decreased (odds ratio 1.76). This argues in favor of treating ADHD first, and only then depression (Chen et al., 2016).

Anxiety disorders, especially those associated with physical symptoms, should be treated prior to ADHD. This is because stimulants may produce the side effect of tachycardia or palpitations, which is interpreted as a return of anxiety or panic. This is so unpleasant that patients refuse to take stimulants again. To prevent this, the anxiety disorder should be diagnosed and treated prior to treatment with medication for ADHD. Based on clinical experience, SSRIs usually reduce anxiety symptoms within a few weeks. Sometimes high doses are needed before the anxiety remits. Clinical experience shows that a stimulant be added to the SSRI without increasing anxiety. It is as yet unknown whether cognitive behavioral therapy affects the anxiety-inducing side effects of stimulants. Some patients will need both treatments to control their anxiety. Although cognitive behavioral therapy (CBT) or interpersonal psychotherapy (IPT) are effective for anxiety and/or depression, the duration of treatment may be a problem for patients with untreated ADHD. They may struggle to complete 12 weeks of therapy, especially if the ADHD is untreated. Combined treatment must therefore also have a rapid effect if it is to have this chance of success.

In case of anxiety or depression + ADHD: first SSRI, then add dexmethylphenidate.

4.20.2 Low Mood Associated with Stimulant Use

Some patients complain of a dip in mood when using stimulants. Owing to the high lifetime prevalence of depressive disorders in adults with ADHD (55%), it can be difficult to determine whether this is a pre-existing, subclinical mood disorder, a missed diagnosis, or truly depressed mood precipitated by the stimulant use (Amons et al., 2006). In clinical practice, euthymic patients are struck by the difference a good treatment response can make to their lives. For patients who have lived without treatment for some forty years, it is a shock to gain clarity suddenly. This insight helps them cope with present challenges, but also gives them a better perspective of the past. Patients make connections between the disorder and the damage they have suffered, such as job losses, broken relationships, and disturbing family bonds. This evokes sadness, anger, and mourning over missed opportunities and lost years. Such a presentation needs to be differentiated from a mood disorder. When mood disorder symptoms present in the short term, it is wise to follow the patient closely and provide support and an explanation of the above processes.

In a study of a group of 45 patients with ADHD treated with methylphenidate, the average mood as measured with the Hamilton Depression Rating Scale did not change before and after treatment. At the individual level, there were minor changes in both directions: improvement as well as worsening of mood (Kooij et al., 2004). Research in ADHD children with and without a history of depression showed that treatment for ADHD had a protective effect on the development of depressive episodes (Daviss et al., 2008). Furthermore, methylphenidate can be used as an adjunctive treatment for severe therapy-resistant depression, in order to increase the antidepressant effect (Buhagiar & Cassar, 2007). While methylphenidate may have mood-enhancing effects, this needs to be systematically researched. In all cases, mood should be monitored in patients with ADHD, with and without stimulant treatment. Regardless of the underlying cause of low mood, it should be treated if the criteria for mood disorder are met.

4.20.3 Combining Stimulants with a Mood Stabilizer

Bipolar II disorder occurs in approximately 10% of adults with ADHD and, conversely, ADHD occurs in 18–30% of patients with bipolar disorder (see also Sect. 2.14.5.4). The combination of stimulants and mood stabilizers is therefore common. In general, it is advisable to treat bipolar disorder first with a mood stabilizer such as lithium or depakine, after which a stimulant can be added. There is now some evidence in the literature that this combination is safe and effective in both children and adults.

In one study, forty ADHD children with comorbid bipolar I- (78%) and II-disorder (22%), aged 6–17 years, were treated for twelve weeks with sodium valproate and a stimulant (mixed amphetamine preparation). No worsening of manic symptoms was seen, and the combination was well tolerated. The researchers concluded that both disorders were effectively and safely treated with sodium valproate and the stimulant (Scheffer et al., 2005). In another study, seven ADHD children aged eight to sixteen years were treated with atomoxetine. Six of them had comorbid bipolar disorder, which was treated with a mood stabilizer. For five of the six children, this combination produced significant improvement in ADHD symptoms, with no increase in depression or (hypo)mania. The treatment duration was one and a half to eighteen months (Hah & Chang, 2005). Children with and without hypomanic characteristics at onset, who participated in the Multimodal Treatment (MTA) study, were compared in their response to and side effects on methylphenidate, in the first month of treatment. For those treated with methylphenidate, no differences were observed in the response or number of adverse events between the two groups (Galanter et al., 2003). A similar study in 75 boys with ADHD with or without bipolar features led to the same conclusion, although the follow-up was longer (11 years). Both groups responded well to methylphenidate and there was no evidence that treatment with methylphenidate led to the development of bipolar disorder in susceptible individuals (Carlson et al., 2000). In the case of eight patients who received adjunctive treatment with a stimulant for bipolar depression or sedation, no mood swings were precipitated (Carlson et al., 2004). A six-year follow-up study of 81 boys with ADHD without mood disorders showed that bipolar disorder developed in 28%. Predictors for this were: more severe dysfunction at the start of the study, recurrent depression in the father and *less* use of stimulants (Tillman & Geller, 2006).

The combination of mood stabilizers and stimulants was evaluated in a study of the patient records of sixteen adults with bipolar I or II disorders, who were taking both a mood stabilizer and methylphenidate. For five, the stimulant was treating ADHD, for the rest, it was being used for therapy-resistant depression. The combination proved to be safe and effective; both mood and attention problems improved, and side effects were mild (Lydon & El-Mallakh, 2006). In Dutch open-label research in ten adult patients with bipolar II disorder and ADHD, methylphenidate was added to the mood stabilizer treatment. After two years, the results in seven patients were as follows: mood was better stabilized, fewer benzodiazepines and a lower dose of lithium was needed, there was more calm, less impulsivity, better concentration, and a better quality of life. The researchers concluded that treatment with methylphenidate is possible and even desirable in bipolar II patients with ADHD, who are on a mood stabilizer. The course of bipolar disorder did not worsen or improve with methylphenidate. The group with ADHD and bipolar II disorder *without* methylphenidate functioned worse than the group with methylphenidate (Seelen & Blom, 2009). This pilot study should be replicated with a larger population of patients. One study contradicts these findings in children and adults. Here, the history of 137 bipolar patients was examined. A quarter of the population had previously used stimulants for ADHD, or bipolar depression. Of these, 43% had also used a mood stabilizer. The percentage of (hypo)mania associated with concomitant stimulant use was 40%. Unfortunately, the researchers did not check for simultaneous use of antidepressants in these patients, which makes the results difficult to interpret. Antidepressants are known to precipitate (hypo)manic episodes, and the combination of an antidepressant and stimulant is widely prescribed. This was also the case in this study (Wingo & Ghaemi, 2008).

In a four-week open-label study with lisdexamphetamine in 45 patients with ADHD and well-controlled bipolar disorder, the ADHD symptoms improved, but there was no increase in manic or psychotic symptoms. Although an open-label study cannot provide definitive evidence of treatment efficacy and safety, the results do confirm previous clinical experience (McIntyre et al., 2013).

A cohort from Taiwan of 145,000 patients with ADHD and an equal number of controls, was followed for eleven years. Here, the effect of methylphenidate and atomoxetine on the risk of developing bipolar disorder was examined. Short- and long-term users were compared with non-users. The ADHD group, as discussed in Sect. 2.14.5.4, had an increased risk of bipolar disorder (odds ratio 2.1), especially the juvenile onset form. Long-term use of methylphenidate in particular protected against this development (odds ratio 0.72). Atomoxetine did not have this effect. More research is needed to elucidate the mechanism of action behind this effect (Wang et al., 2016).

In a Swedish cohort study, 2,300 adults with bipolar disorder who were prescribed methylphenidate with or without a mood stabilizer were followed for eight years. The group without mood stabilization had a greatly increased risk of developing manic episodes (HR 6.7) within three months of the start of the methylphenidate. On the other hand, the group on mood stabilizers had a lower risk of mania after starting with methylphenidate (HR 0.6). In clinical practice, it is therefore recommended that comorbid bipolar disorder is excluded before starting stimulant treatment. Where present, bipolar disorder should be treated with a mood stabilizer before progressing to treat ADHD. With careful monitoring of the patient's mood and other symptoms, combination treatment appears to be safe. However, controlled studies with the combination of mood stabilizer and stimulants are lacking.

In conclusion, there is increasing clinical and early research experience with the combination of a stimulant plus mood stabilizer in both pediatric and adult ADHD populations with comorbid bipolar disorder. Initial results indicate the efficacy of both drugs for the respective disorders, but more and controlled research is needed before definitive conclusions on safety and efficacy can be drawn.

In case of bipolar disorder + ADHD: first mood stabilizer, then add stimulant.

4.20.3.1 Clinical Dilemmas and Experiences

Sometimes it is difficult to distinguish between the return of ADHD symptoms once comorbid depression or hypomania have been successfully treated. Once the depression remits, the patient may suddenly develop hyperactivity or agitation, which may resemble (hypo)mania. The patient and a collateral informant should be questioned as to whether this behavior was before the depression started. If so, it is likely that ADHD symptoms are once again predominant, without the inhibition of a depressive episode. However, if the patient is excessively active, a (hypo)manic episode should be considered.

In patients with ADHD and bipolar disorder, it is crucial to stabilize mood as quickly as possible. The first step is then a mood stabilizer to which methylphenidate is added. In bipolar patients, short-acting methylphenidate is discouraged. Its short duration of action, requires dosing six times daily to avoid rebound. Rebound symptoms include mood swings, which is why these patients should receive long-acting methylphenidate.

According to clinical experience, treatment with methylphenidate alone rarely leads to disinhibition. However, when a stimulant is combined with an antidepressant (especially venlafaxine) or light therapy, it occurs more often. Therefore, all patients with ADHD who are to be treated with an antidepressant and/or stimulant, should first be questioned about a bipolar predisposition or disorder. Those with bipolar I disorder are always protected from subsequently developing mania by starting with a mood stabilizer. Later, an antidepressant, light therapy, and/or stimulant can be added. Opinions are divided on the need to treat patients with bipolar II disorder with a pre-emptive mood stabilizer. On the one hand, a hypomanic episode does not always require treatment, on the other hand, hypomania can develop where light therapy or an antidepressant is used. To avoid this, protection with a mood stabilizer seems to be the safest way.

4.20.4 Stimulants in ADHD with Psychosis

How best are patients with the combination of ADHD and psychosis treated? The safe route of atomoxetine or bupropion can be chosen. However, recently, more information has emerged about using stimulants use in ADHD with psychosis. The medication for both disorders is dopaminergic, but with opposite effects: antipsychotics reduce dopamine metabolism, stimulants increase it. Amphetamines are known to induce psychosis in healthy individuals, but this almost always happens at high or rapidly escalating doses (Berman et al., 2009). The doses of stimulants prescribed for ADHD are much lower than the concentrations of amphetamines used recreationally.

The antipsychotics and the stimulants exert their effects via different brain networks, so that a combination may be possible (Kraguljac et al., 2015; Yang et al., 2016). Antipsychotics influence presynaptic dopamine levels in the meso-limbic system, while stimulants act on dopamine-dependent information processing in the fronto-striatal system (Huber et al., 2007). Another hypothesis is that (low dose) stimulants increase the tonic transmission of dopamine and at the same time decrease the phasic transmission. This results in a calmer patient with enhanced concentration, without provoking psychotic symptoms (Opler et al., 2001). Indeed, the literature describes a case study in which patients were treated with both drugs, without the effect of one drug detracting from that of the other (Blom & Kooij, 2012; Goldberg et al., 1991; Barch & Carter, 2005).

An open-label study was performed where stable schizophrenic patients were treated with lisdexamphetamine. The result was a significant improvement in negative symptoms, with no worsening of positive symptoms. Abrupt discontinuation of stimulant medication did not elicit negative or positive symptoms (Lindenmayer et al., 2013). A large cohort study from Hong Kong followed 20,000 children between the ages of six and nineteen for ten years (Man et al., 2016). Where children were on methylphenidate, there was no increased risk of psychosis. Furthermore, the incidence of psychosis during periods with and without methylphenidate did not vary. However, there was an increased risk of developing psychosis prior to the start with methylphenidate. This finding has been replicated in other studies, and may be due to the behavioral and attentional problems that led to the prescription of the medication (Man et al., 2016; Peralta et al., 2010).

4.20.5 Stimulants in ADHD and Cluster B Personality Disorder

ADHD occurs in 30–65% of patients with borderline or antisocial personality disorder (see Sect. 2.14.8). This means that ADHD should be investigated and treated in patients with cluster B personality disorders. A common question is which disorder should be treated first, ADHD or the personality disorder? The more acute axis I disorders, including anxiety disorders, depressive disorders, addiction, and ADHD, should be addressed before personality disorder. Anxiety and mood disorders and ADHD can be effectively treated with medication within a few weeks, which is clearly to the patient's advantage. Addiction to alcohol and/or drugs also requires immediate treatment. By treating the axis 1 disorder first, there is a greater chance that the patient will be able to comply to the long-term psychotherapy required for personality disorder. Patients with ADHD are restless, impulsive, and easily distracted. These symptoms interfere with the psychotherapeutic process. Many patients with ADHD have had previous psychotherapy that was not either incomplete or very brief. A final reason to treat axis I disorders first is that after ADHD is controlled, impulsivity, mood swings, and anger dissipate and the criteria for the diagnosis of cluster B personality disorders are no longer met.

Sometimes, the treatment order needs to be reversed. For example, patients with cluster B personality disorder may struggle to build up a trusting relationship with the therapist. In such cases, it will be extremely difficult for the prescribing doctor to implement and evaluate pharmacotherapy for ADHD. The working relationship with the practitioner should be the primary focus before effective pharmacological treatment is attempted.

If ADHD and a personality disorder coexist, psycho-education will clarify the reasons for the chosen order of treatment. Subsequently, medication and coaching for ADHD can begin. If symptoms of personality disorder persist and cause dysfunction, targeted psychotherapy can be useful (Multidisciplinary guideline on personality disorders, 2008).

From 1984, a number of cases have been described in the literature, such as that of a 32-year-old woman, who suffered from borderline personality disorder and dependence on drugs and alcohol, and did not respond to treatment. Only after being diagnosed with ADHD and treated with methylphenidate, did the symptoms diminish. She was then able to discontinue alcohol and drug abuse and complete her education (Durst & Rebaudengo-Rosca, 1997; Hooberman & Stern, 1984; Van Reekum & Links, 1994). In an open-label study, adolescent borderline patients with ADHD were treated with methylphenidate for twelve weeks. Not only did the ADHD symptoms improve, but borderline behaviors, such as aggression, also diminished (Golubchik et al., 2008).

In a study of 158 borderline patients where 59 had ADHD, half of those with ADHD received methylphenidate and the other half did not. This pharmacotherapy was in addition to one month of intensive Dialectical Behavioral Therapy (DBT). The medication was prescribed to those patients with the most severe ADHD symptoms. The group with the combination of ADHD and borderline personality was the most impulsive. DBT was effective for borderline symptoms. In the combined treatment group (DBT plus methylphenidate) anger, impulsivity, depression severity, and ADHD improved compared to those without methylphenidate (Prada et al., 2015). This shows that it makes sense to investigate ADHD in borderline patients, and that treatment of ADHD can have an added value to improving the symptoms of personality disorder.

However, more research is needed into effective treatment of ADHD in cluster B personality disorders.

The availability of effective treatment for ADHD may decrease the chronicity of personality disorders (Asherson, 2005; Wolf et al., 2006). Clinical experience shows that the pharmacological treatment of ADHD is not less effective in patients with personality disorders than in patients without axis II diagnosis.

In the case of ADHD + personality disorder: first treat ADHD (and other axes I disorders), then treat personality disorders.

4.20.6 Stimulants in ADHD and Addiction

Many addicts have ADHD and many patients with ADHD use too much alcohol and/or drugs (see Sect. 2.14.7). The treatment of ADHD in addicts is increasingly being investigated (Carpentier & Levin 2017). There is no evidence to suggest that stimulant treatment of ADHD increases the risk of addiction. Rather, the risk lies in the illegal diversion of prescribed stimulants to the population by patients and their family members (Carpentier, 2007; Faraone & Upadhyaya, 2007; Wilens et al., 2003). The non-stimulant atomoxetine is recommended in addicted patients with ADHD, but this is less effective than the stimulants. Addicted patients often have complex problems and multiple comorbid disorders, such as ADHD, mood disorders, and personality disorders. They should be able to use the most effective treatments for their comorbidities, including ADHD (Upadhyaya, 2008). Long-acting stimulants with less risk of abuse have been developed, including the long-acting methylphenidate preparations, a methylphenidate patch, and the long-acting lisdexamphetamine, which is now registered for ADHD in the United States (Upadhyaya, 2008).

In the treatment of ADHD in addicts, it is advised first to minimize substance abuse or ideally, to stop it. Targeted interventions such as lifestyle training and psychotherapy can be helpful here (Merkx et al., 2007). Thereafter, medication for ADHD and other axis I comorbidities can be started. Once the patient is stabilized, it is possible to evaluate treatment effectiveness and to monitor how well the substance abuse is under control (Wilens, 2004a, 2004b). For the question of how many glasses of alcohol or joints per day are permitted during the use of stimulants, see Sect. 4.4.

In early research into ADHD treatment in addicts, the doses of stimulants used were too low. Response to placebo and CBT was high. From this, it could be inferred that treatment had some effect on ADHD symptoms but insufficient impact on substance use. In subsequent studies among addicts with ADHD, higher doses were used, as shown by a recent review (Carpentier et al., 2017). Konstenius (2014) used very high doses of methylphenidate (180 mg Oros-methylphenidate per day) in 54 abstinent prisoners with amphetamine addiction. Treatment was started two weeks before discharge from prison and continued on an outpatient basis for 24 weeks. Oros-methylphenidate showed a significant effect for ADHD, compliance with treatment programs while maintaining abstinence (an increase of negative urine tests). Studies in nicotine addicts showed that Oros-methylphenidate (72 mg per day) effectively reduced ADHD symptoms, but not nicotine addiction, in patients with ADHD who were also treated with a nicotine patch and counselling (Winhusen et al., 2010).

In terms of amphetamine treatment, Levin (2015) showed that 60–80 mg long-acting "mixed amphetamine salts" were significantly effective for ADHD and high rates of abstinence for cocaine addiction were achieved. The highest dose had the greatest effect. In a controlled Dutch study of heroin-addicted patients receiving maintenance treatment with heroin, long-acting dexamphetamine was effective in reducing concomitant **cocaine** addiction (Nuijten et al., 2016). This effect was not observed in a group of cocaine addicts treated with lisdexamphetamine versus placebo (Mooney et al., 2015). In another study of nicotine addicts with ADHD, lisdexamphetamine up to 70 mg per day resulted in a significant decrease in ADHD symptoms, but not in nicotine addiction (Kollins et al., 2014). More research with (dex)amphetamine in addiction is needed. Atomoxetine up to 100 mg per day was not effective for alcohol addiction in recently abstinent patients with ADHD, nor for cannabis or marijuana addiction, but the severity of ADHD decreased (Carpentier et al., 2017). Although atomoxetine is often recommended for ADHD and addiction, its effect on addiction has yet to be demonstrated.

In Table 4.6 difficulties during treatment with stimulants and possible solutions are suggested.

Table 4.6 Treatment strategies for therapy-resistant ADHD in adults[a]

Symptoms	Intervention
• Increase or no change in ADHD symptoms (attention deficit, impulsivity, hyperactivity)	• Increase dosage • Change administration times or give long-acting methylphenidate • Switch from methylphenidate to dextroamphetamine • Consider medication for comorbidity (SSRI/TCA) Check addiction • Consider non-pharmacological treatment, for example (repeat) psycho-education, coaching, behavioral therapy, relationship therapy etc.
• Annoying side effects	• Evaluate overall response • Evaluate if a side effect is due to medication • Actively combat side effects by altering administration times or dose, changing stimulant type or changing to atomoxetine or bupropion • Add (10–40 mg) propranolol in case of persistent palpitations
• Rebound symptoms	• Evaluate overall response and compliance • Change administration times or give long-acting methylphenidate • Change type of stimulant • Dose more frequently (and with lower doses)
• Emergence of dysphoria, anxiety, agitation, irritability	• Evaluate overall response • Evaluate overdose or rebound phenomena • Exclude a return of ADHD symptoms • Evaluate comorbid anxiety/depression and treat with SSRI • Reduce dosage • Change type of stimulant • Stop stimulant, start atomoxetine or bupropion • Consider alternative treatments
• Occurrence of depression, mood swings, severe anxiety symptoms	• Evaluate overdose or rebound phenomena • Evaluate comorbidity • Reduce dosage or stop stimulant • Add SSRI, TCA, or mood stabilizer • Add non-pharmacological intervention
• Occurrence of psychosis	• Stop stimulant • Evaluate comorbidity, including bipolar disorder • Consider antipsychotic

[a]Free to T.E. Wilens et al., (1995)

4.20.7 Stimulants and Sexuality

Methylphenidate increases dopaminergic neurotransmission and thus sex drive, in contrast to SSRIs and ecstasy, which inhibit sexual arousal and function via the serotonergic system. In a double-blind, crossover study of 30 healthy controls, the effect of 40 mg methylphenidate and 75 mg MDMA (ecstasy) on sexual arousal was evaluated. Subjects viewed erotic images of romantic relationships of unknown couples. They were then asked to appraise these intimate relationships. Methylphenidate increased sexual arousal in response to explicit sexual stimuli. Plasma levels of testosterone, estrogen, and progesterone were not associated with the sexual arousal. Neither methylphenidate nor MDMA changed the appraisal of erotic stimuli or the appreciation of romantic relationships of others. This study should be repeated in patients with ADHD (Schmid et al., 2015).

4.21 Treatment with Melatonin in Delayed Sleep Phase Disorder

According to research, three-quarters of adults with ADHD have chronic problems with falling asleep and waking up on time (Van Veen et al., 2010), see also Sect. 2.14.4.3. A similar sleeping pattern was also found in children with ADHD (Van der Heijden et al., 2005). This results in daytime fatigue and drowsiness, which can exacerbate the concentration problems of ADHD. Such a sleeping pattern may be explained by the so-called delayed sleep phase. The appropriate treatment for this condition is melatonin in the evening and/or light early in the morning (Lewy 2007). Based on the most recent research findings, Sect. 4.20 provides advice on the optimal dose and timing of melatonin for these sleep problems.

Chronic delayed sleep phase occurs in 75% of people with ADHD.

4.21.1 Delayed Sleep Phase

Most people sleep between 11 p.m. and 7 a.m. However, "evening" people, or with a delayed sleep phase only fall asleep at 03.00 a.m. They would prefer to sleep until 11 in the morning. If they try to go to bed earlier, they have trouble falling asleep or they do fall asleep, but wake up after a few hours. The circadian rhythm, which is determined by the 24-h rhythm of light and dark, is out of phase *with* respect to the time on the clock. Individual circadian rhythm is genetically determined through clock genes: polymorphisms in clock genes have been identified in ADHD. This is believed to lead to abnormalities in the sleep rhythm. However, much is still unclear about the function and meaning of the different clock genes (Coogan et al., 2017; Mogavero et al., 2018).

Evening people often find it difficult to function in a regular job from 9 a.m. to 5 p.m., and will try to adapt their working hours to their individual circadian rhythm. Indeed, adults with ADHD tend to choose evening and night shifts. When they are self-employed, they can regulate their own pattern of activity. For patients with an extremely late sleep phase, not only does a regular working life come under pressure, but contacts and relationships are also poorly maintained: Furthermore, treatment for ADHD fails when the appointments with the therapist are scheduled in the morning.

The Munich Chronotype Questionnaire is a validated instrument that measures chronotype, i.e., someone's circadian preference for the evening or the morning. The questionnaire can be completed online at www.thewep.org.

4.21.2 Melatonin for Delayed Sleep Phase

The role of melatonin and light treatment in delayed sleep phase and winter depression was extensively investigated by A.J. Lewy, among others. Melatonin and (sun) light are opposites, and both play an important role as Zeitgebers or time indicators in the synchronization of our biological clock. Production of melatonin begins in the evening and ensures that our body synchronizes with the clock time of the environment. In the morning, light entering through the eyes interrupts the production of melatonin, so that we can face the day and wake up (Lewy 2007; Lewy et al., 1992, 2006a, 2006b, 2007). Melatonin is a substance specific to the body, which is produced in the pineal gland of the brain when it gets dark (on average around 9:30 p.m., with a standard deviation of spread of two hours). When melatonin is produced later than average, the term late Dim Light Melatonin Onset (DLMO) is used. DLMO is the biomarker for the Delayed Sleep Phase Syndrome. DLMO indicates when the melatonin level exceeds a certain threshold (3 pg/ml in saliva, or 10 pg/ml in plasma) (see Fig. 4.2). This time is approximately two hours before falling asleep, or fourteen hours after getting up. A late DLMO is associated with a later sleep-onset. As illustrated graphically, the melatonin curve has shifted to the right (Wirtz-Justice et al., 2008).

The melatonin and light are both Zeitgebers, with opposite effects.

Many children and adults with ADHD and delayed sleep onset are prescribed 3 to 5 mg melatonin at night on an experimental basis. All five studies on the effect of melatonin on sleep problems in children with ADHD show an improvement in sleep time (Coogan et al., 2017). Van der Heijden was one of the first to show that 3 mg melatonin before bedtime has beneficial effects on the sleep problems of children

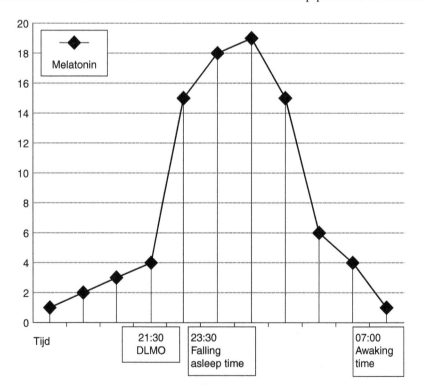

Fig. 4.2 Melatonin curve with a normal circadian rhythm

with ADHD, and that the DLMO curve is indeed shifted to the right (Van der Heijden et al., 2007). Lower doses of melatonin in the late afternoon appear to be equally effective (Lewy et al., 2007), and are preferable. Research is ongoing into low dose melatonin in the late afternoon, with or without light therapy in the morning, for adults with ADHD. Sleep problems are chronic in patients with ADHD, and are often present from childhood. Benzodiazepines should therefore be avoided as much as possible, their use will only lead to dependence and addiction.

The rise in melatonin levels in the evening is delayed in the late sleep phase disorder.

4.21.3 First, Sleep Hygiene

To start with, the questions are asked about daytime and evening behaviors, and in the evening and during the day, and the sleep rhythm is asked:

- Evening activities
- Use of alcohol, cannabis, coffee
- Time spent exercising
- Computer time
- Computer use, TV, iPad, or telephone in bedroom
- Well darkened and ventilated bedroom
- Bedtime (fixed or variable)
- Time of falling asleep
- Waking up time (fixed or variable)
- Time of getting up
- Breakfast time
- Total hours of sleep
- Rest when you get up
- Use of sunglasses during the day;
- Exposure to light during the day
- Naps during the day

Alcohol and coffee should be limited. After 8 p.m., it is generally better to restrict fluids to avoid night-time toilet visits and interrupted sleep. Cannabis should be discontinued, otherwise, the effect of melatonin on sleep problems cannot be evaluated. Patients are advised not to use the computer late at night because light from the computer screen reaching the eyes suppresses melatonin. As a result, the sleep phase is shifted further. Removing the computer from the bedroom can also assist. A good bed, blackout curtains and good ventilation in the bedroom are general measures that contribute to improved sleep hygiene. Exercise increases the level of melatonin, so that one sleeps better after physical exertion (Ronkainen et al., 1986). However, sports at night may delay the sleep phase (Van Reeth et al., 1994).

As a delayed sleep phase with early rising results in few hours of sleep, many patients compensate by taking naps during the day. As a result, the sleep phase is further delayed. So this practice should be discouraged. Exposure to sufficient bright light during the day helps to consolidate the day–night rhythm. Morning or lunchtime walks, when the amount of sunlight is at its maximum, are recommended. In winter, when it is still dark in the morning, a lamp with bright artificial light connected to a timer can help the waking up process. The so-called Wake-Up Light, which is for sale for this purpose, does not provide enough light for everyone to wake up to (75 W), so research is now underway with bright daylight lamps. Frequent use of sunglasses during the day is not recommended for those with delayed sleep phase, as they limit light exposure through the eyes. Nevertheless, almost 70% of adults with ADHD report hypersensitivity to light, so that on average, they wear sunglasses more often and for longer periods in all seasons. This prevents adequate synchronization of the internal biological clock to daylight. It is unclear why ADHD patients are hypersensitive to light. It may be related to the interaction between dopamine and melatonin receptors in the retina, which together with the melanopsin ganglion cells, report directly to the biological clock (Kooij & Bijlenga, 2014). Research into the pupil response to light in ADHD is ongoing.

Many patients with sleep phase problems have no insight into their sleep and rhythm problems. They may worsen their sleep problems in several ways. Patients with chronic debt may try to compensate by going to bed at different times every night, ranging from extremely early to very late. They seem to lack any rhythm or pattern in their sleep. In order to bring their sleep rhythm into phase, they will have to stop these bad habits when starting treatment with melatonin and/or light (see Table 4.7).

The natural sleep rhythm is the rhythm without the compensatory effect of medication, alcohol, or drugs, without the limits of normal working hours and without terminal insomnia caused by comorbid depression. To get an impression of the patient's chronotype (evening or morning person), questions can be asked about the sleep rhythm in adulthood, during free time and holidays, during periods of good health etc. See also Sect. 2.14.4.3.

Table 4.7 Factors influencing sleep rhythm

Deleterious
• Lights and screens on at night
• Coffee, alcohol, cannabis
• Sunglasses during the day
• Waking up late
• Naps during the day

Favorable
• Breakfast early in the morning
• Exercise in the morning or at the end of the afternoon
• After 8:00 p.m., little drinking and eating
• Dark, well-ventilated bedroom
• Direct bright light when you get up
• Go to bed and get up at fixed times

Good questions to ask:

1. Do you usually have trouble falling asleep before midnight?
2. Do you sleep less than seven hours a night on average? If so, how many hours approximately?

4.21.4 Side Effects and Protective Effects of Melatonin

Melatonin has few to no known side effects. Melatonin is considered safe; it has chronobiotic, antioxidant and anti-inflammatory properties, and it captures free radicals (Bruni et al., 2015). Melatonin is involved in bone formation, regulation of fertility, cardiovascular and immunological factors, and BMI. It has protective effects on the brain and gastrointestinal tract in several psychiatric disorders, cardiovascular diseases, and cancer (Tordjman et al., 2017).

Prolonged use of high doses (such as 3–5 mg) can cause drowsiness during the day. Incorrect timing of administration (before 16.00 and after 24.00) may cause the circadian phase to shift in undesirable direction. Incorrect timing of melatonin administration can therefore delay the sleep phase and pose a greater risk of winter depression in susceptible individuals. Seeing that 20 to 30% of adults with ADHD have comorbid winter depression, this is not an insignificant problem (Amons et al., 2006; Levitan et al., 1999; Lewy et al., 2006b). The timing of melatonin intake is therefore very important.

Due to possible virus transmission when using melatonin derived from animals, synthetically manufactured melatonin should be used.

There is evidence of beneficial effects of melatonin on the immune system, however, melatonin can worsen except in the case of rheumatoid arthritis. Melatonin can worsen this disease (Carrillo-Vico et al., 2005). Pregnant and lactating women should not use melatonin. Melatonin protects against DNA damage and cancer through its antioxidant properties (Dopfel et al., 2007; Sliwinski et al., 2007). Research shows that through its anti-oestrogenic effects, melatonin inhibits the growth of breast cancer cells, prevents angiogenesis in tumors, and it reduces the risk of metastases (Hill et al., 2015). Research into the effect of adjunctive melatonin with chemotherapy is ongoing (Nooshinfar et al., 2017).

4.21.5 Melatonin as a Sleep Aid

To facilitate falling asleep, a relatively high dose of melatonin of 3–5 mg is given one hour before the desired bedtime, for example, at 10 p.m. This can have a rapid effect if the patient is exhausted due to sleep deprivation. The duration of treatment with this dose of melatonin is unknown, but if drowsiness occurs during the day, this is a reason to reduce the dose or to switch to a lower dose of 0.5–1 mg. It is advisable to wait a few weeks for the effect of melatonin because the circadian rhythm cannot be reset within a few days. If 3–5 mg is ineffective, one should check whether the melatonin tablets were exposed to light, as this may render them ineffective. Patients should be warned of this in advance. This may also explain why some patients complain that the melatonin has ceased to work after some time. Benzodiazepines are avoided as much as possible in the chronic sleep problems of ADHD to prevent addiction.

4.21.6 Melatonin Resets the Clock

When a low dose of melatonin is administered in the late afternoon, the biological clock receives a time signal. To advance the sleep phase, 0.1–0.5 mg melatonin is given in the late afternoon. To achieve the optimum dosage, several doses should be tried, as this is individually variable. The best time to take the melatonin depends on the time when one's own melatonin production increases (the DLMO). The DLMO can be measured in the saliva during the evening, by getting the patient to chew cotton swabs every hour, under subdued light conditions. In practice, this measurement is not very practical. Therefore, the DLMO is estimated on the basis of the most probable and sustained time of falling asleep. Owing to the fixed period of two hours between DLMO and sleep-onset time, melatonin is given stepwise (see box "Example of how to use melatonin to reset the biological clock." Melatonin is administered six hours before estimated DLMO, or eight hours before the desired sleep-onset time, but *not before 3:30–4 p.m.* (see also Fig. 4.2). If the patient can fall asleep on time, this low dose of melatonin should be continued as a maintenance dose to keep the sleep rhythm in phase.

Example of How to Use Melatonin to Reset the Biological Clock
Where a patient struggles to fall asleep before 3 a.m., the DLMO is probably around 1:00 a.m. The desired sleep onset time is midnight. In theory, a low dose of 0.5 mg melatonin should be given at 4.00 p.m. (24.00 minus 8.00). However, it is better to advance sleep onset in "blocks" of 90 minutes per (the duration of a sleep cycle), until the desired sleep-onset time is reached. If the timed intake was successful in the first week, the desired sleep time is then set at 01.30. Half a mg of melatonin is given 8 hours earlier, i.e., at (25.30 minus 8.00 =) 17:30. After one week, the patient is evaluated in terms of time of melatonin intake and the effect on sleep-onset time. The desired sleep-onset time is once again moved 90 earlier, at midnight. A dose of 0.5 mg melatonin is given at 4 p.m. (24 minus 8). The desired sleep-onset time should be discussed at the consultation, a week later. Once the optimal sleep-onset time has been reached, this regime should be continued (see Table 4.8). Weekly consultations are necessary for practice as they provide chaotic patients with ADHD the structure to achieve a phase shift.

Melatonin is not only a soporific but also resets the biological clock. Timing melatonin intake is crucial for shifting the sleep phase forward or backward.

Table 4.8 Desired sleep-onset time and time of intake 0.5 mg melatonin (= desired sleep onset time minus 8 hours)

Desired sleep-onset time	Time of taking melatonin
01.00	17.00
00.30	16.30
24.00	16.00
23.30	16.00
23.00	16.00

4.21.7 Instructions to the Patient

It is important to tell patients that endogenous melatonin is inactivated through light entering the eyes. In addition, light reaching it through an open or transparent container also renders it inactive. Therefore, tablets should be stored in opaque containers, or the melatonin should be packed in opaque capsules. Many pharmacists are unaware of this, so that when one switches pharmacies, the sleeping difficulties can suddenly return! Melatonin is light sensitive. Being aware of this can help avoid such experiences.

Taking melatonin later than midnight and earlier than 4 p.m. can delay sleep onset and therefore increase the risk of winter depression. An alarm or reminder is absolutely necessary to keep the melatonin intake on time, so that the desired effect is achieved and maintained.

Endogenous melatonin is inactivated by light through the eyes, and melatonin tablets become ineffective when exposed to light.

4.21.8 Tips and Tricks

- If the patient becomes drowsy immediately after taking 0.5 mg melatonin, the dose should be reduced to 0.2 or 0.1 mg.
- If the regime works, every few days, the patient should attempt to fall asleep fifteen minutes earlier, so that after a few weeks the phase shift is complete.
- Getting up fifteen minutes earlier every few days is also extremely helpful. Going outdoors to get sunlight after waking, or applying bright light at wake-up time provides a powerful signal to the biological clock. Morning is signalled, because melatonin is inactivated by light.
- Exercising outdoors and exhausting the dog works as a time signal or *Zeitgeber*.
- Timing of meals is also a useful signal to the biological clock. Having an early breakfast in the morning (almost no ADHD patient eats breakfast!) is not only important for the biorhythm, but also helps prevent obesity (see Sect. 2.14.3.2).
- Sleeping late (also on weekends) is out of the question because it disrupts the rhythm, creating extra difficulty on Monday morning.
- In case of a positive response effect, the same low dose should be continued at the correct time. If melatonin is discontinued, the biological clock returns to its original, probably genetically controlled, position. How quickly the rhythm recovers will vary per individual.

4.21.9 Light Therapy for the Delayed Sleep Phase and Possibly for ADHD

A first open-label study with light therapy in patients with ADHD and winter depression showed not only an effect on mood, but also improvement of ADHD (Rybak et al., 2006). A more extensive pilot study aiming to advance the late sleep phase in ADHD used two weeks of light therapy at 10,000 lux for 30 minutes early in the morning. As a result, melatonin production was 31 minutes earlier. This was associated with a significant decrease in ADHD symptoms, particularly hyperactivity/impulsivity. However, sleep duration and sleep efficiency did not change (Fargason et al., 2017). The significance of the effect of light on the severity of ADHD symptoms is intriguing and may open up new avenues for the treatment of ADHD. Possibly ADHD should no longer be considered exclusively as a disorder of dopaminergic inhibition, but also as a circadian disorder that can be stabilized with light and melatonin.

4.22 Alternative Treatments for ADHD

There are quite a few complementary or alternative treatments that claim to have an effect on ADHD, including certain diets, herbs, homeopathy, St. John's wort, acupuncture, nutritional supplements, the omission of sugars and dyes from the diet, neurofeedback, soothing mattresses, special glasses, fish oil, and even swimming with dolphins. It is often suggested that the dose of the medication can be reduced or even stopped in conjunction with alternative treatments. However, these claims are not scientifically substantiated, or insufficiently so. The safety of alternative treatments has been insufficiently researched (Brue et al., 2001; Coulter & Dean, 2007; Loo & Barkley, 2005; Pelsser et al., 2009, 2011; Raz & Gabis, 2009; Weber & Newmark, 2007; Weber et al., 2008).

Despite the increasing interest in the subject, there is little or no evidence for the effectiveness of complementary and alternative treatment for the core symptoms of ADHD. In a meta-analysis of non-pharmacological treatments for ADHD where strict inclusion criteria for effectiveness were used, the following treatments were unable to be assessed, mainly due to the lack of blinding: the elimination diet, neurofeedback, parental behavioral training, and cognitive behavioral therapy. It is to be expected that both pharmacological and non-pharmacological research have the same strict criteria for blinding. So, final conclusions about therapeutic effectiveness will only be able to be drawn once there is better, blinded research.

The effectiveness of neurofeedback in children and adolescents with ADHD was not significantly better than placebo in a meta-analysis of thirteen studies (Cortese et al., 2016). Omega-3 fatty acids and the omission of food additives in sensitive children did show small, robust effects. (Sonuga-Barke et al., 2013). In meta-analyses of children and adolescents with ADHD, supplementation with EPA-DHA (omega-3 fatty acids) improved aggression, hostility, antisocial behavior, anxiety, impulsivity, and emotional lability (Gajos & Beaver 2016; Patrick & Ames 2015; Gow et al., 2013; Meyer et al., 2015). For the core symptoms of ADHD, low effect sizes have been demonstrated in meta-analyses in children (Bloch & Qawasmi 2011). In healthy adults and elderly, EPA-DHA improves working memory and cognitive performance (Konagai et al., 2013; Witte et al., 2014). These findings can probably be extrapolated to adults with ADHD, but more research is needed.

There is also new evidence for low vitamin D3 levels in ADHD, which can exacerbate executive dysfunction, sensory sensitivity, and impulsive behavior (Rylander & Verhulst, 2013; Anglin et al., 2013). Supplementation of vitamin D3 reduced the severity of attention deficit, hyperactivity, and impulsivity in adults with ADHD (Rucklidge, Frampton, et al., 2014, Rucklidge, Johnstone, et al., 2014).

Parents of children with ADHD seem to opt for alternative treatments, more often than average (Chan et al., 2003). In addition, negative publicity about stimulants and a lack of clarity about possible long-term effects of the medication may together have led to an increase in the use of alternative treatments (Brue & Oakland, 2002; Sawni, 2008). It, therefore, seems advisable to discuss the use of alternative therapies with the patient. Often the practitioner is unaware of this parallel therapy, so that it may later be unclear to the patient which effect is due to which treatment, and also which treatment should be continued.

It is striking that alternative treatments are very time consuming, and just as expensive or more expensive than medication, while effectiveness and safety have not been established. Of course, any approach that may be effective should be explored, but until then, the advice is to prescribe treatments whose effect has been scientifically proven. Supplementation of vitamin D3 and use of omega 3 fatty acids in ADHD appear to be the most rational so far.

4.22.1 Gaming and Exercise in Young Children with ADHD

The so-called TEAMS study showed the benefit of therapeutic computer games and exercise for young children with ADHD (4–5 years). Where these fun games were played for at least 30 minutes per day, in addition to 30 minutes per day of physical activity intensively supervised by the parent (dancing, cycling, jumping), after five weeks there was a significant effect on the ADHD symptoms. Medication was more effective, but the effects of gaming and exercise persisted after discontinuation of the medication. These effects are explained by "early environmental enrichment," i.e., brain development can be stimulated by intensive daily exercise and gaming with parental support, and may bring about symptom reduction, also in the longer term (Halperin et al., 2014). More research is in progress.

Treatment: Coaching of Adults with ADHD

5

In cooperation with M.H. Francken, M.P.T.M. Pennings

5.1   What Is Coaching?

This chapter is based on the literature on coaching and cognitive behavioral therapy in adults with ADHD, and on experiences from clinical practice. The aim is to provide clinicians with tools for the practical application of coaching in adults with ADHD.

The literature regularly distinguishes between coaching and psychotherapy (particularly cognitive behavioral therapy) in ADHD (Ramsay & Rostain, 2008). With coaching, the patient is supported in achieving practical goals, for example, in work or training. In psychotherapy, more attention is paid to the patient's overall function and diagnostics are an important part of the treatment. Some coaches use cognitive behavioral interventions, although this is uncommon.

There are some differences in the treatment focus of various models of cognitive behavioral therapy in adults with ADHD . For example, Ramsay and Rostain focus relatively more on the cognitive component, while Safren pays more attention to learning practical skills (Ramsay & Rostain, 2008; Safren, Sprich, Perlman, & Otto, 2006a, b).

The concept of coaching in this chapter is used flexibly. On the one hand, more formal cognitive behavioral therapy techniques may be used, for example, in patients with a negative self-image as a result of persistent failure. For other patients, the focus may be on learning practical skills and support in achieving goals, possibly supplemented by practical guidance in the home situation. For many patients, coaching contains both elements. The focus of the treatment, therefore, depends on the presenting problems of the patient. In all patients, an important condition for the start of treatment is diagnosis, including that of comorbid disorders. Treatment as

J. J. S. Kooij, *Adult ADHD*, https://doi.org/10.1007/978-3-030-82812-7_5

discussed further, will be more in line with cognitive behavioral therapy than coaching in a narrower sense. In this chapter, the term "coach" will be alternated with "practitioner."

5.2   Similarities and Differences in Cognitive Behavioral Therapy in ADHD and Other Disorders

What exactly is different about cognitive behavioral therapy for ADHD as opposed to other disorders, such as depression or anxiety?

Similarities
- The treatment is transparent; an explanation is given of what is being done and the reasons behind it.
- The treatment is structured and targeted.
- The treatment focuses on the here and now, and on the past only if it is relevant to the present.

Differences
- Coaching makes use of more limited homework assignments, to avoid patient failure.
- For this reason, assignments are discussed in more detail during the consultation.
- Due to forgetfulness of patients, repetition of previously discussed issues is important.
- Coaching is more practical in the sense that learning how to plan and structure is emphasized.
- The lack of hierarchy between practitioner and patient is more important in coaching to prevent the patient from dropping out or resisting treatment.

5.3   Rationale of the Treatment

ADHD in adults is still a relatively young diagnosis. As a result, there is little research data available in the field of psychosocial treatment, although the number of publications is clearly increasing. Based on the data available so far, cognitive behavioral therapy (individually or in a group) appears to be a useful addition to medication for patients still experiencing symptoms and limitations (Ramsay, 2007; Safren et al., 2006a, b; Solanto, Marks, Mitchell, Wasserstein, & Kofman, 2008; Weiss et al., 2008).

One of the first studies on the effect of cognitive behavioral therapy in adults with ADHD showed promising results (Safren et al., 2005). The model on which the treatment is based is shown in Fig. 5.1. The treatment covers the following subjects: psycho-education, learning skills in the area of planning and organizing,

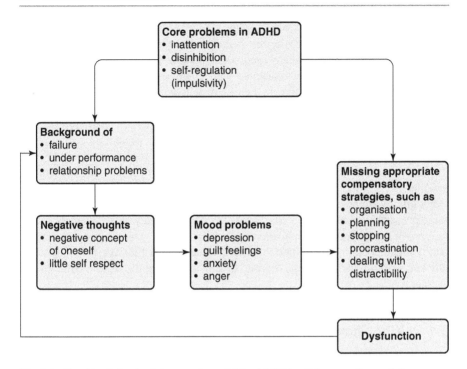

Fig. 5.1 Cognitive-behavioral therapeutic model for ADHD in adults according to Safren

problem-solving skills, dealing with distractibility and procrastination, cognitive training, and preventing relapse.

According to this model, the core symptoms of ADHD are neurobiological in nature. In addition, cognitions and behavior influence the severity of the symptoms. First of all, medication is used to treat the core symptoms. As a result, the core symptoms improve in a large number of patients. However, underdeveloped skills (e.g., in the field of planning) remain unchanged. In addition to medication, cognitive behavioral therapy is used to increase (practical) skills and to tackle problems such as avoidance behavior and negative self-concept.

Coaching is an important addition to pharmacological treatment. The practitioner's approach is directive and uses homework assignments. Coaching also focuses on frequently occurring problems such as fear of failure, negative self-image, and depressive complaints that can result from ADHD. Attention is also paid to relationships, social and financial problems, and to acceptance of the diagnosis. In individual treatment, comorbid disorders are discussed in addition to ADHD-related problems.

Group coaching has developed rapidly in recent years. The advantage of coaching in a group is that patients meet each other and derive support from the recognition of their life stories. Speaking openly about an ADHD diagnosis was found to reduce the risk of social rejection in a study among young adults (Jastrowski, Berlin,

Sato, & Davies, 2007). However, it is questionable whether this applies to every situation and to every person. For the time being, psychiatric disorders, including ADHD, are taboo. There are many ignorant laypersons and professionals with prejudices who deal with those who disclose their diagnoses. This is why "coming out of the closet" is most safely done in a group of fellow sufferers.

Usually, the group begins with psycho-education. An example of such a group can be found in "Introduction Course" in Appendix, the so-called Introductory group. This group consists of four sessions and provides psycho-education about ADHD and treatment, as well as contact with fellow sufferers.

Furthermore, many patients find a group teaching practical planning and organizational skills extremely useful. This can be supplemented by cognitive training. Other groups are possible, for example, in the fields of impulse control, self-image, sleep phase problems, and specific groups for students and women. Patients can be referred to these groups on indication by the practitioner. A group for partners and family members is another important addition (see Table 6.1 in Sect. 6.1). The structure and working method of these group treatments are not discussed further in this chapter.

5.4   Who Should Provide the Coaching?

Individual coaching in ADHD should be given by care providers with knowledge and experience in the field of cognitive behavioral therapy, who are also trained in the diagnostics and treatment of adults with ADHD. These may be psychiatric nurses psychologists or social workers. The coach is matched to the patient's comorbidity and social problems. If there are many psychosocial problems (e.g., finance, housing, family problems), a psychiatric nurse or social worker may be preferred. When an anxiety disorder, depression, or personality problems occur in addition to ADHD, or when perfectionism and a negative self-image are at the forefront, a psychologist may be more appropriate.

5.5   (Contra) Indications for Coaching

Before starting with specific ADHD coaching, it is important that comorbid disorders are sufficiently (pharmacologically) treated. In addition, ADHD medication should be optimal and stable to provide the most benefit from coaching. However, if coaching and medication start simultaneously, the treatment plan is drawn up and psycho-education is started. During coaching, prescription medication and substance use are always discussed. Where a patient refuses ADHD treatment, it is useful to agree to a clear term within which progress must be made. If this goal is not met, coaching should be discontinued and the use of medication becomes a prerequisite to continuing coaching. Experience shows that only a small proportion of patients benefit from coaching without medication; the majority only to a very limited extent. Therefore, this should be clarified to the patient beforehand.

In some situations, coaching for ADHD is not the preferred treatment. This is particularly the case in crisis situations, where suicidality, lack of motivation, or when another axis I or II disorder are at the forefront. In crises situations, crisis intervention is the first step. When the patient and his/her circumstances are more stable, coaching for ADHD can be started.

If a personality disorder such as borderline or antisocial is at the forefront, coaching often does not get off the ground. Where the therapeutic relationship is under pressure, or the patient has difficulty trusting the practitioner, the interaction between patient and coach is hindered. If it is not possible to build a relationship of trust with the coach, it becomes difficult for the prescriber to stabilize and optimize the ADHD medication. When self-mutilation or suicidal ideation are at the forefront, coaching often fails. In such cases, it makes sense to refer the patient first for specialist treatment of the personality disorder. In many cases, however, ADHD is in the foreground and it is addressed before referring the patient on. Sometimes, if medical treatment of ADHD is successful, the diagnostic criteria for personality disorder are no longer met.

When there is dependence on alcohol and/or drugs, a patient will first have to reduce use. If addiction is the primary problem, coaching will not stop use and targeted treatment of the ADHD symptoms will most likely be unsuccessful. ADHD medication is not advised in the presence of significant substance use. Patients should first be referred to specialist addiction care. Mild-to-moderate substance abuse can usually be reduced in agreement with the doctor and coach, plus with the help of medication. If this does not succeed within a few weeks, it is wise to refer the patient again.

With a history of traumatic experiences or PTSD in addition to ADHD, it can be difficult to determine what takes priority in treatment. ADHD medication is likely to improve concentration. As a result, the patient is less distracted and has a better overview, so that traumatic memories may surface more. If a patient has previously failed to address the trauma, this sudden change can lead to decompensation. On the other hand, many patients cannot work on their trauma if their lives are chaotic and unstructured. In such cases, it is preferable to discuss the best treatment approach with PTSD specialists.

ADHD and bipolar-II disorder frequently co-occur. Prior to starting treatment, it is important to determine whether this is a bipolar type I or II, the previous history, and any (hypo)manic episodes and/or past characteristics. When bipolar disorder is at the forefront, in most cases it is best to refer the patient first to specialist treatment for mood disorders.

Where patients lack motivation and commitment, long-term coaching treatment may fail or stagnate.

Patients who deny their diagnosis, who externalize their problems, or those who are pushed into treatment by someone else, need to undergo a preliminary phase before the actual treatment for ADHD starts. This should be used to motivate the patient as much as possible.

5.6   Motivation for Treatment

Some patients do not make a clear choice of treatment, cannot accept the diagnosis, or do not want medication. In these cases, the treatment often remains without much result. A lot of time, money, and effort is wasted if patients do not accept their diagnosis or refuse medication. An unmotivated patient may complain that the treatment is ineffective. This can be prevented by providing realistic expectations of the patient's required commitment, before treatment starts. Patients should also be aware of what can be expected from the various components of treatment. Ineffective treatments are pointless. For this reason, the patient's motivation should be assessed during the initial stages. Those who are not motivated should not be treated; they may return once they are ready for treatment.

The starting point for the research into motivation is that everyone is offered the best treatment available, namely medication and coaching. Those who wish to follow only a part, are letting themselves down and will receive inadequate treatment. These patients may receive treatment for a limited period of time. If during that period they do choose for the entire treatment offer, or if they clearly benefit from the (limited) intervention, the duration can be extended. Patients often struggle with making the best choice. The practitioner should therefore inform them, discuss fears and prejudices and, if necessary, refute them. Only a well-informed person can decide about future management, having weighed the advantages and disadvantages of the treatment offer. Providing clarity promotes patients being empowered to make a conscious choice and encourages their involvement in the treatment process. Hopefully, it leads to better and faster treatment results.

5.6.1   What Is Motivation all about?

It is important to pay attention to these questions at the beginning of the treatment, especially for those with:

1. An unclear request for help (I am not struggling with anything, it is my partner who is whining).
2. Doubts about the accuracy of the diagnosis (Is it ADHD?).
3. Without willingness to try medication (I am not taking any chemical junk).

When in doubt about the motivation for treatment, delving into the background of motivation, as listed above, can be useful. In a maximum of five appointments, the request for help/diagnosis/motivation for treatment should have been clarified, and the decision whether or not to progress with treatment taken. Doubts about the diagnosis and difficulty with acceptance, and difficulty in taking medication are issues that are common in many patients.

5.6.2   Where Does Motivation Begin?

A motivational process starts with the patient. The patient has an idea, feeling, experience, fear, or doubt about the diagnosis or treatment, and the practitioner can join in. Without this, there is no entrance to a conversation about motivation. The following examples of unmotivated patients come from clinical practice and can serve to address the problem.

1. The Patient Perceives no Problem, Rather the Environment Is at Fault
A patient who does not experience any problems him/herself and externalizes everything is not ready for treatment, unless common ground can be found. For example, the patient says that the partner is complaining, and it is the partner rather who should be treated. In this case, the only way to assess whether there is an inroad to treatment is to assess whether the patient acknowledges the partner's complaints, i.e., are there relationship problems? If the patient admits to having difficulties in the areas identified by the partner, there is a problem. If that problem can be related to the diagnosis, the symptoms, and if treatment could improve the relationship, then motivation for treatment may develop. All other attempts at motivation will fail if there is no entry point through a problem that the patient him/herself acknowledges.

2. Doubts about the Correctness of the Diagnosis
When a patient doubts the accuracy of the diagnosis, s/he tends to postpone appointments and feels it is necessary to think, read and talk about it with others. These patients refuse medication or treatment as they do not accept the disorder. Here, the patient's difficulties with the diagnosis should be explored and clarified first. Helpful questions include:

- What would it mean to him or her if it was ADHD? (I am not like those hyperactive kids).
- How would the partner or family respond to the diagnosis? (If you have ADHD, then don't we all?).
- What does a psychiatric diagnosis or help seeking imply to him or her? (Such a failure, such a loser).

These thoughts and feelings determine the patient's behavior and should be openly addressed. Where there is a misunderstanding about ADHD, the motivation techniques focus on providing information: about the different presentations, comorbidities, differences between children and adults, between men and women, etc. Where the family has rejected the diagnosis, one needs to explore what this means for the patient and what can help to make the right choices. The following fears can be addressed: a psychiatric diagnosis implies failure, not finding a job, losing control of one's own life. By unravelling these fears, one can help the patient assess how their life has been so far, without adequate help. Undertaking this process emphasizes that the patient has little to lose and possibly a lot to gain from treatment. It can also be stressed that the patient will be in control of all decisions; the practitioner provides information and guides, based on knowledge and experience. If the approach or the medication is not to one's liking, one can stop anytime. This discussion may just give the patient the space needed to dare to embark on treatment.

3. Unwilling to Try Medication

If the patient is not prepared to try medication, the underlying thought or fear must be explored. Is medication considered "poison" or "chemical waste" have family members or friends had bad experiences with medication, did they become "hooked," did they suffer from side effects? The exact cognition needs to be exposed, otherwise, it is impossible to educate, to address fears, and to provide motivation. So ask the patient! What does it mean for you to take medication? What adverse effects do you fear? After which, targeted information can be given. The following stories about medication can help to provide clarity.

- Of course, you can treat ADHD without medication. However, experience has shown that many people with ADHD are unable to benefit properly from the coaching because their attention is insufficient. Homework assignments may fail as a result. Often they drop out after three months, and get distracted by something else. As a result, treatment programs do not get completed, with no benefit or outcome. Do you recognize that? Is that what you want for yourself? With medication, concentration is increased, so that the coaching has a much faster effect. As a result, treatment often takes less time.
- You can try the medication once, if you do not like it, you can stop it in consultation with the doctor. Give it a chance, you are the boss.
- If you have ADHD, you need to be at the top of your game to get everything done on a daily basis. ADHD is like a top sport. People who want to treat their ADHD without medication could be compared to top athletes who run on the racetrack, but sprint while wearing rubber boots. It works, you move forward, but not as fast and easily as with sports shoes.

The message is clear: ADHD is a top sport, do not do yourself short for fear of medication (= sports shoes). NB Most people do not like to do themselves short.

5.7   Attitude and Tasks of the Coach

5.7.1   Active Structuring

Generally, ADHD patients have little structure. The coach will therefore have to structure the conversations and keep control. One way of doing this is by keeping an agenda for the session, to which both patient and practitioner can add items for discussion. One important agenda item is the discussion of homework assignments that were completed or not completed. Compared to the treatment of other psychiatric problems, the coach plays a very active role in ADHD. Where this does not occur, the patient can get bogged down in details, and lose sight of the finish line (along with the coach). At the end of the consultation, much may have been discussed, but no progress has been made.

5.7.2   Acceptance

If the homework has not been done, the patient should not be criticized. The coach names the tasks that have been achieved. Together with the patient, the coach explores a way in which the goals can be met. A pitfall is that patients may avoid admitting a task was not done so as to avoid the confrontation with (supposed) failure.

5.7.3   Information

Psycho-education is extremely important. It gives the patient a framework from which to explain the problems experienced. This allows patients to distance themselves from their difficulties and understand themselves more objectively. Getting a diagnosis may provide an explanation for longstanding difficulties. This makes it easier for patients to accept the diagnosis of ADHD. In addition, patients harbor many prejudices and misunderstandings with regard to ADHD. The coach can help put these into perspective or refute them.

5.7.4   Motivation

Many patients are ambivalent toward treatment. For example, on the one hand, they welcome structure, they view it positively and recognized that they need it. On the other hand, having structure means they can fail again, which may have happened in the past. So, as long as there is no appointment or assignment, it cannot be forgotten or avoided. In addition, some patients steer clear of boredom or drudgery. The role of the coach is to motivate patients to confront these difficult issues, which may also relate to the use of medication.

5.7.5   Case Management

Since many patients with ADHD experience various comorbid disorders and sometimes have serious problems in the home situation, it may be necessary to involve several care providers in the treatment. In the case of problems in the home situation, additional help at home may be necessary. Providing outpatient help alone may be inadequate. It is the coach's task to estimate what help is needed at home and to request it in consultation with the patient. Subsequently, the coach coordinates with the patient's health care givers. The home situation should be a part of the individual coaching. The coach can make an initial appointment with the patient and the homecare provider to discuss these matters, give information about ADHD and determine the support needed in the home situation. In addition, in consultation with the patient, the coach should be in contact with the prescribing doctor, refer for additional group therapy, make contact with the support system and identify any crises.

5.7.6 Giving Insight

Learning practical skills is often insufficient. It is also important to tackle negative thoughts and negative self-images and to provide patients with insight as to how these can hinder learning. ADHD is present from childhood, which means that there is often a backlog of deficient organizational and social skills that cannot be made up in the short term. As a result, patients may approach new tasks with a negative attitude, or the patient has become so pessimistic about the chance of success that he or she does not even start. Avoidance, fear of failure, resistance, shame, high demands, and perfectionism often play a role. The coach tries to make patients aware of these processes.

5.7.7 Supporting

As with all patients with psychiatric disorders, a supportive attitude is very important. Patients with ADHD usually have extensive experience of failure and they often feel rejected and misunderstood. Therefore, the coach sets manageable goals and takes into account the patient's difficulties and strengths. The coach searches for a form and structure that suits the patient and his/her daily life. Without criticizing, the coach should dare to set limits and demands. An optimal balance between empathy and confrontation, enables a patient to move forward. If this succeeds, the patient will feel understood and supported.

5.7.8 Changing Role of the Coach

If all goes well during treatment, a role change occurs for the coach. In the beginning, the coach acts as a teacher. When teaching various skills, one should not assume that the patient has the correct approach. For example, the coach describes the theory of how to use an agenda and how to plan. During treatment, the coach will increasingly stimulate and encourage the patient to persevere. Giving positive feedback about tasks that have been successfully accomplished is essential. The aim of the treatment is that the patient learns personalized skills so that they can be applied in daily life. In addition, the goal is that the patient gains insight into his or her own pitfalls and knows how to deal with them.

5.7.9 Relationship between Individual Coaching and Group Treatment

The personal coach is the main caregiver and continues to supervise the patient throughout the treatment, including during group activities, although at this point, the frequency of individual consultations may be reduced. The personal coach signs up the patient for a group, gives information and with the patient, formulates the goals for this specific group. The coach should refer to an appropriate group, making sure that the patient has the time and motivation to participate. Discussing expectations of the outcome will help to avoid disappointment. Groups often follow a specific protocol when teaching. During the group, the coach should check for obstacles the patient experiences in order to increase participation and motivation. The coach can also provide support with the homework assignments that the patient receives. At the end of the group, it is important that the patient continues to apply the skills learned, so this should be monitored by the coach. In the individual coaching sessions, the skills learned can also be addressed, for example, dealing with negative cognitions when working on certain goals. The coach can also go deeper into other issues that were brought up in the group.

5.7.10 Cooperation with the Doctor

In the treatment of adults with ADHD, there are often several health care workers involved. For this reason, coordination is important. The coach is the main treatment provider and works together with all disciplines within and outside the team. The coach should manage the treatment and ensures that the patient is not overburdened by too many therapies and appointments at the same time. The first liaison is with the prescribing doctor. The coach, therefore, needs to be aware of the effects, duration of action, and side effects of the various medications. The result of the treatment largely depends on adherence and a good attitude to medication. Therapy compliance, as well as problems and questions of the patient about medication, are important topics in coaching. The coach can give tips and teach skills to remember taking the medication, for example, a timer, mobile phone with alarm, and keeping the medication in a fixed place. In addition, the coach can pay attention to the psychological side of "obligatory" medication use. Pharmacological treatment for ADHD often brings about a rapid and drastic change. Complaints can quickly diminish and the patient's head clears. Suddenly, it becomes necessary to find a new balance. The supportive and informative attitude of the coach plays an important role in this. Guidance in the use of medication supports the doctor's pharmacological treatment.

5.7.11 Digital Coaching

Super Brains is a newly developed application, where patient and practitioner can work together. Together, they define the most important goals for treatment, after which the patient begins to receive agenda planning, lifestyle tips, support, and reminders in the app. The practitioner follows the progress of each patient in the app and can show informative videos on topics that are discussed. Questions can be asked in between consultations by using the secure chat function. The treatment is thus much more intensive between consultations, and this is likely to shorten the duration of treatment (www.superbrains.nl). Patients can also use the app without a practitioner, or after treatment. This maintains goals that were achieved during treatment, such as day and night rhythm, therapy compliance, etc.

5.7.12 Cooperation with External Organizations

In the case of serious psychosocial or work problems, outpatient care alone may be insufficient. Home-based help or reintegration into the workplace may be indicated. The role of the coach is to coordinate all care and to check whether it is effective. This can be done, for example, by having regular consultations with the patient and the external health care provider.

Help in the home situation may be indicated, where the patient:

- Fails to get goals and assignments done at home due to lack of overview, not knowing where to start, causing the treatment to stagnate.
- Has a poor support system and lives alone.
- Needs practical help in bringing up the children.
- Does not (independently) manage the administration and finances, leading to serious problems such as debt, attachment of possessions, or homelessness.

Help in the home situation can be provided by various home care agencies and agencies that may or not have experience with ADHD. In case of lack of knowledge about ADHD, the coach may consider informing the organization before referring the patient. Assistance in resuming work after unemployment or work incapacity may be required. Employment agencies, company and insurance doctors, job coaching agencies may provide help in finding a new or more suitable job.

5.8   The Structure of Coaching

5.8.1   Patient Expectations

Many patients are unclear about what it means to be in treatment and what is expected of them. It is therefore important to discuss this subject with the patient at the very beginning. There needs to be agreement on the importance of arriving on time, what to do if this fails, completing homework assignments, etc. In addition, it is important to make clear what the patient's (implicit) expectations are with regard to the outcome of the treatment, in order to avoid unrealistic expectations and thus a disappointment.

5.8.2 Duration and Frequency of the Coaching Sessions

Usually, 30 to 45 minutes are available per coaching session. The frequency is once every two weeks at the beginning of the treatment. Later, this frequency is reduced to once every three weeks because the patient starts group treatment in addition to individual coaching. At the end of the treatment, appointments are less often. The planning of the sessions is done on the basis of the treatment plan established for the patient. If necessary, the frequency can be adapted to the individual situation of the patient. Additional appointments can also be scheduled in the event of a crisis.

5.8.3 Duration of Treatment

The duration of treatment depends on the ADHD severity, comorbidity, psychosocial problems, the effect of the medication, and the patient's commitment. In patients who have no comorbid disorders and few social problems in addition to ADHD, the duration of treatment is approximately six months. On average, treatment takes one to one and a half years. For patients with complex problems, the treatment duration can be two to three years. The aim of the treatment is for the patient to be able to function independently in daily life with as little help as possible. The optimal medication dosage should be prescribed by the general practitioner after the treatment.

5.8.4 Use of a Session Agenda

In order to structure the conversation, it is useful to use a so-called session agenda. At the start of the conversation, the coach examines what needs to be discussed during that specific session. These can be parts of the treatment goals as agreed upon in the treatment plan. Both the coach and the patient have room to introduce points for discussion and the priority can be adjusted. In general, the goals of the previous session will be reiterated in each session and new goals will be formulated at the end of the current session.

5.8.5 Common Treatment Objectives

Treatment goals that are regularly determined in consultation with the patient are the following:

- Increase structure
- Learn to use a diary

- Punctuality
- Order in finances and administration
- Reducing depressive and/or anxiety symptoms
- Reducing substance use
- Finding suitable employment
- Reducing perfectionism
- Improving self-image
- Bettering study techniques
- Improving relationship with partner
- Learning to set boundaries
- Going to bed on time

5.8.6   Setting Targets

As discussed earlier, coaching involves working with goals and homework assignments. These assignments differ in content from those that are drawn up for cognitive behavioral therapy. Assignments that require patients to keep track of things are very demanding for a patient with ADHD (e.g., monitoring anxiety symptoms that occur several times a day). Creating a daily CBT inventory of the activating event, beliefs about the event and its consequences (ABC), is required by the protocol for depression. This is not feasible for most ADHD patients (even those taking medication). At the beginning of treatment, it is therefore important to keep the homework assignments limited so that the patient succeeds. Once small goals are met, they can be extended if necessary. For example, an ADHD homework assignment could be that the patient fills in a CBT inventory between two consultations. Discuss one situation for this CBT inventory. This makes it easier to start the assignment. Keep the goals concrete and ask the patient whether they are clear. Many patients with ADHD tend to set too many, overly optimistic goals. Therefore, check with the patient whether their target is achievable in the set time period. Goals often have to be broken down into smaller intermediate steps because resistance or difficulties are encountered. For example, the major goal of "fixing teeth" is divided into: making an appointment with the dentist, noting the appointment in the agenda, setting a reminder on the mobile phone for the appointment, etc.

5.8.7   Dealing with Being Late

Symptoms of ADHD include forgetfulness and difficulty with planning. For this reason, patients are often late for appointments, especially at the beginning of treatment. For patients who have problems with being punctual, this should be the first treatment goal. It helps to schedule the appointment always at a fixed time. If necessary, the support of the partner or parent can be requested at the start of the treatment, to remind the patient of upcoming appointments. However, the aim is to make the patient responsible as early as possible. When the ADHD symptoms improve, for example, with pharmacotherapy, punctuality becomes less difficult for the patient. If a patient arrives late, it is preferable not to focus on this and not to label it as therapy resistance. Many patients with ADHD have been criticized during their lives for tardiness. They may experience it as a failure, and may be ashamed, so they keep it hidden from the coach. If the patient apologizes, it is enough for the coach to say that he or she is indeed late, but that it is helpful that the patient is still there to make the best use of the remaining time together. The consequence is that there is less time to discuss things with the patient. If arriving late occurs often, punctuality can become a primary treatment goal, as discussed earlier.

5.8.8   Dealing with no-Show

In view of the chaotic style of patients with ADHD, it is advisable to have a clear no-show policy. This aims to set limits for poorly motivated patients or not yet ready for treatment. The aim is for patients to prioritize their treatment. If the patient fails to value treatment, as evidenced by missing two appointments, the patient should in principle be deregistered from treatment. If desire and motivation return after some time, the patient can re-register. Patients should be informed about this rule at the intake session. The background to the strict policy is that, prior to treatment, clear information is given about what the treatment involves and also about what is expected of the patient in terms of commitment. Successful treatment can only be achieved through the commitment of both patient and practitioner. Continuation of unsuccessful treatments is thus avoided. Regular, frequent cancellation of appointments by patients also leads to poor treatment outcomes, so this should be included in the no-show policy. Cancellation due to illness (where this cannot be checked) also counts as a no-show. Exceptions are permitted, for example, when motivated patients occasionally miss sessions because of serious chaos or illness. Exceptions to the no-show policy should always be discussed in the team.

When patients regularly miss their appointments, it is important to find out the reason. Missing can be the result of ADHD symptoms, but can also occur for completely different reasons such as dissatisfaction with treatment, disappointment in the practitioner, avoidance of reporting on incomplete homework assignments. If the no-show or lateness results from problems with planning and/or forgetfulness, punctuality should of course be the first treatment goal.

5.9   Structure of the Treatment

Although each patient is unique and each treatment is therefore different, there are certain shared phases and components of ADHD treatment. Several of these have already been or will be discussed.

- Motivation (possibly preliminary) (see Sect. 5.6)
- Psycho-education (see Sect. 4.2)

- Medication (see Sect. 4.3)
- Acceptance (see Sect. 5.9.1)
- Coaching for comorbidity (see Sect. 5.9.2)
- ADHD skills (see Sect. 5.9.3)
- Cognitive training (see Sect. 5.13)
- Psychotherapeutic deepening (see Sect. 5.14)
- Relationship therapy (see Sect. 5.16)
- Prevention of relapse (see Sect. 5.17)
- Completion (see Sect. 5.18)
- Aftercare (see Sect. 5.19)

5.9.1   Acceptance

The diagnosis of ADHD has a lot of impacts. For some patients, the diagnosis is a huge relief. The problems appear to be related to a disorder that they have had all their lives. At that moment, or a little later, sadness and anger arise over everything that has gone wrong in their lives. The process of diagnosis causes a patient to examine his or her life retrospectively. This can be confronting, as patients have often had to deal with failure. Diagnosis and treatment lead to a better perspective, so that patients get an overview of the repetitive nature of their problems. The pieces of the puzzle begin to fall into place. It takes time to process things and give them a place; this also applies to acceptance. One's whole life may be viewed from a different perspective because of the diagnosis. For many patients, everything changes at the same time; their vision of themselves, of their present situation, the past and their questions, and possibilities for the future. Once these issues have been grappled with, can the changes begin (Kooij, 2003a, b).

The coach guides patients through this acceptance process by providing information and support. The meaning of the diagnosis and the proposed treatment should be examined in each patient. If the diagnosis has brought relief and provides a good explanation for years of problems, this has different consequences for acceptance than if the diagnosis is seen as a sign of weakness. When ADHD is experienced as appropriate to the self (egosyntonic), it can be a challenge for the patient to separate the consequences of ADHD from the self. Here, the problems caused by ADHD can be made egodystonic by teaching the patient techniques to view ADHD as distinct from the self. For example, in the statement "I am … I have ADHD. For me, this means …." By making it clear that ADHD is a neurobiological disorder that can be addressed, patients are given hope. This is a powerful intervention. Patients should be asked what his or her image of ADHD is. Psycho-education can be linked to this paradigm.

It is important to make it clear to a patient that the acceptance process can be accompanied by strong feelings (sadness, anger, shame, fear, perhaps relief) and that these reactions are normal. Information about emotional reactions gives a patient more control. The fact that the coach is aware of and experienced in dealing with these processes, is reassuring for many patients. The coach emphasizes that the acceptance process can be cyclical: previously experienced emotions of sadness or anger may return at a later stage. The coach takes a supportive and non-condemnatory stance.

5.9.2 Coaching for Comorbidity

Three-quarters of adults with ADHD have another axis I disorder, often a sleep, anxiety, or mood disorder and/or substance abuse.

5.9.2.1 Reducing Substance Abuse

If there is an addiction to drugs, the patient should be referred for specialized assistance. Where substance abuse can be reduced under the guidance of the coach, a referral is not necessary. Substance abuse should be stopped or phased out as much as possible before treatment with medication starts. The role of the coach in the cessation of substance abuse focuses mainly on motivation. The short- and long-term advantages and disadvantages of substance use and of cessation, are inventoried by the coach and patient. In addition, use is monitored. Let the patient keep a written record of how much is used, and at what times. Next, find out together what the function of the use is, what the risk moments, in which environment, and whether the use is related to certain events, such as wearing off of the ADHD medication (rebound), or to the mood fluctuations? Finally, look for alternative behavior together: for example, going out, playing sports, calling a friend. It is especially important that the coach offers support.

5.9.2.2 Anxiety Disorders

If there is a comorbid anxiety disorder, it is advisable to treat it with medication first (see Sect. 4.19.1) and only then to treat the ADHD. Reasons for this are that patients with an untreated anxiety disorder often experience an increase in anxiety symptoms in response to ADHD medication. This is understandable because stimulants can produce an accelerated heartbeat or palpitations. These can be misinterpreted as anxiety symptoms by a patient with (previous) anxiety complaints. Clinical experience has shown that when using a serotonin reuptake inhibitor (SSRI), this side effect is better tolerated. Psychological and cognitive factors should be taken into account during the coaching.

If a patient still suffers from anxiety complaints, or if these remain in the foreground after treatment with medication, cognitive behavioral therapy can be started. If comorbid ADHD is untreated, the success of comorbid anxiety complaints with CBT is limited (see, e.g., Keijsers, Minnen, & Hoogduin, 2004). CBT requires a lot from the patient (e.g., doing homework assignments). An anxious patient with untreated ADHD is often less able to perform because of concentration problems, forgetfulness, and chaos.

5.9.2.3 Depression and Bipolar Disorder

Depression should be treated pharmacologically before ADHD is treated (see Sect. 4.19.1). Firstly, severe depression results in a stagnation of daily life and poor response to the treatment of ADHD. In addition, it is easier to assess the effect of medication for ADHD if the mood disorder is in remission. Depression can be significantly reduced in four weeks with medication. Antidepressants (usually the SSRIs) can be co-prescribed with medication for ADHD.

Coaching should aim to raise the activity level. The relationship between activity level and mood can be demonstrated by means of self-report (a diary) in which the patient keeps daily records (if feasible) of:

- What activities were undertaken?
- How much these were enjoyed on a scale of 0–10?
- Mood score on a scale of 0–10.

Patients should then be motivated to increase the level of activity gradually. For most patients, increasing activity leads to an improvement in mood. In addition, where activities take place in a group, social skills will improve.

Detecting and challenging dysfunctional thoughts can provide patients with much insight. These negative cognitions can result from the problems the patient experiences or has experienced because of ADHD. See Safren's cognitive-behavioral therapeutic model of ADHD in adults (see Fig. 5.1). Changing these cognitions can as well improve mood. It may be helpful to refer a patient to specific cognitive training aimed at challenging negative cognitions. If necessary, patients can be referred for specific treatment of depression, such as interpersonal psychotherapy (IPT), cognitive behavioral therapy (CBT), or pharmacotherapy. An exercise group with running activities can also be considered for depressed patients.

When there is a bipolar disorder or (hypo)mania, psychopharmacotherapy is necessary (see Sect. 4.19.3). If the patient is overtly manic, admission may be necessary. Bipolar II disorder can often be treated in the outpatient clinic. Coaching focuses on psycho-education (e.g., the distinction between ADHD and bipolar disorder), therapy compliance, and the prevention of recurrence. If necessary, a patient can be referred for treatment of bipolar disorder.

5.9.2.4 Seasonal Affective Disorder

The incidence of winter depression in adults with ADHD is estimated at 27% (Amons, Kooij, Haffmans, Hoffman, & Hoencamp, 2006). The following signs and symptoms are observed in the autumn and winter:

- The patient has a low mood for at least two consecutive years, which improves in the spring, and is not exclusively due to recurring seasonal stress factors, such as family meetings at X-mas dinner.
- There are atypical symptoms.
- More need for sleep: sleeping for longer, not getting out of bed, wanting to sleep in the afternoon.

- Increase appetite, especially carbohydrate-rich foods.
- Weight gain.

If necessary, a QIDS-SR questionnaire can be used to measure mood. The patient can be enrolled in light therapy between September and April, if the score on the QIDS-SR list is 12 or higher.

Atypical symptoms predict a positive reaction to light therapy, but even if they are less pronounced, a patient can benefit from this treatment. Light therapy consists of a course thirty minutes of intense light (10,000 lux) reaching the eyes, for five consecutive days. Patients sit 20 cm away from a light box, which has been placed at eye level. The patient does not have to look directly into the light. Reading or listening to music with occasional glances at the light is sufficient. This treatment is effective in 50–80% of cases. Rapid treatment at the onset of winter depression helps to prevent relapse during the rest of the season. There may be side effects such as headache, nausea, dry and irritated eyes and mucous membranes, slight skin burns, overactivity, irritation, emotional lability, change of menstrual pattern, and insomnia. Where patients show such sensitivity, there may be an underlying tendency for hypomania.

It is still unknown exactly how light therapy works. There are several hypotheses: light is the opposite of melatonin. Melatonin is the hormone that determines the day and night rhythm and is secreted in the evening. In ADHD, the production of melatonin is delayed, causing patients to fall asleep too late and have difficulty getting up (Van Veen, Kooij, Boonstra, Gordijn, & Van Someren, 2009). This phase shift in the day and night rhythm (circadian rhythm) is probably also related to the rhythm of the seasons, which manifests in winter depression (Lewy et al., 2006).

5.9.2.5 Sleep Phase Problems
A late sleep phase can be pharmacologically treated with melatonin. This substance is made in the pineal gland in the brain when it gets dark, and has few or no side effects. The effect of giving melatonin in tablet form is to send an earlier time signal to the brain, so that the biological clock registers nighttime. Melatonin production is suppressed by light (through the eyes). There are indications that the light from a computer screen late at night also breaks down melatonin, causing the sleep phase to shift even further. Patients should therefore be discouraged from using screens at night. The coach helps the patient to improve his sleep hygiene (see Sect. 4.20.3).

5.9.2.6 Personality Disorders
If, during the treatment, a personality disorder is suspected, a patient can be referred for further diagnostics and treatment.

5.9.3   ADHD skills

Before dealing with other content, the coach should ensure that basic, practical skills have been mastered. After all, basic goals should be achievable if the coaching is to be effective. A good grasp of some (basic) skills is often the first step in treatment. These include planning, setting priorities, reducing distractions, learning to deal with procrastination, creating routines, and managing administration. When teaching these skills, it is important to pay attention to negative attitudes and cognitions that may influence the process of learning. Resistance to acquiring structure may be present due to previous negative experiences, and in turn lead to mood symptoms or avoidance behaviors. Together with the patient, the coach should look for a structure that suits him or her. The theory should be relevant to the patient's daily life. Goals should not be set too high. It should be clarified that these skills are not an end in themselves, but a means to achieve the desired goal. For example, the use of an agenda can help to prevent forgetting appointments, which will prevent negative reactions from others about missed appointments.

Skills can be learned through both individual and group coaching. In comparison with group coaching, individual coaching pays more attention to dysfunctional cognitions when learning skills. In addition, it is more personalized so attention can be individual skills relevant to the patient. Less attention needs to be paid to skills that the patient has already mastered. However, a "skills gap" of years cannot be made up in a training course lasting several weeks. Skills training in the group context is especially helpful for patients who experience shame and difficulty in accepting the diagnosis. After all, a number of core problems of ADHD such as poor planning will emerge clearly in the group. Patients become aware of not being the only one experiencing such difficulties. This sharing provides much support and can contribute to the motivation for change.

This section discusses a number of practical issues that many patients with ADHD have problems with. Specific tips for patients are given for a number of topics.

5.9.3.1 Planning and Agenda Management

Many people with ADHD use neither watch nor calendar. This is remarkable because these tools can really benefit them. A watch reminds you of the time and a calendar can be used to make a schedule. People with ADHD live as if time does not exist. They seem to have little awareness of it, often arrive late, they cannot properly estimate the time needed for certain tasks. As a result, tasks take more time than they should and they are always running late for appointments. An agenda can help here, but people with ADHD rarely use them. If the agenda is there and the appointment has been noted, this sometimes happens on the wrong date or time. After all, all these actions require concentration.

Working with an agenda is taught step by step. First a diary is purchased, then it is given a fixed place and is always taken along. Viewing the diary twice a day should be taught, as well as going through the weekly structure (possibly with a partner) and learning to make notes of appointments. Finally, entering tasks into the agenda is taught.

5.9.3.2 Tips for Patients when Using a Diary
The following tips can be discussed with patients to help them choose an agenda and how to use it.

Target Agenda
- Find out what you want to use a diary for. It is often useful to be able to take notes as well as appointments.

Format
- What size diary is convenient for you? You should be able to fit them in a bag or jacket pocket. Or choose an electronic diary/handheld electronic organizer (pda).

Layout
- Which layout is most convenient? A diary with a weekly overview per two pages is useful, so you can check the week at a glance.

Agenda in Mobile Phone
- Many people find it useful to put appointments in their phone and use them as an agenda. Reminder alarms can be set in advance. This option should be used, especially for important appointments.

Fixed Place
- Where do you leave your diary? Make a routine out of this and possibly add it to an already existing routine. For example, the diary should be placed at home next to the mobile phone and keys. Choosing a fixed place for the items most often needed creates less chance of losing them or forgetting to take them along.

Notice Board
- In addition to a diary, you can put up a notice board in a place where you can look at it often. For example, in the kitchen or the toilet. Here you can put up appointment cards, invitation letters, etc.

Fixed Appointments First
- First, fill in all the fixed appointments and obligations on your agenda. This will give you an overview of how much time you have left.

Plan Relaxation Time
- Also make time to relax, to talk to your partner in the evening, spend time with friends or do something for yourself.

Possible Pitfalls
- Do not wait to devise a perfect system before starting to use a diary. If you want perfection, you will not use a diary at all.

- Do not give up if you do not (immediately) succeed in using your calendar properly. Give yourself time to get used to it. Find out what the problem is and find a solution. It takes time to develop a routine. Success occurs through trial and error.

5.9.3.3 Make Time to Plan Ahead

Patients can use a so-called "planning time," which is a fixed time in the evening and/or the morning when the plans can be made for that day. This moment is also used to check the diary. It gives the patient a better overview of his or her day. Let the patient make a routine of this, so discuss a convenient time for each specific patient.

5.9.3.4 Learning Routines

Learning routines can help patients not to forget things, such as looking at the diary. Many people with ADHD are forgetful, but most of them will not forget their cell phones. The reason is that it has become a routine to think about this and therefore requires less concentration. A routine is best developed by making it as simple as possible and identifying possible pitfalls when using it in advance. After that it is important to improve the routine, this takes time.

Example

A patient wants to learn to check the agenda for the coming week every Sunday evening, after her family dinner. She discusses this with her partner and asks him to help remind her of this. She also writes it on the chalkboard in the kitchen so she can see it every day. With her children, she discusses why she wants to do this every Sunday evening and she actively involves them in it. She makes it a cozy family ritual.

When learning routine, the following are important:

- Think carefully in advance about what suits a patient and what does not: good preparation is half the job.
- Do not make it too complicated.
- Do not choose a specific time, but match a certain activity. So not: "I look in my diary at 7 p.m.," but "Before I go to sleep I look in my diary." This reduces the chance of forgetting.
- Connect to an existing routine, such as eating or brushing your teeth.
- At the start, ask family members to help you remember.
- Something that occurs regularly is learned more quickly. Something that needs to be done once a month will probably not become routine very quickly. Not every activity lends itself to becoming a routine.

5.9.3.5 Weekly Schedule

The weekly schedule is an A4 sheet of paper where the days of the week are listed, as are the hours of the day. This format has been chosen because it allows the weekly schedule to be hung up in a place where it encountered on a daily basis. For example, on a kitchen cupboard or door. People with ADHD do not automatically look in their diary, hence this tool is also helpful.

The purpose of the weekly schedule is to get an overview of the fixed daily activities, such as getting up, eating, travel time to and from work, and working hours. Once the schedule has been completed, color or shading can be used to indicate which "time blocks" are full. Then it is immediately clear how much time is left for other desired activities. Some people then reach an important conclusion. For example, given time restrictions, a renovation is not an option at present. Realistic time planning can prevent a lot of misery.

Next, the weekly schedule can be used to add additional activities in the blank spaces. The weekly schedule can be copied a number of times, showing the fixed activities. Once a week, (e.g., on Sunday evening) the planning for the coming week is reviewed and noted, possibly together with the partner. The current overview of the coming week is then hung up somewhere clearly visible. See section "Week Schedule" in Appendix for the weekly schedule with instructions.

5.9.3.6 Noting activities by Using the Weekly Schedule

A weekly schedule can also be used as an assignment to note how time is allocated. Here, the patient records how much time has been spent on various activities over a week (or longer). This gives a better overview of how much time everything takes and brings bottlenecks to light. Based on the record, the patient can discuss with the practitioner how the week can be filled in more efficiently, for example, by combining certain activities. The record can also reveal issues such as a disturbed day–night rhythm or excessive Internet use. It will often become apparent that a patient is simply overscheduled in a week, which makes it impossible for him or her to relax and to plan properly.

5.9.3.7 Tips for Patients Using the Weekly Schedule

Extra Time
- Allocate extra time for when you run late, where things go wrong or unexpected activities develop. Optimistic planners should always factor in extra time.

Travel Time
- Plan in travel time as well. For example, set the leaving home time in your diary. Carefully consider how much travel time you need, instead of making an (overly optimistic) estimate.

Fixed Time
- Plan a fixed time for daily things, for example, for doing your administration or recurring household chores. The goal is to make this a routine as well. Choose a convenient time.

Plan Activities in Blocks of Time
- Plan a block of time to do different tasks. It is often easier to do many things once you are up and running, rather than to do one task at a time.

Give yourself Time
- Give yourself the time to improve the planning and do not expect yourself to be able to do this perfectly from the start. The skills discussed here can first be applied to a certain area (e.g., household chores) and later be extended to other areas. You cannot do everything at once.

Make Success Likely
- Choose an enjoyable task to begin with. Do not start with something you really detest. By choosing an easy job, you avoid problems with getting going.

Make it More Fun
- Make doing a certain task (e.g., in the household) more fun by, for example, putting on loud music.

Stop in Time
- Avoid continuing for too long once you have gotten going. You should not be getting overly tired or losing track of time. Consider in advance how long you want to work on a task and set off an alarm clock, or have someone tell you to stop.

5.9.3.8 Task List
In addition to using a calendar, it is useful to have specific tasks kept in a task list or *to-do booklet*. Tips for patients when using this are:

- Create a to-do list for everyday things and a separate list for other tasks.
- If you have not been able to do all the tasks on your list, create a new list for the next day. Use the "planning time," for example.
- Cross out the tasks you have done.

5.9.3.9 Setting Targets
It is important not to let patients set targets that are too high. Many people with ADHD tend to set very ambitious goals and then fail to meet them. By setting small and achievable goals, a successful experience can be gained and the patient can possibly start a new routine. Ultimately, the aim is to ensure that these tasks can be sustained in the long term. Planning can be compared to keeping to a diet to lose weight. It is generally not fun, but it is good for you. If you go on a crash diet and lose a lot of weight, then the benefit is limited if the weight loss cannot be sustained. If you plan to lose ten kilos in a month, and you only lose four, it is demotivating. While four kilos is a good result, the diet may be abandoned because the goals were not achievable.

The theory of goal setting can be useful to discuss with the patient. For example, the distinction between short- and long-term goals and how these relate to each other. When setting goals, the following tips can be discussed:

Specifically
- Describe your goals in concrete behavioral terms, so that you know exactly what you need to do to achieve your goals.

Verifiable
- Make sure your goal is described in such a way that it is verifiable, i.e., that you can evaluate it.

Positively Formulated
- Formulate your goals in positive terms: do not name what you do not want, but name what you do want.

Timetable and Steps
- Make sure there is a time schedule: divide the long-term goal into short-term goals and, if possible, into even smaller steps.

Feasible
- Make sure your goal is achievable. While the goal may be a challenge, in principle, it should be reachable.

No Vague Description
- Avoid vague targets.

Personalize the Goal
- Make sure it is within your power to reach the goal and that you are not dependent on someone else's (unpredictable) contribution.

Because you Want it
- Be convinced that you stand behind your goal, do not try to reach a goal because it is fun for others or because you think others want it.

Smart
- In short, targets must be SMART: Specific, Measurable, Acceptable, Realistic, and Time bound.

5.9.3.10 Goals target

The goals target is a form where one can fill in a maximum of three concrete and achievable targets for the coming week. The date and time of the planned execution are listed, and there is a space to note the result. The goals target helps to limit the number of goals and reminds you of your aims. This form can also be posted in a visible place, for example, next to the weekly schedule. The practitioner helps formulate three achievable and verifiable goals the first few times and evaluates whether they have been achieved the next time. If a goal has not been achieved, the reasons why are assessed (were there too many steps?). Thereafter, new or adjusted goals are drawn up and the process is repeated (see section "Chart of Objectives" in Appendix).

5.9.3.11   Overscheduling and Planning
In some adults with ADHD, their time scheduling problem seems to overscheduling rather than an inability to plan. Focussing merely on improving planning skills does not solve this problem.

Overscheduling has several causes. Sometimes the problem is related to a lack of overview and a lack of time, but often other factors are involved. Some patients need constant challenges, others promise too much because they are reluctant to disappoint. Some find it difficult to miss an opportunity to get involved or get carried away with enthusiasm. To diminish overscheduling, the motives why it is being done need to be elucidated. These should be discussed with the patient and then ways of tackling them can be explored.

The background to overscheduling may be a negative self-image. It is useful to teach the patient to set boundaries. It is important that the patient has an overview of the tasks he or she already has to complete, and of how much time is left. The tips from Sect. 5.9.3.12 can be discussed with the patient.

5.9.3.12   Patient Tips

Agree Only under Certain Conditions
- You do not have refuse to take on all new tasks. But you can also teach yourself to consider that certain conditions are met before taking on something new. An example: "Yes, I would like to do that, if I can ask sometime to take on the responsibility for my current project." Or: "Yes, I would like to go with my mother to the hospital if you can do the shopping for me."

Exchanging Tasks
- For each new task, you should drop two old tasks (by mutual agreement). After all, new duties can turn out to be bigger than you had anticipated. An example: at work, your manager asks if you want to become a mentor for a new colleague. You indicate that you like this very much, but you ask whether a colleague can take over your current task of checking incoming email.

Take the Time to Decide
- For example, you say to your supervisor: "I might want to do it, but I have to think about it." After consultation with your coach, for example, you report: "I already have too much work to do at the moment. But when project X is completed in three months" time, I can start working on it." When asked whether you would like to do something, always say: "I need some time to think about it."

5.9.3.13 E-Mail, Forms, and Mail

Failure to open e-mail, post, and invoices can create problems with the income tax authorities or result in getting into debt. At that point, more forms will have to be read and completed and that takes even more effort. In this phase, the patient panics, as the finances start to fall apart. A satisfactory system can be devised by coach and patient. If necessary, extra help can be called in to clear up an administration that has fallen behind, for example, from family, friends, social workers, or specialized family care.

For example, the following email ordering system can be discussed with the patient:

- Create digital folders for storing and organizing e-mail.
- Mark messages that are urgent.
- Schedule a fixed time daily for handling email.

Then get to work on the mail from the post:

- Gather your mail in one place.
- Open your mail every day and sort it into one of two categories: deal with immediately or handle within a week. The advantage of this is that there is no backlog and the job is done quickly.
- Sort through magazines, newsletters, and catalogs, which take up a lot of space. Keep catalogs only if you want to order something from them right away; otherwise, throw them away.
- Sort through junk mail. Only open advertising mail if you want to read it. For example, if it is an offer on a new mortgage and you were just about to transfer your mortgage, open it. If not, throw it away immediately. You can also put a NO sticker on your mailbox to stop receiving this kind of mail.
- Choose a fixed day during the week to pay bills and store papers in folders; this can be included in your weekly schedule or agenda. Connect this time to other routines. Of course, the frequency of how often you do this depends on how many bills and other administrative matters you receive per week and how much is automatically debited. Keep in mind that it is more motivating to do this regularly than having to clean up a pile every now and then.

5.9.3.14 Financials

Impulsive spending, shopping sprees, or gambling all lead to red tape and debt. Where there is a good salary, the damage is manageable. Where one is unemployed and receives benefits, immediate problems arise because there is insufficient cash to spend on the daily necessities of life. In the event of major financial problems, a debt restructuring institution can be called in. If this facility has already been used in the past, one cannot simply go back to debt restructuring. If the debt rescheduling approach has no chance of success, the practitioner should contact this institution to request a different approach to clear the debts. In addition to these problems, adults with ADHD often have financial difficulties as a result of having no overview of their expenses, losing or forgetting to pay their bills.

People with ADHD can manage their finances well by using just a few simple principles:

- Use only one debit card. Spend as little as possible on credit and pay immediately. This way it is easier to keep track of what you spend.
- Make sure you cannot get into debt, reduce your credit facility.
- Have as many transactions done electronically as possible. Have your salary deposited into a bank account. Rental, gas and electricity, insurances, subscriptions, and contributions should be automatically debited by your bank, preferably a few days after you receive your salary. Open an automatic savings account so that you can save a fixed amount each month.
- Avoid impulsive (online) purchases. Withdraw cash once a week and use the money over the week. Leave your credit card at home and take enough cash with you when grocery shopping. Do not go to town for shopping. Try to find out the lowest price of an item online before spending the money. When shopping, make sure you have written down what you need and buy only what you intended to buy.
- Regularly take stock of your income and expenses, so you can see what you have to spend.

Possible Pitfall
- Avoid an administration system that is too complicated. This is time consuming to maintain and awkward to use, so eventually you abandon it. Try to come up with a system that is as simple and effective as possible. Discuss this with your partner, a family member, or friend.

5.9.3.15   Distractions
To reduce the risk of distractions, external stimuli are avoided as much as possible. Timers, alarms and the like help the adult with ADHD to re focus. Where there is hyper-focus (remaining too long on a task due to overconcentration) an alarm clock or mobile phone reminder can be used to warn when the time is almost up.

Tools that have been developed for setting targets and keeping track of time are the so-called weekly schedule and target schedule, see Sects. 5.9.3.5 and 5.9.3.10.

5.9.3.16   Procrastination
Many adults with ADHD postpone tasks, with all the negative consequences that this entails. Reasons to postpone things can include:

- Perfectionism, or fearing criticism if the outcome is not perfect.
- Difficulty with getting started, unless there is time pressure.
- The job is too big, not knowing where to start.
- The task is boring or the activity requires continuous concentration.
- Believing that it is better to wait for the perfect conditions (which never materialize).

Delay may have more advantages than disadvantages in the short term, but not in the long term. To clarify this to the patient, to motivate him/her to postpone less, it is useful to explore the pros and cons of postponing. In this way, the issues underlying procrastination become clearer. Discuss any additional negative consequences of procrastination:

- The stress of waiting until the last moment.
- A boring task grows in your mind, because you are constantly thinking that you still have to do it.
- The risk of missing a deadline.
- Feeling worse about yourself afterward.
- The final product is often not as good as it could have been if you had started earlier.
- Ignoring a problem only worsens it and makes solving it later more difficult.

Some causes of endless deferring of tasks can be solved. For example, if a patient does not know where to start, the task can be broken down into smaller steps so that the patient knows where to begin. A boring chore can be turned into a routine or a reward can be promised when the task is completed. Other reasons for postponement can be addressed with cognitive behavioral techniques, for example, in the case of perfectionism or where the patient believes s/he will not succeed because of (many) past failure experiences.

5.10   Pitfalls and Tips for the Coach

The practitioner may encounter a number of pitfalls when coaching a patient with ADHD.

5.10.1 The Coach Is Too Active

If the coach is too active, there is a risk that the patient gives too little input. The coach may lose touch with the wishes and problems of the patient. In addition, the overall responsibility for the treatment should not lie with the coach.

5.10.2 The Coach Is Too Passive

The treatment of ADHD is clearly different from other psychiatric disorders such as anxiety and depression, in the sense that the patient needs much more structure. If the coach is too hesitant, asks too many open questions, or gives the patient exclusive responsibility for the process, there is a risk that the patient will get bogged down in details or irrelevancies. It is the coach's task to keep the patient focussed on progress and the big picture. The coach should not assume that the patient understands everything or that s/he has mastered certain skills.

5.10.3 The Coach overestimates the (Intelligent) Patient

Many patients with ADHD who seek help have found creative solutions to their problems. As a result, a considerable group of patients have completed their education and have a decent job. This does not always mean that they have well-developed practical skills. For intelligent patients particularly, shame plays a major role. These patients are aware of their difficulties in completing practical tasks such as planning and administration, but frequently they will fail to mention it. They may have the theoretical know-how, but they cannot translate this into practice. This issue should be raised with the patient.

5.10.4 Tips for the Coach

- Have patients write down their homework/goals and keep them on file.
- Give clear instructions and inform comprehensively, do not assume that people think of things themselves (e.g., calling to reschedule an appointment, details about the treatment, or how long a conversation will take).
- Assume that patients will forget many things, so repetition and patience are important.
- Let the patient make their own choices, challenge them instead of imposing restrictions on them.
- Be clear and predictable (e.g., when you are available and when you are not, and how you can be reached).
- Stick to appointments with the patient. Do not overreact, this can lead to reduced confidence in the practitioner.
- If the practitioner is disappointed, the patient may quit rather than discuss the problem. Discuss this point in case of a no-show, for example.

5.10.5 Handy Questions to Ask

- With a patient who says s/he knows how to plan or who says s/he can make a plan: But do you also manage to carry out your planning?
- For homework that is forgotten: Did you know how to do it, did you know what to do?
- For an appointment that is been forgotten: Were you dreading something? For patients who avoid appointments, shame or fear of a negative reaction from the coach about not having done homework may play a role.

- With a patient who says s/he already has an agenda: How often do you look in it? How much do you write in it? How many diaries do you have? Is the diary clear and practical enough? Does this diary suit you? Where do you put your diary? Does the diary fit in your bag?

5.11   Patient Characteristics

Patients who sign up for ADHD treatment may have the following characteristics, which can make coaching difficult.

5.11.1 Impatient and Enthusiastic

Impatient and enthusiastic patients are often highly motivated for the treatment. Initially, they may be happy and relieved with the diagnosis and the new perspective it has given them. Typically, they are enthusiastic and want to change everything at the same time. Possible pitfalls are that their expectations of the treatment are too high: they overestimate how quickly they can achieve results. It is important to provide information about what can be expected in the short term and that the coaching works by taking small steps to get a lasting result in the end. This is preferable to rushing in the beginning but not being able to maintain the pace. These patients may also lose focus later in the coaching process, once their initial goals have been met. After the initial positive phase, negative feelings and difficulty accepting the diagnosis also play a role.

5.11.2 Complaints that Cause Minimal Distress

Some patients indicate that they do not really experience any problems with their ADHD. If this is actually the case, then it is not a problem. However, it is often a denial of the situation. Here it can be useful to provide psycho-education and to indicate which problems can occur with ADHD and what can be done about them. Alternatively, the DIVA interview that was done at intake can be checked; specifically, which concrete examples were mentioned under"Dysfunctioning due to the symptoms"? These examples can provide a starting point for treatment, because without them, the patients are unable to specify what they would like to achieve. They may have little insight into what ADHD entails and what can be done about it. For them, ADHD symptoms feel normal, they have experienced them life-long. After psycho-education, if a patient still insists that s/he has no treatment goal, the treatment cannot be started. A follow-up appointment at a later stage is useful, after which treatment can be initiated or stopped. Patients have had time to decide whether they will benefit from treatment and may be more motivated (for more information, see also Sect. 5.6).

5.11.3 I Have no Problem (but Others Have a Problem with me)

Another group of patients are those who are 'directed' by their partner, parents or an institution to seek help. This is tricky, especially for those patients who have been told by others that there is something "wrong" with them. This may result in resistance and limited intrinsic motivation for the treatment. Before treatment can be started, a common basis must first be formulated. The patient can be motivated to undergo treatment with psycho-education and discussing what being "directed" means for the patient. A useful starting point is why those around the patient have a problem with him/her, so that the patient feels invested in the process.

In the case of patients who have something to gain from treatment (e.g., receiving a payout, benefits, or having a partner who will not leave as long as s/he is being treated), it is important to agree that the treatment depends on sufficient commitment from the patient. Where patients are poorly motivated, it should be a simple process to rejoin a treatment program once their desire to do so improves. This "second chance" should be discussed with the patient. Here, too, an accepting attitude is important (see also Sect. 5.6).

5.12   Problems in the Treatment

5.12.1 The List of Problems Is Overwhelming

In some patients problems exist in several areas of life. These patients can be very demanding. The role of the coach is to make an inventory of the various problems and, together with the patient, to determine what takes priority. The coach should be aware that not all problems need to be solved at the same time. This should be communicated to the patient. Certain problems may be solved on their own when the patient has been medicated and is able to structure him/herself better. Discuss the patient's expectations and adjust them if necessary. Do not forget to identify and encourage the patient's strengths. Additional help can be sought for these patients in the home situation. Here, the coach has the role of coordinator or case manager.

5.12.2 Resistance to Structure

Many adults with ADHD are ambivalent about structure. On the one hand, they realize that structure can help them deal with the chaos they experience. On the other hand, they have experienced problems precisely because of the structure imposed on them by others, or by society in general (which they could never meet). They have learned to avoid structure, for example , "by not agreeing on a time, you can't come too late." During coaching, it is important to look for a structure that suits the patient. In this way, a middle ground can be found that offers few disadvantages and many advantages. A good approach is "to make use of ADHD, not to fight it." Developing your own strategies that suit your ADHD. Do not copy others who seem to be doing so well. This takes into account the structure is not the goal; rather, it is a means to achieve another goal. The use of an agenda is not in and of itself the goal. Being punctual or preventing appointments from being forgotten and the subsequent negative reactions of others is the goal. The use of an agenda is a means to this end.

The structure offered by the coach during individual coaching or in a group can also provoke resistance. This can be negotiated by asking the patient if s/he agrees to be interrupted if s/he digresses too much or strays from the subject.

5.13   Cognitive Behavioral Therapy

Cognitive behavioral therapy is the most widely used form of psychotherapy in mental health care. Its effectiveness in treating various forms of anxiety, depression, and eating disorders has been convincingly demonstrated. Most programs are based on learning skills, such as learning to organize and plan, problem solving, emotional regulation, cognitive strategies to improve attention and impulsivity, techniques such as cognitive restructuring, identifying automatic negative thoughts, cognitive errors, and mindfulness. These methods can also be helpful for the problems and consequences of ADHD.

There is increasing research into the effectiveness of cognitive behavioral therapy (CBT) in adults with ADHD who are treated with medication. Research into the effectiveness of CBT alone versus CBT with medication is recent and shows that after twelve sessions of CBT, the group with CBT and medication improved more than the group with CBT alone. This was true for ADHD symptoms, organizational skills, and self-esteem. The CBT group further improved during the six-month follow-up, while the combined group remained stable (Cherkasova et al., 2016). Both groups received coaching booster sessions after the CBT treatment. At the endpoint, the differences between the two groups had decreased and were no longer significant.

Although this study was not blinded and needs to be replicated, the differences between medication and CBT over time are interesting for clinical practice. In German multicenter research into the effect of twelve weeks of intensive group CBT versus "clinical management" with methylphenidate or placebo, there was no difference between CBT and clinical management after one year. Methylphenidate was superior to placebo in both groups (Philipsen et al., 2015a, b). A meta-analysis of nine studies in which CBT was compared with a waiting list or with an active control group, shows that CBT is more effective than the other two groups, with a moderate to large effect size, respectively, compared to individual treatment and versus waiting list (Young, Moghaddam, & Tickle, 2016). The effect of CBT compared to "treatment as usual" in adults with ADHD was systematically reviewed. Based on the patient's ratings, CBT was effective in reducing ADHD symptoms, but not according to the clinician's ratings. Symptoms of anxiety and depression did decrease significantly according to both ratings. The conclusion was that CBT is effective for certain symptoms but not for all, and that more research is needed (Jensen, Amdisen, Jørgensen, & Arnfred, 2016).

Based on these preliminary findings, the conclusion seems justified that CBT is more effective than a waiting list group, but clearly not more effective than "treatment as usual" or "clinical management." Medication is more effective, and more rapid than CBT, but CBT still adds slightly to follow-up after six months, after which the differences between groups are no longer significant. For the time being, the combination of CBT and medication seems to be the best approach in ADHD.

5.14 Schema therapy for Adults with ADHD

Research on maladaptive schedules from Young's Schedule focussed therapy model in adults with ADHD, compared to controls, shows that patients with ADHD score significantly higher on almost all schedules. Schema domains such as "Failure," "Defectiveness/Shame," "Subjugation," and "Emotional Deprivation" are most common. These fit well with the history of learning problems and with the consequences of ADHD. This research suggests that schema therapy for adults with ADHD can be a good addition to the therapeutic arsenal, but research is still lacking (Philipsen et al., 2017).

5.15 Mindfulness

Mindfulness is a form of meditation derived from Buddhism. Initially, mindfulness was applied for chronic pain, stress, and chronic disease. Mindfulness focuses on posture, behavior, cognitive-emotional processes, and their relationship with health. Important aspects are observing without judgement, acceptance of inner experiences such as thoughts and feelings, and being aware of these. Research confirms the efficacy of mindfulness in stress, anxiety, and depression (Khoury et al., 2013).

In research among Dutch adults with ADHD, 53 patients receiving "mindfulness-based cognitive therapy" (MBCT) were compared with a waiting list group. The study lasted twelve weeks. Patients with more depressive symptoms dropped out earlier ($n = 12$). The results of 41 patients could be reported: for 43% ($n = 16$), there was a 30% decrease on the ADHD Rating Scale. Executive functioning and mindfulness skills also improved. In this study, there was no improvement in anxiety and depressive symptoms, nor in functioning. Medication was used in about half of the participants in both groups, but this did not change the results.

In a study of 54 adolescents with ADHD treated with MBCT or placed on a waiting list, after six weeks, ADHD symptoms, anxiety and depressive symptoms, and mindfulness skills improved significantly more in the MBCT group than in the waiting list group (Gu, Xu, & Zhu, 2018).

In a meta-analysis of ten small studies, MBCT was effective for both attention problems and hyperactivity/impulsivity in adults with ADHD. The effect sizes were − 0.5 to −0.6 (Cairncross & Miller, 2020). More comparative research with larger populations is needed with MBCT in ADHD.

5.16   Relationship Therapy

The influence of ADHD on relationships is considerable. Where patients have difficulty with meeting their responsibilities, being punctual, planning, or being irritable, the relationship suffers, particularly where they lie to cover up mistakes. The partner is often overburdened and exhausted by the time the diagnosis is made. Sometimes the partner also needs help. The diagnosis and treatment of ADHD may become a power struggle between the two. There may also be sexual problems. Violence in intimate partner relationships is also more common with ADHD, especially in women (Guendelman, Ahmad, Meza, Owens, & Hinshaw, 2016).

Couples with and without ADHD were compared in terms of relationship quality, maintenance of the relationship, and symptoms of attention deficit and hyperactive/impulsive behavior: couples with ADHD experienced significantly more relationship problems. Attention deficit was associated with having multiple partners, and less constructive responses to negative behavior of the partner. Hyperactive-impulsive behavior with negative responses to bad behavior of the partner. Cognitive relationship therapy may be helpful in this respect (VanderDrift, Antshel, & Olszewski, 2017).

Explaining which problems result from ADHD is crucial to create insight and overview. In this way, understanding is created, for both the patient and the partner. Problems caused and sustained by disability rather than unwillingness are better tolerated and can be addressed in a different way.

Form
Relationship therapy can be offered by a systems therapist in a series of four to ten sixty-minute relationship sessions with the ADHD patient and the partner.

Inclusion Criteria
ADHD may be comorbid with other disorders, but this must be in a stable phase of treatment. There must be a lasting relationship. The relationship problems should be related to the symptoms and consequences of ADHD. Patient and partner must have previously received psycho-education about ADHD and its treatment.

Method
Common systems strategies are used, in line with a model that takes into account the limitations of ADHD as a chronic disorder. Psycho-education plays an important role.

Attention is also paid to communication patterns from the family of origin and their influence on the current relationship (transmission). The aim is to improve the communication and negotiation skills of both partners. If applicable, the parenting style(s) and the division of tasks and roles are also discussed. Homework assignments are recommended.

5.17   Prevention of Relapse

At the end of the treatment, an overview of the known reasons for relapse is made together with the patient. Strategies to deal with these are discussed. A summary of the treatment is made, so that the patient has tools to fall back on later. Issues that can be addressed here are: signalling an increase in substance use and the risk factors for this, therapy compliance, stopping medication (for ADHD and/or anxiety/depression), and a change in the sleeping pattern, (as sleep deprivation can lead to an increase in ADHD symptoms). The Super Brains app can be used; in particular the "Digital coach." This part of the app is specially designed for aftercare and relapse prevention. Patient and practitioner then keep in touch via the app.

With the so-called Self Monitor app, ten different complaint domains can be monitored over time, with tips on what to do if things get worse in each domain. In addition, it is important to discuss what can be done in case of a return of winter depression, as these complaints recur annually. Solutions include re-registration for light therapy or timely application of light in the home situation.

5.18   Conclusion

Evaluations using questionnaires at the end of treatment provides the patient with insight into the areas in which s/he has made progress. This also serves as a useful overview of treatment. Upon completion of treatment, further management of medication is referred to the general practitioner. The patient should be informed that, if necessary, s/he can re-enter a therapeutic program for ADHD.

5.19   Aftercare

Despite good motivation and treatment, a small group of patients will continue to have considerable complaints. Usually, this is the result of complex comorbidity or serious ADHD in which medication has insufficient effect or is not tolerated because of side effects. These patients need extensive treatment to stabilize their symptoms. The aim of treatment in these situations is no longer to bring about change, but to maintain the level of functioning. Other goals are: to provide easy access to a therapeutic group to prevent relapse, to provide structure and support contacts. For this group of patients, intermittent group therapy can also be effective, possibly supplemented by practical home care. Patients can also receive a number of supportive conversations.

In the group of patients with relatively many problems, it is important to find out whether a diagnosis may have been missed. For example, a disorder in the autistic spectrum. In that case, the patient may be referred to a department or colleague who treats this disorder.

5.20   Contact with Fellow Experience Experts

Patients who have been diagnosed with ADHD should be informed about the existence of support groups for adults with ADHD and related disorders, as well as parent associations, for parents of children with learning and behavioral problems, including ADHD.

A feeling of sharing and fellowship occurs because experienced patients tell newcomers about their experiences. Experienced patients will have first been trained by a professional. The Internet also offers enormous opportunities for exchanging information via chat rooms and platforms.

Set up and Organization of an Outpatient and Life Course Clinic for ADHD

6.1 Introduction

Experience over the past decades has shown that the demand for care for ADHD in adults in The Netherlands and Europe is high. This is related to improvements in diagnostics and treatment in this age group. ADHD is a lifelong, persistent disorder in the majority of the children who receive the diagnosis. This has consequences for the organization of adult care and care for the elderly in psychiatry. At PsyQ in the Hague, the Netherlands a specialized adult ADHD department was set up in 2002. In Table 6.1 an overview of the increase per year in the number of patients and employees since the start is shown.

Assuming a prevalence of ADHD of 5% in the adult population, the PsyQ Department adult ADHD in The Hague treats only about 2% of the prevalence annually (about 1200 patients). Every large city and every region should be able to meet the same demand. ADHD is common and is increasingly recognized by both general practitioners and second-line practitioners. To give an idea of how the demand for care for ADHD can direct the growth of a department, Table 6.1 shows the data from PsyQ in The Hague.

Table 6.1 shows that the number of employees doubled in the first half of the year due to the explosive increase in the number of referrals. After one year, the number of staff and patients almost doubled, followed by annual growth of around four staff members and one hundred patients. The total number of employees includes the secretariat, management, and trainees. On average, a coach treats about forty patients and a doctor about one hundred, at a given time.

Initially, patients were mainly referred by general practitioners, but better recognition and detection of ADHD in patients with other psychiatric disorders has increased the number of referrals from mental health care facilities, and with it the complexity of the patient population. ADHD occurs as a comorbid disorder in approximately 20% of psychiatric patients, making it impossible to have all patients

© The Author(s), under exclusive license to Springer Nature Switzerland AG 2022
J. J. S. Kooij, *Adult ADHD*, https://doi.org/10.1007/978-3-030-82812-7_6

Table 6.1 Development of the department adult ADHD PsyQ, The Hague

Year	Number of employees	Number of patients
2003	5	150
2003 (3 months later)	10	350
2004	20	600
2005	24	700
2006	28	800
2007	32	900
2008	36	1100
2009	42	1200
2017	45	1300

with ADHD in a city or region treated by a single specialized team or department. ADHD is so prevalent in psychiatry that all psychiatrists and psychologists should be able to recognize and treat the disorder. Specialized wards can then focus on difficult and complex cases. This means that ADHD in adults should be taught by default to trainee physicians, psychologists and psychiatric nurses, and then be the subject of systematic in-service training for established professionals.

6.1.1   Starting a Life Course Clinic for ADHD

ADHD often runs in families because of its hereditary nature. In order to give parents with ADHD quick access to help for their children with the same disorder, (and vice versa for the children of adult patients with ADHD), a life course clinic was established. This offers systems interventions that can be designed jointly by the child and adult units. There was a parenting course that focuses on increasing the parents' sense of competence. FlexCare ADHD was being developed for the group of adolescents who are at risk for dropping out of treatment around the age of 15 years. This treatment offer was developed together with the target group. It uses digital platforms as much as possible and is used flexibly (short or long term).

Given the persistence of ADHD in older people after the age of 60 years, and the increasing demand for treatment of this group, a psychiatrist specializing in geriatric patients is a valuable addition to a life course clinic. Together with a psychologist, an inventory of the treatment needs of elderly people with ADHD was established so that the treatment offer can be tailored to these needs. The next step was research into the response to and safety of medication in the elderly (Michielsen et al., 2020). The QbTest, which objectively measures attention, hyperactivity, and impulsivity, was validated in the elderly (Bijlenga et al., 2019) (see Sect. 1.1.9).

This approach was chosen to allow adults with ADHD reaching the age of 65 years to get help. In this way, the life course clinic serves people with ADHD of all ages; anyone can return when symptoms increase. Unfortunately, the different funding streams of child and adult psychiatry complicate the collaboration.

6.2   Employees

Successful treatment starts with the quality of the employees. A prerequisite for all practitioners who want to work with adults with ADHD is that they are trained in the diagnosis and treatment of this disorder.

In a new team, the following five disciplines at least are required to start multidisciplinary treatment of adults with ADHD:

1. Psychiatrist
2. Physician assistant or medical resident
3. Registered psychologist
4. Nurse practitioner
5. Secretary

The management of the department is not the responsibility of these five full-time employees. The team cannot function with fewer than these 5 professionals. Approximately, 150 patients can be treated by the team described above, and the 3 major pillars of the treatment can be offered: medication, individual coaching, and groups.

6.2.1   Tasks and Responsibilities of Treatment Staff

Table 6.2 shows the activities and responsibilities of the various disciplines, and what supervision should be offered.

Table 6.2 Overview of tasks and responsibilities of treatment staff

Work	Implemented by	Under the supervision of
Intake	Nurse practitioner, psychologist, physician assistant	Independent qualified practitioner (psychiatrist, psychologist)
Intake supervision	Psychiatrist, psychologist	N/A
Consultation	Nurse practioner psychologist, physician assistant	Independent qualified practitioner (psychiatrist, psychologist)
Prescribing medication for ADHD and comorbidity, physical and laboratory testing, psychiatric examination	Psychiatrist, nurse practitioner, and physician assistants	Physician assistants and nurse practitioners are supervised by a psychiatrist
Individual coaching and coordination treatment	Nurse practitioner, psychologist	Inexperienced psychologists are supervised by a specialized psychologist
Group coaching	Psychologist, nurse practitioner and, if necessary, physician assistant	N/A

As Table 6.2 shows, all disciplines do intakes, except the psychiatrist. The reason for this is that psychiatrists are few and have to devote themselves to complex (differential) diagnosis, pharmacological treatment, and supervision. To a lesser extent, this applies to the assistant physician. The participation of all other employees in the intake ensures that it occurs rapidly and efficiently. The weekly intake supervision by a psychiatrist or psychologist provides the necessary support and also serves as training for all staff involved. This is the best way to guarantee that the quality of the intake for all staff is of a similarly high level.

6.3   Inclusion and Exclusion Criteria

The inclusion and exclusion criteria for referral to a department for ADHD in adults can be:

- Suspicion of ADHD, or confirmed diagnosis
- No other (more) prominent axis I or II disorder
- Age between 17 and 65 years
- IQ > 70

This means that, if a different disorder that needs to be treated first is more prominent, referral for this disorder takes place first (for instance in the case of a severe depression, addiction, or bipolar disorder). Depending on the organization of the mental health care organisation into specialized teams or departments, or in general outpatient clinics, choices can be made on this matter.

6.4   Intake

In adults, the diagnosis of ADHD and any additional disorders is either established or rejected during the intake phase. This is done on the basis of information obtained during the intake interview from the patient, partner, and parents, or other family members. Treatment begins if the patient has been diagnosed with ADHD and he or she continues to meet the criteria for treatment on the basis of the inclusion and exclusion criteria.

The duration of the intake interview is three hours and the complete interview is conducted in one day for a smooth procedure. Although this is tiring for both the patient and the staff, having several appointments may lead to untreated patients with ADHD missing their next appointment and permanent uncertainty about the diagnosis. Treatment cannot get started without a diagnosis. For this reason, at the end of the intake session, a short summary of the diagnosis should be given to the patient. The intake is performed using the standardized instruments including: the structured Diagnostic Interview for ADHD, the DIVA (see section "Self-report Questionnaire on Attention Problems and Hyperactivity for Adulthood and Childhood" in Appendix), instruments to diagnose comorbid disorders, and a history taking. Comorbid conditions are almost always present and include addiction, mood, anxiety, sleep, and personality disorders, as well as dyslexia, autism spectrum disorder, psychosis, and possible neglect or abuse in the past. Ascertaining whether these are present is necessary to be able to differentiate other disorders from ADHD and to be able to offer treatment(s) for comorbidities in the correct order.

Patients and families may be asked in advance to complete a questionnaire for ADHD (Self-report questionnaire on attention problems and hyperactivity, (see section "Self-report Questionnaire on Attention Problems and Hyperactivity for Adulthood and Childhood" in Appendix). The total score of this questionnaire serves as a baseline measurement for the evaluation of treatment for ADHD, with Routine Outcome Monitoring (ROM) (see section "ADHD Rating Scale, Self-Report" in Appendix and Sect. 4.7.2).

6.5   Staff Discussion

The psychiatrist or other independently qualified practitioner discusses the findings with the staff after the intake interview with the patient. He or she sees the patient in order to assess the quality of the diagnostics and the treatment plan. Treatment advice is also discussed with the patient and possibly family members.

During this counselling interview, the patient, partner, and any family members are given psycho-education about the diagnosis(es). The treatment plan and diagnoses are explained. Other subjects discussed are: expectations of the treatment, symptom reduction, duration and content of the treatment, procedures, and rules for crisis and file management, complaints procedure, evaluation of treatment, no-show policy (see also Sect. 5.8.8), and feedback on the scores of the questionnaires submitted during the intake interview. In some cases, it is necessary to examine the patient further, for example, a psychiatric, physical, or psychological examination.

At the end of the counselling interview, the patient is asked whether he or she can agree to the treatment proposal and therefore decides to start treatment. If the request for help and/or motivation for treatment is unclear, the patient is not immediately taken into care, but first follows a limited number of interviews to examine motivation (see also Sect. 5.6).

After the intake, the patient is assigned a doctor, a coach, and a path of care. The coach acts as an individual and coordinating practitioner. There is a general treatment path with three standard components that are used because of their synergistic effect. These are: medication, individual coaching (including digital), and group work.

6.6   Range of Treatment

The entire treatment range consists of the parts described below:

- Psycho-education or information giving.
- Discussion about medication.
- Individual or group coaching.
- Group programs.
- Cognitive behavioral therapy, individual or group
- Digital coaching via app.
- Relationship therapy with a psychotherapist (after stabilization, if there is a need to process the past or if there is any indication).
- Light therapy for seasonal affective disorder and delayed sleep phase disorder
- Support group for partners and family members.

6.6.1   Minimum Treatment

The minimum treatment of a starter department could consist of the following parts:

- Psycho-education or information
- Information about medication and a protocol for starting it
- Individual coaching
- Three basic groups: Introduction group, ADHD skills training, cognitive, or behavioral training (see Table 6.3)

The resulting treatment path is shown in Fig. 6.1.

6.6.2   Treatment Objectives and Plan

Starting during the intake, treatment goals and the treatment plan are drawn up in consultation with the patient. Completion of the baseline questionnaires from the intake is checked. If incomplete, they are filled in again. The policy with regard to no show at appointments is also discussed. The treatment is carried out according to the treatment plan. Here, the practitioner can register the patient for digital coaching, and for groups addressing certain treatment goals. The group program is a supplement to the individual treatment. In addition to the group program of the ADHD department, a patient can also be referred for external treatment. This could be a treatment group for another condition, light therapy for winter depression, or guidance at home.

Table 6.3 Overview of ADHD groups at PsyQ, The Hague

Group	Purpose of the group	Target group	Contraindications
Introduction group	Psycho-education and peer-to-peer contact	General target group	General group criteria (i.e., no crisis or suicidality)
ADHD skills training	Learning practical planning and organizational skills; reducing distractibility and procrastination behavior	There should be basic knowledge of skills such as planning, agenda management, and dealing with distractions, but patients have difficulty applying these in practice	Patients in crisis
Target group	Further development of ADHD skills	Members desire help in setting concrete and achievable goals, following ADHD skills training NB patient and practitioner set goals together in advance	General group criteria
Study skill training	Increasing study skills such as planning, dealing with procrastination and distractibility	Students who find it difficult to structure their studies, get an overview of a topic and experience planning problems	General group criteria
CBT training	Learning to recognise and change negative thinking patterns, improving cognition	Complaints such as perfectionism, fear of failure, lack of self-confidence, difficulty in dealing with criticism. Some insight was necessary. Patient is motivated to be intensely involved in the course and homework	Lower average intelligence, in crisis
Partner relationship group	Providing information, contact with peers, support, and tools for the relationship	Partners who experience problems within their relationship due to ADHD symptoms. Partners must have followed the support group	General group criteria

(continued)

Table 6.3 (continued)

Group	Purpose of the group	Target group	Contraindications
Self-image group	Thinking and feeling more positively about oneself	Indication: Negative self-image. The CBT training is a prerequisite for participation in self-image group. In addition, the patient is prepared to be open and to do homework N.B. self-image is assessed on intake, prior to participation	Incomplete mastery of CBT training, below-average intelligence, in crisis
Impulse control group	Learning to gain more control over impulsive tendencies; recognising situations that provoke impulsivity; learning to think about the consequences of one's own behavior and learning to find behavioral alternatives	Impulsive, make hasty decisions, substance abuse, greed, binge eating, reckless driving in traffic, gambling, impulsively saying things and hurting people; willingness to work on behavioral change and do homework	In crisis
Sleep group for delayed sleep phase	Increase knowledge and insight regarding ADHD and sleep problems	Patients with delayed sleep phase disorder associated with disturbed circadian rhythm N.B. sleep is assessed on intake, prior to participation	General group criteria
Parenting course for parents who have ADHD	Learning more skilful in parenting behavior, dealing with boundaries, punishing and rewarding, keeping impulses under control, applying structure, and fixed routines in family life. In addition, the goal is to increase the feeling of competence as a parent	Patients are on medication, have completed the introductory training, followed the ADHD skills training. Children should be aged at least 5 years. Possible anxiety and mood disorders are under control. It is important to be able to involve a partner or buddy in the training	General group criteria and in crisis
Women's group	Exchange experiences with other women with ADHD in role expectation, life stages, communication, relationships, and sexuality	Women with ADHD	General group criteria

Table 6.3 (continued)

Group	Purpose of the group	Target group	Contraindications
Professionals with ADHD	Exchanging experiences of ADHD as a professional and patient in a safe environment; dealing with acceptance and shame; training in executive functioning	Doctors, psychologists and other professionals with ADHD	General group criteria
Support group	Information about ADHD and treatment; exchanging experiences and tips on dealing with someone with ADHD	Partners and relatives of patients with ADHD	General group criteria
Experiential peer counselling (EPC)	Independent learning to investigate cognitive schemes in a structured way, to gain insight into desired behavioral changes	Patients are on medication and have followed the CBT training and introductory group.	General group criteria and in crisis
Maintenance group	Maintain and possibly increase the stability acquired during treatment. Offers support and recognition by means of a peer group	Patients who have acquired certain stability through the treatment, but where it is desirable to keep a 'finger on the pulse' in connection with sensitivity to relapse	General group criteria

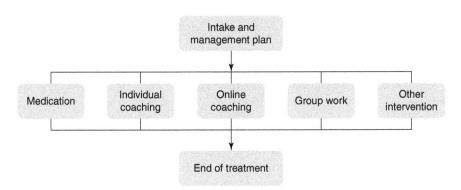

Fig. 6.1 Treatment route

6.6.3 Groups

At PsyQ a varied group program has been developed. In a starting department, the range would be more limited. See Sect. 6.6.1 for the recommended minimum group offer. Groups are intended for patients with ADHD who are motivated to participate. In general, the condition is that patients who follow groups should be able to function adequately in a group setting. Possible limitations include: serious impulsivity, inability to listen, disinterest in fellow group members, severely autistic, externalizing, oppositional, or aggressive behavior. Another general contraindication is not showing up at appointments. In order for the group to have optimal effect, it is preferable that patients have already started with medication. The Introductory group is an exception to this. This group is seen as a first experience, and a prerequisite for following other groups.

Table 6.3 gives an overview of the ADHD groups that have been developed. It describes the goal of the group, the target participants and the contraindications. Group participants receive a printed manual, and PowerPoint presentations improve the attention of patients with ADHD in the transfer of information.

6.7   Evaluation and Impact Measurement

6.7.1   Objective of the Evaluation

The aim of the evaluation is to gain insight into the degree of effectiveness of the treatment. The result should be a guideline for the continuation of treatment. This means that if progress stagnates in one or more areas, the treatment plan needs to be adjusted. In addition, the evaluation can be used to decide about continuation or termination of treatment. This is the case when evaluating the first year of treatment.

6.7.2   Evaluation of the Treatment Plan

After several months of treatment, there is an evaluation session to check how the therapy is progressing. In principle, the treatment is evaluated every 6 months and at the end of the treatment.

At this session, the treatment objectives from the original treatment plan are evaluated. The reduction in the severity of ADHD symptoms is measured using the ADHD Rating Scale (see section "ADHD Rating Scale, Self-Report" in Appendix and Sect. 4.7.2). The reduction in the severity of comorbid disorders is also evaluated, as is the improvement in functioning. The latter can be done with the Sheehan Disability Scale (Sheehan, Harrett-Sheehan, & Raj, 1996). The presence of the patient at appointments and motivation for treatment are also discussed. Specific goals of the patient are evaluated. The outcome of each evaluation should lead to adjustment of the treatment plan and to targeted action to further improve the outcomes.

6.7.3   Discussion of Evaluation in Patient Consultations

The outcome of the evaluation should be discussed at the next patient meeting. During this meeting, discussion revolves around whether objectives were met, whether it is time for discharge or if further treatment is necessary.

6.8   End of Treatment

The treatment is terminated when the treatment objectives have been achieved, after repeated no-shows, referral to another department, or at the patient's request. The general practitioner is informed about the outcome of the treatment and is tasked with the continuation of the medication prescribed.

Appendix A: Instruments for Diagnostic Assessment

Ultrashort Screening List for ADHD in Adults (J.J.S. Kooij)

1. **Do you usually feel restless?**
   (*for example: hurried, difficulty in sitting still, fidgeting, doing a lot of sports, or being agile*)
   Yes/No
2. **Do you usually tend to do first and then think?**
   (*for example: flapping things out, spending too much money, or being impatient*)
   Yes/No
3. **Do you usually have concentration problems?**
   (*for example: being quickly distracted, not finishing things, quickly bored, forgetful, or chaotic*)
   Yes/No
   If the answer to questions 1 and/or 2 and/or 3 is yes:
4. **Have you always had this?**
   (*as long as you can remember, or have you been like this most of your life*)
   Yes/No

If the answer to question 4 is yes, consider further diagnostics of ADHD.

Further diagnostics of ADHD can be carried out using the Self-Report Questionnaire for attention problems and hyperactivity for adulthood and childhood (see Appendix A.2) and/or the Diagnostic Interview for ADHD in adults (DIVA-5).

Self-Report Questionnaire on Attention Problems and Hyperactivity for Adulthood and Childhood

J.J.S. Kooij and J.K. Buitelaar © 1997 and adapted to DSM-5.
Name: _____ Date of birth:___ Date:___
Circle the number that best describes your behavior over the *past six months*.
Always give one score per sentence (0, 1, 2, or 3).

© The Editor(s) (if applicable) and The Author(s), under exclusive license to
Springer Nature Switzerland AG 2022
J. J. S. Kooij, *Adult ADHD*, https://doi.org/10.1007/978-3-030-82812-7

0 = never or rarely 1 = sometimes 2 = often 3 = very often					
1.	I don't pay enough attention to details in my work.	0	1	2	3
2.	When I sit, I fiddle with my hands or feet.	0	1	2	3
3.	I make sloppy mistakes in my work.	0	1	2	3
4.	I'm wiggling and turning in my chair.	0	1	2	3
5.	When I'm working on something, I can't keep my eye on it.	0	1	2	3
6.	I quickly get up from my chair in situations in which I am expected to stay neatly seated.	0	1	2	3
7.	I don't listen well when others say something to me.	0	1	2	3
8.	I feel restless.	0	1	2	3
9.	I'm bored fast.	0	1	2	3
10.	I'm having trouble following directions.	0	1	2	3
11.	I don't finish chores or work I start.	0	1	2	3
12.	I find it hard to relax in my spare time.	0	1	2	3
13.	In my holiday or leisure time I look for an environment with hustle and bustle.	0	1	2	3
14.	I find it difficult to organize my activities or tasks.	0	1	2	3
15.	I'm constantly "busy," as if I'm "powered by an engine."	0	1	2	3
16.	I'm trying to get out of activities that I need to concentrate on for a longer period of time.	0	1	2	3
17.	I'm talking in one piece.	0	1	2	3
18.	I'm losing things I need for chores or pursuits.	0	1	2	3
19.	I answer before questions are finished.	0	1	2	3
20.	I'm easily distracted.	0	1	2	3
21.	I find it hard to wait my turn.	0	1	2	3
22.	I'm forgetful in everyday activities.	0	1	2	3
23.	I interrupt others or interrupt them.	0	1	2	3

Would you please answer the follow-up questions?
The following questions are about the same characteristics, but now *in childhood*.
Circle the number that best describes *your behavior as a child (0–12 years)*
Always give one score per sentence (0, 1, 2, or 3)

0 = never or rarely 1 = sometimes 2 = often 3 = very often					
1.	I didn't pay enough attention to details in schoolwork.	0	1	2	3
2.	I fiddled with hands or feet.	0	1	2	3
3.	I made sloppy mistakes in schoolwork.	0	1	2	3
4.	I was wiggling and turning in the chair.	0	1	2	3
5.	I couldn't keep my eye on things.	0	1	2	3
6.	I quickly got up from my chair in situations where I was expected to stay properly seated.	0	1	2	3
7.	I listened badly when others said something.	0	1	2	3
8.	I felt restless.	0	1	2	3
9.	I was bored fast.	0	1	2	3
10.	I had trouble following directions.	0	1	2	3
11.	I started chores or work, but I didn't finish them.	0	1	2	3

0 = never or rarely 1 = sometimes 2 = often 3 = very often					
12.	It was hard for me to relax.	0	1	2	3
13.	I had trouble playing quietly.	0	1	2	3
14.	I had a hard time organizing activities or tasks.	0	1	2	3
15.	I was constantly "busy," like "powered by an engine."	0	1	2	3
16.	I was trying to get out of activities I had to concentrate on for a long time.	0	1	2	3
17.	I was talking in one piece.	0	1	2	3
18.	I lost things needed for tasks or pursuits.	0	1	2	3
19.	I answered before questions were finished.	0	1	2	3
20.	I was easily distracted.	0	1	2	3
21.	I found it hard to wait my turn.	0	1	2	3
22.	I was forgetful in everyday activities.	0	1	2	3
23.	I interrupted others or interrupted them.	0	1	2	3

Criterion DSM-5	Scoring form, childhood and adulthood. Self-report questionnaire on attention problems and hyperactivity	Child:		Adult:	
		Yes	No	Yes	No
1a	Question 1 or question 3 = score $\geq$ 2				
1b	Question 5 = score $\geq$ 2				
1c	Question 7 = score $\geq$ 2				
1d	Question 10 or question 11 = score $\geq$ 2				
1e	Question 14 = score $\geq$ 2				
1f	Question 16 = score $\geq$ 2				
1g	Question 18 = score $\geq$ 2				
1h	Question 20 = score $\geq$ 2				
1i	Question 22 = score $\geq$ 2				
2a	Question 2 or question 4 = score $\geq$ 2				
2b	Question 6 = score $\geq$ 2				
2c	Question 8 or question 9 = score $\geq$ 2				
2d	Question 12 or question 13 = score $\geq$ 2				
2e	Question 15 = score $\geq$ 2				
2f	Question 17 = score $\geq$ 2				
2g	Question 19 = score $\geq$ 2				
2h	Question 21 = score $\geq$ 2				
2i	Question 23 = score $\geq$ 2				
Childhood score				**Yes**	**No**
A:___/9 characteristics	Is the number of A-characteristics $\geq$6?				
HI:___/9 characteristics	Is the number of HI characteristics $\geq$6?				
Adulthood score				**Yes**	**No**
A:___/9 characteristics	Is the number of A-characteristics $\geq$5?				
HI:___/9 characteristics	Is the number of HI characteristics $\geq$5?				

The self-report questionnaire on attention problems and hyperactivity is based on the DSM criteria for ADHD (APA), by J.J.S. Kooij and J.K. Buitelaar © 1997, and adapted to the DSM-5

*The cut-off point for ADHD in the DSM-5 is set for current childhood symptoms at six out of nine criteria; the retrospective number of characteristics in early childhood before age 12, is set at "several" symptoms, that has been operationalized as 3 or more symptoms; the cut-off point for current symptoms in adolescents and adults is set at five out of nine criteria

Appendix B: Instruments for Treatment Medication and Coaching

List of Symptoms and Side Effects of ADHD

Name: _____Date of birth: _____

Instruction: Start stimulating medication (methylphenidate/dexamphetamine)*
Fill in 1 week before the start, continue until the effect is clear (about 2–4 weeks).
Delete where not applicable
    Symptoms (severity: 0 = not, 1 = occasionally, 2 = clearly and frequently present, 3 = continuously dominant).
With/without medication*
Delete where not applicable

Date						
Tense						
Quickly distracted						
Mood changes						
Don't finish things						
Poor concentration						
Forgetful, chaotic						
Irritable, quickly irritated						
Physical aggression (indicate number of times)						
Flapping things out, acting impulsively						
Restless, fidgeting, difficulty sitting still						

Adverse reactions (severity 0–3)

Date						
Palpitations						
Difficulty falling asleep						
Too little appetite						
Tired						
Nervous						
Headache						

ADHD Rating Scale, Self-Report

Patient's name: Date of birth:
   Date: Intaker:
   Evaluation 0/6/12/18/... months/final evaluation.
   Circle the number that best describes your behavior.
   Always give one score (0, 1, 2 or 3).

0 = never or rarely	1 = sometimes	2 = often	3 = very often		
1.	I don't pay enough attention to details in my work.	0	1	2	3
2.	When I sit, I fiddle with my hands or feet.	0	1	2	3
3.	I make sloppy mistakes in my work.	0	1	2	3
4.	I'm wiggling and turning in my chair.	0	1	2	3
5.	When I'm working on something, I can't keep my eye on it.	0	1	2	3
6.	I quickly get up from my chair in situations in which I am expected to stay neatly seated.	0	1	2	3
7.	I don't listen well when others say something to me.	0	1	2	3
8.	I feel restless.	0	1	2	3
9.	I'm bored fast.	0	1	2	3
10.	I'm having trouble following directions.	0	1	2	3
11.	I don't finish chores or work I start.	0	1	2	3
12.	I find it hard to relax in my spare time.	0	1	2	3
13.	In my holiday or leisure time I look for an environment with hustle and bustle.	0	1	2	3
14.	I find it difficult to organize my activities or tasks.	0	1	2	3
15.	I'm constantly "busy," as if I'm "powered by an engine."	0	1	2	3
16.	I'm trying to get out of activities I have to concentrate on for a long time.	0	1	2	3
17.	I'm talking in one piece.	0	1	2	3
18.	I'm losing things I need for chores or pursuits.	0	1	2	3
19.	I answer before questions are finished.	0	1	2	3
20.	I'm easily distracted.	0	1	2	3
21.	I find it hard to wait my turn.	0	1	2	3
22.	I'm forgetful in everyday activities.	0	1	2	3
23.	I interrupt others or interrupt them.	0	1	2	3

Total Score

After you have answered all items, add up the total score. For items 1 + 3, 2 + 4, 8 + 9, 10 + 11, 12 + 13 per pair, take the highest score. So a score 1 on item 10 and a score 3 on item 11 becomes a score 3.

This ADHD Rating Scale (ADHD-RS) self-reporting is based on the DSM-5 criteria for ADHD (APA, 2013). By J.J.S. Kooij and J.K. Buitelaar © 1997.

Individual Target Symptom List

Example of an Individual Target Symptom List:

Target	Frequency now	Frequency after treatment
1. Being able to read for longer periods of time without being distracted	3 min	_____
2. Less irritable in family	Quarrel 4 times a week	_____
3. Less effort with tidying up	1x per month with a lot of effort and reluctance	_____

Weekly Schedule

	Monday	Tuesday	Wednesday	Thursday	Friday	Saturday	Sunday
7.00							
7.30							
8.00							
8.30							
9.00							
9.30							
10.00							
10.30							
11.00							
11.30							
12.00							
12.30							
13.00							
13.30							
14.00							
14.30							
15.00							
15.30							
16.00							
16.30							
17.00							
17.30							
18.00							
18.30							
19.00							
19.30							
20.00							
20.30							
21.00							
21.30							

	Monday	Tuesday	Wednesday	Thursday	Friday	Saturday	Sunday
22.00							
22.30							
23.00							

Instruction week schedule:

1. Make a schedule of the activities per day that return every week, for example: 7.30 a.m. getting up, 8.00 a.m. breakfast, 8.15 a.m. cycling to work, 9.00 a.m. work, 12.30 p.m. lunch, and so on.
2. Make clear blocks by giving the different activities a different color or shading.
3. Do this for every day and evening of the week, including weekends.
4. Copy the list a number of times.
5. See how many "empty" spots there are in the weekly schedule.
6. Then plan the variable activities of the coming week in the weekly schedule, for example: to the movie with Marie on Wednesday the 12th.
7. Do the planning for the coming week on a fixed day, e.g. Sunday evening.
8. Hang the weekly schedule in a place where you often come across it, for example on the fridge or kitchen door.
9. Always replace the old with the new weekly schedule.
10. Do not make appointments until you have an overview of the available time.
11. Make realistic choices from your list of priorities based on the weekly schedule.

Goal Schedule (Maximum 3 Goals per Week)

Targets for the next week:

	What	When	Result +/−
1.			
2.			
3.			

Evaluation (after one week).
Date: Time: _____ With Whom:
Instruction goal schedule:

1. A goal must always be concrete, achievable, and measurable. Choose the three most important goals to work on in the coming week under "What."
2. For example: target 1 = create standard weekly schedule, target 2 = copy weekly schedule, target 3 = adjust weekly schedule for next week.
3. Plan the day and time you can work on the target under the heading "When."
4. Hang the target schedule next to the weekly schedule in a visible place, for example on the fridge or kitchen door.

5. Indicate under "Result" whether the goal has been achieved or not. If the goal has been reached, a next goal can be chosen. If the goal has not yet been reached, it can be re-entered in the goal schedule. See what is needed to reach the goal now.

6. At the end of the week, evaluate whether the goals have been achieved, possibly together with the partner or an acquaintance. Plan this appointment! Then make three new goals.

Appendix C: Introduction Course

Program ADHD in Adults, PsyQ

- Introduction
- Structure of the meetings.
- Group participation rules.
- Meeting 1 What is ADHD?
- Meeting 2 Neurobiology and medication.
- Meeting 3 What does ADHD do with your life?
- Meeting 4 How to proceed?
- Other group offers.

Introduction

This is the script of the Introduction group ADHD in adults. This group is part of the treatment offer of Program ADHD in adults of PsyQ, the Hague, The Netherlands.

After the diagnosis of ADHD, it is important that you learn what ADHD means to you and how you can deal with it. In addition, it can be very pleasant to exchange experiences with others. The two starting points of the Introductory group ADHD in adults are therefore education and contact with fellow sufferers.

The script consists of four double meetings of one hour each. For each meeting a theme is dealt with. In order to meet the demand for information, articles are distributed per meeting.

We wish you lots of success and fun during the group!

Team ADHD in adults. PsyQ, psycho-medical programs, the Hague, the Netherlands.

Structure of the Meetings

- The group consists of four weekly meetings. The duration of the meetings is twice 1 hour, with a break of 15 minutes between the two parts.
- There are 8–10 participants per group.

J. J. S. Kooij, *Adult ADHD*, https://doi.org/10.1007/978-3-030-82812-7

- The group is accompanied by two coaches.
- The goals of this group are: information, psycho-education, and contact with fellow sufferers.
- There will be opportunity for discussion and questioning.
- The meetings of the Introductory group ADHD in adults will be held according to a fixed schedule:
  1. Opening
  2. Discussing homework assignment (if applicable)
  3. Information
  4. Homework assignment next meeting (if applicable)
  5. Continue reading
- The following themes will be covered in the course:
  - Meeting 1 What is ADHD?
  - Meeting 2 Neurobiology and medication
  - Meeting 3 What does ADHD do with your life?
  - Meeting 4 How to proceed?

Group Participation Rules

The following arrangements apply to the group:

- It is important that you arrive on time and are present all the time. If you do have to unsubscribe, you are requested to contact the secretariat.
- In connection with your and other people's privacy, personal information is expected to be discussed only during the meetings.
- It's important that you let each other talk it out.
- During the meetings, the mobile must be switched off. If an alarm is required for the use of medication, leave it on as still as possible.
- You're not allowed to smoke in the building, you can smoke outside during the break.
- Alcohol and drug use are not allowed.
- If you know one of the participants privately, it is better to join the next group.

Late arrival and absence policy:

- If you're late, wait in the waiting room or in the hallway. After 15 minutes there is another possibility to come in, the group coach will come and get you. If, due to circumstances, you are more than 15 minutes late, you can come in the second hour (after the break) if the coach agrees.
- When you are absent for the first time without a message you will be contacted by the group coach and you will receive a warning. After the second absence without a message you can no longer join the group.
- Even if you are absent with a message, you may miss a maximum of two meetings.

- In general, absence is a consequence:
  - For *yourself* that you are missing information that cannot be caught up with and that the effect of the group treatment will be less.
  - For *the department* that there is no reimbursement of costs for every absent for that meeting, while the time is reserved.
  - For *the group* that regular absence of group members is demotivating and negatively affects the safety and atmosphere in the group.

Meeting 1 What Is ADHD?

Agenda Meeting 1

- Opening
  - *Introducing the coaches*
  - *Discussion group rules*
- Brief introduction
  - *Introducing the participants to each other:*
    Name, age, social situation, work;
    Since when the diagnosis of ADHD;
    Expectations of the group;
    Own complaints/symptoms of ADHD.
- Information about ADHD and the diagnosis
  - *You've been diagnosed with ADHD, but what is it?*
  - *Where did you get ADHD?*
  - *ADHD and the functioning of the brain*
  - *How common is ADHD?*
  - *ADHD and concomitant disorders*
- Homework assignment
- Continue reading

You've Been Diagnosed with ADHD, But What's That Supposed to Mean?

The abbreviation ADHD stands for Attention Deficit/Hyperactivity Disorder. There are a number of core symptoms that have to be present since childhood in order to be diagnosed.

- *Concentration deficit/attention problems*
  - Quickly distracted: internal/external;
  - No overview. Too late;
  - No overview: debts rising;
  - Poor planning and organization;
  - Start a lot (enthusiastically), finish little;
  - Dreamy, slow, and vague;
  - Chaotic and forgetful;
  - Great ability to delay.

- *Hyperactivity*
  - All the time, restless;
  - Constantly "running engine";
  - Inwardly restless, "storm in your head";
  - Always fiddling or tapping;
  - Don't stop talking.
- *Impulsiveness*
  - … Flapping things out;
  - First acting, thinking later;
  - Interrupting conversations;
  - Impatient;
  - Make impulsive purchases, gamble, establish or break relationships or jobs.

With These Core Symptoms, Three Types of Presentation Emerge

1. Attention deficit hyperactivity disorder, combined presentation type, also known as ADHD. This is the most common form. It includes attention deficit, hyperactivity, and impulsivity.
2. Attention deficit hyperactivity disorder, predominantly inattentive type of presentation, also known as ADD. These are the dreamy introverted adults, distracted and quickly distracted, who are not busy and impulsive. This type is more difficult to diagnose because concentration problems are difficult for others to perceive. Approximately 10% of people diagnosed with ADHD belong to this presentation type of ADHD.
3. Attention deficit hyperactivity disorder, predominantly hyperactive/impulsive presentation type. These are busy people without attention problems. This type is the least common, about 3–5% of people diagnosed with ADHD belong to this type of presentation.

Complaints that People with ADHD May Experience Are, for Example

- Functioning below your level of performance: it's in there but it's not coming out;
- Chaos in the head;
- Fast-changing moods;
- Outbursts of anger;
- Scattered;
- Be absent/dreamless;
- Many doubts;
- Starting enthusiastically but struggling to finish things;
- If you're interested, you don't have problems concentrating, otherwise you do;
- Trouble relaxing;
- Alcohol and/or drug problems;
- Gloominess;
- Relationship problems.

In order to be able to speak of ADHD, the typical symptoms must occur from childhood (based on information from family, among other things). At school and at home (information from school reports, partner), at work or elsewhere, these symptoms must have given rise to problems, and they must still be present in several situations. Everyone recognizes the symptoms in themselves at some point, but this is temporary, following an event and it goes away again.

Someone with ADHD has these symptoms 24 h a day, throughout his/her life, and this leads to dysfunction.

In adulthood, the manifestation of symptoms changes. It may be that you learn to deal with your disability and that you have developed all kinds of tricks. It may be that others take them into account. Then you will probably suffer less from your symptoms than when you were a child.

It can also be the other way around. In a structured environment, the complaints are less noticeable. If as a child you have been given a lot of structure at home and/ or at school, it is possible that the complaints only become apparent later, for example when you start living on your own and are given more responsibilities.

Also a good intelligence can compensate a lot, but this cannot replace concentration.

Where Did You Get ADHD?

ADHD used to fall under the collective name Minimal Brain Damage (MBD), because it was thought that minor brain damage was the cause of the complaints. However, this does not appear to be the case.

The cause of ADHD is heredity. This is shown by twin, adoption, and family research. If one of the identical twins has ADHD, the chance is 60–80% that the other also has it. Oxygen deficiency just after birth only explains the onset of ADHD in 2% of cases. Even with low birth weight or preterm birth, the chance of developing ADHD is increased. Problems during (early) pregnancy, such as high blood pressure and bleeding, are considered to influence the development of ADHD. This also applies to prenatal unfavorable factors such as the mother's use of drugs, alcohol and nicotine during pregnancy. Finally, lead poisoning can play a role in the development of ADHD.

ADHD and the Functioning of the Brain

Most experts assume that ADHD is a neurobiological disorder. This means that ADHD is heritable in many cases and runs in families, and there are differences in the functioning of the brains of people with and without ADHD. The frontal cerebral cortex (the area behind your forehead) and the basal nuclei function less well:

- ADHD brains are 5% smaller than normal in children (but no longer in adults);
- Reduced blood flow in the frontal cortex;
- More blood flow in sensorimotor cortex;
- Reduced sugar metabolism in the brain.

The brains of people with ADHD mainly function differently in the frontal lobe. The brain consists of billions of nerve cells that are constantly connected to each other. Neurotransmitters are substances that transmit messages from one nerve cell to another.

In ADHD, something goes wrong in conveying those messages. People with ADHD probably have a shortage of the neurotransmitters dopamine and norepinephrine. It is suspected that this deficiency has consequences for the anterior part of the brain: the part responsible for planning and organizing activities and for inhibiting impulses. This can lead to learning and memory disorders, impulsivity, and hyperactivity. The drugs used in the treatment of ADHD increase the amount of dopamine and norepinephrine. They improve the functioning of the brain cells.

ADHD remains lifelong, you can't cure it (like a broken leg), but you can learn how to live well with it (compare diabetes).

How Common Is ADHD?
ADHD occurs in 4–8% of children of primary school age. More than 50% of these suffer from ADHD in adulthood. ADHD occurs in adulthood in approximately 3–5% of people.

There Is a Difference in the Occurrence of ADHD in Boys and Girls
- Distribution boys–girls 3–4:1
- Male–female distribution 1½:1

There Are Several Reasons for these Differences
- The GPs are insufficiently familiar with the diagnosis of ADHD in girls and women; ADHD is still too often seen as a typical "male disorder." As a result, girls and women are less recognized and referred for help.
- Women tend to express their additional complaints differently from men. Women generally focus more on the inside (internalize) and men generally focus more on the outside (externalize). For example, in women you more often see anxiety complaints and in men more often behavioral problems in addition to ADHD.
- The diagnostic criteria for ADHD were originally drawn up on the basis of ADHD characteristics as they often occur in boys.

Misunderstandings
- If you were good at school, you can't have ADHD.
- Being highly educated/university degree would argue against ADHD.
- Dyes or sugar as the cause of ADHD.
- ADHD is caused by laziness, disinterest, or lack of motivation.
- ADHD comes from a traumatic childhood.

NB: ADHD is an explanation, not an excuse!

ADHD and Concomitant Disorders
Someone who has ADHD since childhood usually has to contend with consequences for their school career, emotional development, performance, chances of promotion, and difficult relationships with others.

ADHD is associated with one or more other psychiatric disorders in three quarters of the patients:

- Depression 20–55%
- Anxiety disorders 20–30%
- Addiction problems (alcohol, drugs) 25–45%
- Personality issues 25%
- Bipolar disorder 10%
- Sleeping problems 75%

Meeting 2 Neurobiology and Medication

Agenda Meeting 2

- Opening
- Information about effects and side effects of medication for adults with ADHD
- Discussion
- Homework next meeting
- Continue reading

Opening
Are there any questions about last time?

Discussion
- Do you have any questions about ADHD medication?

Discussion
- What are your experiences with medication?
- What are your expectations of medication for ADHD?
- How do you think about taking (or having to take) medication in general?

Homework Assignment
- Think about what influence (both positive and negative) ADHD has had in your life.

Meeting 3 What Does ADHD Do with Your Life?

Agenda Meeting 3

- Opening
- Consequences of ADHD
- Communication and relations
- Self-image

- Meaning ADHD
- Homework assignment
- Continue reading

What Does ADHD Do with Your Life?

Opening

Today's program and answering any questions from the previous meeting.

Consequences of ADHD

In meeting 1, the core symptoms and additional problems of ADHD were briefly discussed. But how do these symptoms express themselves and what are the consequences for daily life?

A distinction can be made between different types of problems. For example, there are problems that are an expression of the core symptoms of ADHD. For example, being quickly distracted and as a result having difficulty reading a book, flipping out impulsively, experiencing inner turmoil, etcetera. Certain problems can also be caused by compensation. For example, being extremely tidy and always wanting to keep everything tidy (in order to avoid distraction and unrest) and not being able to manage your finances independently (because your partner always does this for you).

Situations can also arise as a result of the core symptoms of ADHD. For example, having completed a lower education than is appropriate for your intellectual abilities and therefore having a lower level of work. Or being quickly fed up with a relationship and therefore having a pattern of many short-term relationships; drug or alcohol abuse to make you feel calmer, debts as a result of impulsive purchases, etcetera. Keeping the housekeeping and administration in order can be very difficult. In addition, social problems can arise due to (regular) forgetting appointments, not keeping promises, the impulsive flapping out of remarks that others do not appreciate.

Communication and Relations

The problem in contact with someone with ADHD is that this person can quickly be distracted by internal and external stimuli. For example, someone is quickly bored, doesn't listen well, talks pressure, has difficulty sitting still, flaps things out, tends to interrupt, and is hypersensitive to criticism.

These problems make communication difficult. It is important that these issues remain negotiable, taking into account the capabilities and limitations of someone with ADHD.

ADHD can also have a major impact on a relationship and cause many problems if the disorder is not recognized, understood, and accepted by both partners. Acceptance is probably the most important and often the most difficult step to take. Once acceptance has taken place, the partners can work together to find solutions to the problems they encounter.

Discussion

In hindsight, in which problems do you have the idea that ADHD plays or has played a role? Think of problems in the field of school, work, relationships, social contacts, etcetera.

Self-Image

Many people with ADHD suffer to a greater or lesser extent from a negative self-image. Incidentally, this is not something that only occurs with ADHD. Because ADHD is a disorder that occurs from childhood, ADHD does have a relatively greater influence on the development of self-image than, for example, a problem that does not develop until adulthood. As a result of negative experiences and criticism from others over many years, people can develop negative opinions about themselves. Examples of this are, "I'm lazy," "I can't do anything."

The way you see yourself also has consequences for how you see your surroundings. If you yourself think you are lazy (because you may have heard it many times before), you will think "you see, he thinks I'm lazy" more quickly when someone else says "you see, he thinks I'm lazy," while the person might not even think that. Because of this, dealing with criticism can become a problem and you can react more vehemently than is appropriate.

Previous negative experiences can also increase the chance of a new negative experience. For example, if you think "there is no point in learning for this exam, I can't do it anyway," the chance of passing the exam will also increase, purely because you didn't learn it. This can create a vicious circle.

In the treatment it is therefore important that you pay attention to this and that you have positive experiences. If you are able to concentrate better by taking medication, you will hopefully notice when studying, for example, that you will be able to do this better than before.

Discussion

How have your ADHD symptoms affected your self-image?

Meaning of ADHD

You were recently diagnosed with ADHD, now you know what's going on. On the one hand, this can be a huge relief (finally I know why some things are not going well), on the other hand, it can also lead to grief and anger (why didn't they know much earlier and why have I been struggling for so long? How would my life have been different if I had been on medication sooner?).

Getting diagnosed with ADHD can also raise all kinds of questions. Because you basically have the symptoms of ADHD all your life, it is also something that suits you and that makes you who you are. Distinguishing between "what is ADHD" and "what is who I am" is often difficult. That is why it is important to know what ADHD means, so that you can better give it a place. It is also often the "too much" of a trait that can bother you. An example: being spontaneous is generally a positive quality. However, it can be too spontaneous, then it is called impulsive.

Group Discussion

- What was your first idea about what ADHD means and how do you feel about it now?
- What does your environment think about ADHD?
- What positive and/or negative aspects of being diagnosed with ADHD have you experienced?
- What does taking medication mean to you?

Homework Assignment

In the next meeting we will discuss the treatment possibilities and the result of the treatment. Think for yourself what your expectations are regarding the treatment.

Meeting 4 How to Proceed?

Agenda Meeting 4

- Opening
- Acceptance process
- How to proceed: the treatment
- Treatment options for ADHD
- How fast improvement?
- Evaluation
- Continue reading

After the Diagnosis, How to Proceed?

Opening

Today's program and answering any questions you may have about the previous meeting.

Acceptance Process

The consequences of ADHD were discussed earlier. There could be a lot of them. In the diagnostic phase all kinds of things emerge that may have gone less well in your life. It can be difficult to be confronted with these.

Acceptance of *life-events* (important life events), including getting a diagnosis, is a process. You can compare it to learning to cope with a loss. In order to cope with ADHD properly, you must first learn to accept that some aspects of your life have turned out differently by having ADHD and will continue to turn out differently in the future.

Acceptance is hard work, after all, you have been diagnosed with a diagnosis that definitely has an impact on your life. It can also happen that you are on your own in acceptance, that the environment thinks it's not so bad or that ADHD is just a fashionable disease while you are extremely angry or sad.

Ideas you have about what ADHD means and about treatment can also hinder acceptance. For example, if you think that medication use is a sign of weakness or that you only associate ADHD with busy boys running around all day.

Acceptance is a subject about which much has been written, the most famous author is Elisabeth Kübler-Ross. She has written a lot about the acceptance process of the so-called life-events, she distinguishes a number of steps in this process:

- Denial;
- Anger and/or resistance;
- Haggle, or negotiate with yourself;
- Depression/disappointment;
- Acceptance.

This process of acceptance is certainly not static, you do not have to start with denial and end with acceptance. On the contrary, you often see strong changes between the different phases. In addition to strong changes, there is also the repeated return to a certain phase of the process. There is also no "standard" to be given for the duration of the acceptance process and when you "must" be finished accepting!

However, acceptance is important, it helps you to be able to change things. For example, if you have the idea "there is nothing wrong with me, others have a problem with me," you yourself will have less motivation to get started. With the result that things stay the way they are.

Acceptance can also give peace of mind: after all, every person has strengths and weaknesses. Then you can try to use your strong points as much as possible and learn to deal with your less strong points.

Discussion
Are there any positive sides to having ADHD? And how can you make the best use of it?

How to Proceed: The Treatment
What are your expectations of the treatment?

Ask
- What are your expectations regarding the treatment of ADHD?
- Where do you expect improvement and what do you think your life will be like after treatment?

Treatment Options for ADHD
Treatment of ADHD consists of: information, medication, individual (digital) coaching, and group coaching. Coaching means that you will work on your goals under supervision. This can, for example, be agenda management, learning to plan, finding a suitable job, or developing a more positive self-image. It is also possible that you want to learn to think in a different way or learn to behave in a different way. Your coach will evaluate the course of the treatment together with you.

In the group you learn with and through others to increase your organizational skills, you learn certain habits and get support and recognition and many tips. Different groups are possible, consultation which is most suitable for you with your coach.

On Indication: Cognitive Behavioral Therapy and/or Relationship Therapy

In addition to the coaching sessions and the groups, you can make use of cognitive behavioral therapy for additional complaints such as anxiety or depression or a negative self-image. It is also possible to follow relationship therapy. If you think this is applicable, you can discuss this with your coach.

Cooperation with Other Organizations
- Debt counseling;
- Home care;
- Basic care agency;
- Outpatient residential counseling.

Ask your primary caretaker what the possibilities are for a specific problem. Often more is possible than you think.

The treatment is regularly evaluated by means of questionnaires. The duration of treatment varies from six months to three years. If necessary, the treatment can be prolonged if not all treatment goals have yet been achieved.

How Fast Improvement?

If you have relatively few diagnoses, are motivated and keep your appointments, the complaints diminish the quickest (within six months to a year). If, in addition to ADHD, you also suffer from other disorders, such as anxiety, depression, or addiction, these are often treated first. It may then take a little longer before the treatment of ADHD itself can be started, but even then, clear improvement is possible.

The effect of the treatment depends, among other things, on the choice you make whether or not to take medication. Not everyone benefits equally from medication. The chance of clear improvement with the use of the first choice medicine methylphenidate is between 50 and 70%. That is a lot, but it also means that there is a group of 30–50% who experience no or insufficient effect with this medicine. For them there are some alternatives. If this is the case, you can discuss this with your doctor.

Furthermore, it is not the case that all the problems you experience will be solved by the treatment. It is important to have realistic expectations to avoid disappointment.

In short: with treatment a clear improvement of your complaints and functioning is possible. For some people this effect will be greater than for others. You can achieve the optimal result yourself by working as hard as possible.

Evaluation

Themes that have been discussed are discussed and wishes and tips for improving the program are inventoried.

Other Group Offers

Groups at Program ADHD in Adults PSYQ

- *ADHD skills training (8 meetings)*
  The ADHD skills training is aimed at learning practical skills and applying them in your daily life. Themes are: planning and agenda management, setting and planning priorities, problem solving skills, finance and administration, reducing distractions, dealing with procrastination.
- *Study skill training (open group)*
  This group resembles skill training. However, the skills are focused on your studies. Think, for example, of planning and prioritizing, study skills, and dealing with perfectionism.
- *Target group (open group)*
  In this group each participant works on his or her own goals. You will learn to distinguish between short- and long-term goals and to set concrete and achievable goals.
- *Pulse control group (7 meetings)*
  In a number of steps you will learn a number of skills to better deal with certain impulsive behaviors.
- *G-training (8 meetings)*
  A goal of the G-training is to learn to recognize and change negative thinking patterns. The connection between thoughts, feelings, and behavior and the distinction between them are discussed.
- *Self-image group (7 meetings)*
  This group is a possible continuation of the G-training. The goal is that during the group you will try to think more positive about yourself, in a way that is credible for you. Visualization, body posture, and self-talk will be used.
- *Women's group (8 meetings)*
  You learn to deal better with your symptoms and exchange experiences with other women with ADHD. Themes discussed in this group include role expectancy, life phases, communication, relationships, and sexuality.
- *Self-therapy course (also called EPC)*
  During the course you will gradually learn a method for self-therapy in the area of contacts and relationships. The advantage of this method is that you can continue to apply what you have learned after the treatment. Your personal experiences with events in your life are central to the self-therapy.

- *Course parenting (6 meetings)*
  During the course, you will learn, in consultation with your partner, to identify and address problems you experience during your upbringing.
- *Sleep education course (8 meetings)*
  In this course for people with a late sleep phase, you keep track of your sleep pattern and learn to influence your sleep rhythm. Treatment with melatonin and/or light is part of this group.

Groups for Partners, Family Members, and Children

- *Support group (10 meetings)*
  Group for partners, family members, or those directly involved in adults with ADHD. Within this group information and exchange of experiences are central.
- *KOPP (children of parents with psychiatric problems)*
  Group for children (of different ages) of parents with psychiatric problems.

Internet Sites

www.chadd.org *American patient organization for children and adults with ADHD*
www.add.org *Organization for adults with ADHD in the USA*
https://www.additudemag.com *Online magazine on ADHD.*
https://adhdeurope.eu *European patient organization on ADHD*
www.addiss.co.uk *Patient organization on ADHD in the UK*
https://adhdfoundation.org.uk *Health and education service for those with ADHD.*

J. J. S. Kooij, *Adult ADHD*, https://doi.org/10.1007/978-3-030-82812-7

Useful Addresses

European Network Adult ADHD

Carel Reinierszkade 197.
2593 HR Den Haag.
Tel. 088–3,572,040.
E-mail i.vankasteren@psyq.nl
www.eunetworkadultadhd.com

The European Network Adult ADHD is an international network of professionals and scientists from 28 countries in Europe and beyond. The Network was founded in 2002 by Sandra Kooij, aiming to increase knowledge and information about adult ADHD in Europe, to organize symposia, to stimulate research, and to improve access to care for patients. The European Network published two *Consensus Statements* on diagnostics and treatment of ADHD in adults in Europe (in 2010 and in 2019), stimulates the start of national networks of professionals and organizes international symposia and courses.

ADHD Europe

ADHD-Europe aims to advance the rights of, and advocate throughout Europe for, people affected by ADHD and co-morbid conditions in order to help them reach their full potential. ADHD Europe facilitates the efforts of national ADHD organizations in Europe. www.adhdeurope.eu

APSARD, American Professional Society of ADHD and Related Disorders

APSARD is an organization consisting of a broad spectrum of allied mental health experts working to improve the quality of care for patients with ADHD through the advancement and dissemination of research and evidence-based practices. APSARD will fill unmet education and training needs for healthcare professionals helping patients with ADHD, from childhood through adulthood. www.apsard.org

J. J. S. Kooij, *Adult ADHD*, https://doi.org/10.1007/978-3-030-82812-7

EUNETHYDIS, European Network for Hyperkinetic Disorders

EUNETHYDIS is a network of scientists (animal and human research), clinicians and clinical researchers, cardiologists, pharmacologists, and neuroscientists dedicated to the study and treatment of children with Attention Deficit Hyperactivity Disorder (ADHD) or Hyperkinesis. EUNETHYDIS has 40 full members and 120 junior members throughout the EU countries and has held an annual meeting for the last 20 years. Full members of EUNETHYDIS usually hold positions as chairs or heads of department and research institutions. They have all individually contributed both clinically and scientifically to the study of ADHD. Usually members of EUNETHYDIS have at least 20 international peer-reviewed papers on or related to ADHD. EUNETHYDIS has been extremely influential in the care and management of ADHD in European countries and is recognized by institutions such as "'The American Academy of Child and Adolescent Psychiatry," "European Child and Adolescent psychiatry," and the "American Psychiatric Association" as the key European organization on ADHD. https://eutnethydis.eu

World Federation of ADHD

The objective and mission of the World Federation of ADHD is to support and promote worldwide clinical and scientific study projects, including training activities in the field of ADHD (Attention Deficit Hyperactivity Disorder) and related disorders. To also support the exchange of information between scientists, physicians, health experts, ADHD lay organizations, self-help groups, and the public; to collaborate with other related professional and lay organizations. www.adhd-federation.org

References

Adams, Z., Adams, T., Stauffacher, K., Mandel, H., & Wang, Z. (2015). The effects of inattentiveness and hyperactivity on posttraumatic stress symptoms: Does a diagnosis of posttraumatic stress disorder matter? *Journal of Attention Disorders, 24*(9), 1246–1254. https://doi.org/10.1177/1087054715580846. Epub 2015 Apr 16.

Adisetiyo, V., & Gray, K. M. (2017, March). Neuroimaging the neural correlates of increased risk for substance use disorders in attention-deficit/hyperactivity disorder-A systematic review. *The American Journal on Addictions, 26*(2), 99–111.

Adler, C. M., Delbello, M. P., Mills, N. P., Schmithorst, V., Holland, S., & Strakowski, S. M. (2005). Comorbid ADHD is associated with altered patterns of neuronal activation in adolescents with bipolar disorder performing a simple attention task. *Bipolar Disorders, 7*(6), 577–588.

Adler, L., Kunz, M., Chua, H., Rotrosen, J., & Resnick, S. (2004). Attention-Deficit/Hyperactivity Disorder in adult patients with Posttraumatic stress disorder (PTSD): Is ADHD a vulnerability factor? *Journal of Attention Disorders, 8*(1), 11–16.

Adler, L. A., Liebowitz, M., Kronenberger, W., Qiao, M., Rubin, R., Hollandbeck, M., et al. (2009). Atomoxetine treatment in adults with attention-deficit/hyperactivity disorder and comorbid social anxiety disorder. *Depression and Anxiety, 26*(3), 212–221.

Adler, L. A., Spencer, T., Faraone, S. V., Kessler, R. C., Howes, M. J., Biederman, J., et al. (2006). Validity of pilot adult ADHD Self-Report Scale (ASRS) to Rate Adult ADHD symptoms. *Annals of Clinical Psychiatry, 18*(3), 145–148.

Agnew-Blais, J. C., Polanczyk, G. V., Danese, A., Wertz, J., Moffitt, T. E., & Arseneault, L. (2016, July 1). Evaluation of the persistence, remission, and emergence of attention-deficit/hyperactivity disorder in young adulthood. *JAMA Psychiatry, 73*(7), 713–720.

Agranat-Meged, A., Ghanadri, Y., Eisenberg, I., Ben Neriah, Z., Kieselstein-Gross, E., & Mitrani-Rosenbaum, S. (2008). Attention deficit hyperactivity disorder in obese melanocortin-4-receptor (MC4R) deficient subjects: A newly described expression of MC4R deficiency. *American Journal of Medical Genetics Part B Neuropsychiatric Genetics, 5*, 5.

Alpert, J. E., Maddocks, A., Nierenberg, A. A., OíSullivan, R., Pava, J. A., Worthington, J. J., et al. (1996). Attention deficit hyperactivity disorder in childhood among adults with major depression. *Psychiatry Research, 62*(3), 213–219.

Altfas, J. R. (2002). Prevalence of attention deficit/hyperactivity disorder among adults in obesity treatment. *BMC Psychiatry, 2*, 9.

Aman, M. G., Armstrong, S., Buican, B., & Sillick, T. (2002). Four-year follow-up of children with low intelligence and ADHD: A replication. *Research in Developmental Disabilities, 23*(2), 119–134.

Aman, M. G., Buican, B., & Arnold, L. E. (2003). Methylphenidate treatment in children with borderline IQ and mental retardation: Analysis of three aggregated studies. *Journal of Child and Adolescent Psychopharmacology, 13*(1), 29–40.

Amiri, S., Farhang, S., Ghoreishizadeh, M. A., Malek, A., & Mohammadzadeh, S. (2012). Double-blind controlled trial of venlafaxine for treatment of adults with attention deficit/hyperactivity disorder. *Human Psychopharmacology, 27*, 76–81.

Amiri, S., Mohammadi, M. R., Mohammadi, M., Nouroozinejad, G. H., Kahbazi, M., & Akhondzadeh, S. (2008). Modafinil as a treatment for attention-deficit/hyperactivity disorder in children and adolescents: A double blind, randomized clinical trial. *Progress in Neuropsychopharmacology and Biological Psychiatry, 32*(1), 145–149.

Amons, P., Kooij, J., Haffmans, P., Hoffman, T., & Hoencamp, E. (2006). Seasonality of mood disorders in adults with lifetime attention-deficit/hyperactivity disorder (ADHD). *Journal of Affective Disorders, 91*(2-3), 251–255.

Andrade, R. C., Silva, V. A., & Assumpção, F. B., Jr. (2004, August). Preliminary data on the prevalence of psychiatric disorders in Brazilian male and female juvenile delinquents. *Brazilian Journal of Medical and Biological Research, 37*(8), 1.

Anglin, R. E., Samaan, Z., Walter, S. D., & McDonald, S. D. (2013). Vitamin D deficiency and depression in adults: Systematic review and meta-analysis. *The British Journal of Psychiatry, 202*, 100–107.

Angst, J., Gamma, A., Benazzi, F., Ajdacic, V., & Rossler, W. (2008). Does psychomotor agitation in major depressive episodes indicate bipolarity? Evidence from the Zurich study. *European Archives of Psychiatry and Clinical Neuroscience, 19*, 19.

Antalis, C. J., Stevens, L. J., Campbell, M., Pazdro, R., Ericson, K., & Burgess, J. R. (2006). Omega-3 fatty acid status in attention-deficit/hyperactivity disorder. *Prostaglandins, Leukotrienes, and Essential Fatty Acids, 75*(4-5), 299–308.

Antshel, K. M., Faraone, S. V., Maglione, K., Doyle, A., Fried, R., Seidman, L., et al. (2008). Is adult attention deficit hyperactivity disorder a valid diagnosis in the presence of high IQ? *Psychological Medicine, 24*, 1–11.

Antshel, K. M., Phillips, M. H., Gordon, M., Barkley, R., & Faraone, S. V. (2006). Is ADHD a valid disorder in children with intellectual delays? *Clinical Psychology Review, 26*(5), 555–572.

APA. (1994). *Diagnostic and statistical manual of mental disorders* (4th ed.). APA.

APA. (2013). *Diagnostic and statistical manual of mental disorders* (5th ed.). APA.

APA. (2014). *Beknopt overzicht van de criteria DSM-5.* Uitgeverij Boom.

Applegate, B., Lahey, B. B., Hart, E. L., Biederman, J., Hynd, G. W., Barkley, R. A., et al. (1997). Validity of the age-of-onset criterion for ADHD: A report from the DSM-IV field trials. *Journal of the American Academy of Child and Adolescent Psychiatry, 36*(9), 1211–1221.

Arnold, L. E. (2001). Alternative treatments for adults with attention-deficit hyperactivity disorder (ADHD). *Annals of the New York Academy of Sciences, 931*, 310–341.

Arnold, V. K., Feifel, D., Earl, C. Q., Yang, R., & Adler, L. A. (2014, February). A 9-week, randomized, double-blind, placebo-controlled, parallel-group, dose-finding study to evaluate the efficacy and safety of modafinil as treatment for adults with ADHD. *Journal of Attention Disorders, 18*(2), 133–144.

Asherson, P. P. (2004). Bridging the service divide. Invited commentary on: Attention-deficit hyperactivity disorder in adults. *Advances in Psychiatric Treatment, 10*(4), 257–259.

Asherson, P. (2005). Clinical assessment and treatment of attention deficit hyperactivity disorder in adults. *Expert Review of Neurotherapeutics, 5*(4), 525–539.

Babinski, L. M., Hartsough, C. S., & Lambert, N. M. (1999). Childhood conduct problems, hyperactivity-impulsivity, and inattention as predictors of adult criminal activity. *Journal of Child Psychology and Psychiatry, 40*(3), 347–355.

Bagot, K. S., & Kaminer, Y. (2014, April). Efficacy of stimulants for cognitive enhancement in non-attention deficit hyperactivity disorder youth: A systematic review. *Addiction, 109*(4), 547–557.

Baird, G., Simonoff, E., Pickles, A., Chandler, S., Loucas, T., Meldrum, D., et al. (2006). Prevalence of disorders of the autism spectrum in a population cohort of children in South Thames: The Special Needs and Autism Project (SNAP). *Lancet, 368*(9531), 210–215.

Banaschewski, T., Hollis, C., Oosterlaan, J., Roeyers, H., Rubia, K., Willcutt, E., et al. (2005). Towards an understanding of unique and shared pathways in the psychopathophysiology of ADHD. *Developmental Science, 8*(2), 132–140.

Bangs, M. E., Emslie, G. J., Spencer, T. J., Ramsey, J. L., Carlson, C., Bartky, E. J., et al. (2007). Efficacy and safety of atomoxetine in adolescents with attention-deficit/hyperactivity disorder and major depression. *Journal of Child and Adolescent Psychopharmacology, 17*(4), 407–420.

Bangs, M. E., Jin, L., Zhang, S., Desaiah, D., Allen, A. J., Read, H. A., et al. (2008). Hepatic events associated with atomoxetine treatment for attention-deficit hyperactivity disorder. *Drug Safety, 31*(4), 345–354.

Bangs, M. E., Tauscher-Wisniewski, S., Polzer, J., Zhang, S., Acharya, N., Desaiah, D., et al. (2008). Meta-analysis of suicide-related behavior events in patients treated with atomoxetine. *Journal of the American Academy of Child and Adolescent Psychiatry, 47*(2), 209–218.

Barch, D. M., & Carter, C. S. (2005, September 1). Amphetamine improves cognitive function in medicated individuals with schizophrenia and in healthy volunteers. *Schizophrenia Research, 77*(1), 43–58.

Barkley, R. A. (1997a). *ADHD and the nature of self-control*. The Guilford Press.

Barkley, R. A. (1997b). Age dependent decline in ADHD: True recovery or statistical illusion? *The ADHD Report, 5*, 1–5.

Barkley, R. A., & Biederman, J. (1997). Toward a broader definition of the age-of-onset criterion for attention-deficit hyperactivity disorder. *Journal of the American Academy of Child and Adolescent Psychiatry, 36*(9), 1204–1210.

Barkley, R. A., & Cox, D. A. (2007). Review of driving risks and impairments associated with attention-deficit/hyperactivity disorder and the effects of stimulant medication on driving performance. *Journal of Safety Research, 38*(1), 113–128.

Barkley, R. A., Murphy, K. R., O'Connell, T., & Connor, D. F. (2005, April). Effects of two doses of methylphenidate on simulator driving performance in adults with attention deficit hyperactivity disorder. *Journal of Safety Research, 36*(2), 121–31. https://doi.org/10.1016/j.jsr.2005.01.001. Epub 18. PMID: 15896352.

Barkley, R. A., & Fischer, M. (2005). Suicidality in children with ADHD, grown up. *The ADHD Report, 13*(6), 1–6.

Barkley, R. A., Fischer, M., Smallish, L., & Fletcher, K. (2006). Young adult outcome of hyperactive children: Adaptive functioning in major life activities. *Journal of the American Academy of Child and Adolescent Psychiatry, 45*(2), 192–202.

Barkley, R. A., Guevremont, D. C., Anastopoulos, A. D., DuPaul, G. J., & Shelton, T. L. (1993). Driving-related risks and outcomes of attention deficit hyperactivity disorder in adolescents and young adults: A 3-to 5-year follow-up survey. *Pediatrics, 92*(2 I), 212–218.

Barkley, R. A., & Murphy, K. R. (2006). *Attention-deficit hyperactivity disorder, 3rd ed.: A clinical workbook*. Guilford Publications.

Barkley, R. A., Murphy, K. R., & Fischer, M. (2007). *ADHD in adults. What the science says*. The Guilford Press.

Barkley, R. A., Murphy, K. R., & Kwasnik, D. (1996). Motor vehicle driving competencies and risks in teens and young adults with attention deficit hyperactivity disorder. *Pediatrics, 98*(6 Pt 1), 1089–1095.

Bartsch, H., Buchberger, A., Franz, H., Bartsch, C., Maidonis, I., Mecke, D., et al. (2000). Effect of melatonin and pineal extracts on human ovarian and mammary tumor cells in a chemosensitivity assay. *Life Sciences, 67*(24), 2953–2960.

Bauer, M., Beaulieu, S., Dunner, D. L., Lafer, B., & Kupka, R. (2008). Rapid cycling bipolar disorder--diagnostic concepts. *Bipolar Disorders, 10*(1 Pt 2), 153–162.

Bekker, E. M. (2004). *Inhibitory control and adults with ADHD*. Thesis, University of Utrecht, Utrecht.

Bekker, E. M., Kooij, J. J. S., & Buitelaar, J. K. (*2008*). Sleep and quality of life in ADHD. In J. Verster (Ed.), *Sleep and quality of life in medical illness*. Humana Press.

Bekker, E. M., Overtoom, C. C., Kooij, J. J. S., Buitelaar, J. K., Verbaten, M. N., & Kenemans, J. (2005). Disentangling deficits in adults with attention-deficit/hyperactivity disorder. *Archives of General Psychiatry, 62*(10), 1129–1136.

Berkey, C. S., Rockett, H. R., Gillman, M. W., Field, A. E., & Colditz, G. A. (2003). Longitudinal study of skipping breakfast and weight change in adolescents. *International Journal of Obesity and Related Metabolic Disorders, 27*(10), 1258–1266.

Berman, T., Douglas, V. I., & Barr, R. G. (1999). Effects of methylphenidate on complex cognitive processing in attention- deficit hyperactivity disorder. *Journal of Abnormal Psychology, 108*(1), 90–105.

Berman, S. M., Kuczenski, R., McCracken, J. T., & London, E. D. (2009, February). Potential adverse effects of amphetamine treatment on brain and behavior: A review. *Molecular Psychiatry, 14*(2), 123–142.

Bernfort, L., Nordfeldt, S., & Persson, J. (2008). ADHD from a socio-economic perspective. *Acta Paediatrica, 97*(2), 239–245.

Biederman, J. (1998). A 55-year-old man with attention-deficit/hyperactivity disorder. *JAMA Journal of the American Medical Association, 280*(12), 1086.

Biederman, J., Arnsten, A. F., Faraone, S. V., Doyle, A. E., Spencer, T. J., Wilens, T. E., et al. (2006). New developments in the treatment of ADHD. *Journal of Clinical Psychiatry, 67*(1), 148–159.

Biederman, J., Ball, S. W., Monuteaux, M. C., Mick, E., Spencer, T. J., McCREARY, M., et al. (2008, April). New insights into the comorbidity between ADHD and major depression in adolescent and young adult females. *Journal of the American Academy of Child and Adolescent Psychiatry, 47*(4), 426–34. https://doi.org/10.1097/CHI.0b013e31816429d3. PMID: 18388760.

Biederman, J., & Faraone, S. V. (2006). The effects of attention-deficit/hyperactivity disorder on employment and household income. *Medgenmed: Medscape General Medicine, 8*(3), 12.

Biederman, J., Faraone, S. V., Mick, E., Williamson, S., Wilens, T. E., Spencer, T. J., et al. (1999). Clinical correlates of ADHD in females: Findings from a large group of girls ascertained from pediatric and psychiatric referral sources. *Journal of the American Academy of Child and Adolescent Psychiatry, 38*(8), 966–975.

Biederman, J., Faraone, S., Milberger, S., Curtis, S., Chen, L., Marrs, A., et al. (1996). Predictors of persistence and remission of ADHD into adolescence: Results from a four-year prospective follow-up study. *Journal of the American Academy of Child and Adolescent Psychiatry, 35*(3), 343–351.

Biederman, J., Faraone, S., Milberger, S., Guite, J., Mick, E., Chen, L., et al. (1996). A prospective 4-year follow-up study of attention-deficit hyperactivity and related disorders. *Archives of General Psychiatry, 53*(5), 437–446.

Biederman, J., Faraone, S. V., Spencer, T., Wilens, T., Norman, D., Lapey, K. A., et al. (1993). Patterns of psychiatric comorbidity, cognition, and psychosocial functioning in adults with attention deficit hyperactivity disorder. *American Journal of Psychiatry, 150*(12), 1792–1798.

Biederman, J., Faraone, S. V., Spencer, T., Wilens, T. E., et al. (1994). Gender differences in a sample of adults with attention deficit hyperactivity disorder. *Psychiatry Research, 53*(1), 13–29.

Biederman, J., Faraone, S. V., Wozniak, J., Mick, E., Kwon, A., Cayton, G. A., & Clark, S. V. (2005). Clinical correlates of bipolar disorder in a large, referred sample of children and adolescents. *Journal of Psychiatric Research, 39*(6), 611–622.

Biederman, J., Melmed, R. D., Patel, A., McBurnett, K., Donahue, J., & Lyne, A. (2008). Long-term, open-label extension study of guanfacine extended release in children and adolescents with ADHD. *CNS Spectrums, 13*(12), 1047–1055.

Biederman, J., Mick, E., & Faraone, S. V. (2000). Age-dependent decline of symptoms of attention deficit hyperactivity disorder: Impact of remission definition and symptom type. *American Journal of Psychiatry, 157*(5), 816–818.

Biederman, J., Mick, E., Faraone, S. V., Braaten, E., Doyle, A., Spencer, T., et al. (2002). Influence of gender on attention deficit hyperactivity disorder in children referred to a psychiatric clinic. *American Journal of Psychiatry, 159*(1), 36–42.

Biederman, J., Newcorn, J., & Sprich, S. (1991). Comorbidity of attention deficit hyperactivity disorder with conduct, depressive, anxiety, and other disorders. *American Journal of Psychiatry, 148*(5), 564–577.

Biederman, J., Petty, C. R., Dolan, C., Hughes, S., Mick, E., Monuteaux, M. C., et al. (2008, July). The long-term longitudinal course of oppositional defiant disorder and conduct disorder in ADHD boys: Findings from a controlled 10-year prospective longitudinal follow-up study. *Psychological Medicine, 38*(7), 1027–1036.

Biederman, J., Makris, N., Valera, E. M., Monuteaux, M. C., Goldstein, J. M., Buka, S., et al. (2008, July). Towards further understanding of the co-morbidity between attention deficit hyperactivity disorder and bipolar disorder: a MRI study of brain volumes. *Psychological Medicine, 38*(7), 1045–56. https://doi.org/10.1017/S0033291707001791. Epub 2007 Oct 15. PMID: 17935640.

Biederman, J., Petty, C. R., Spencer, T. J., Woodworth, K. Y., Bhide, P., Zhu, J., et al. (2014, January). Is ADHD a risk for posttraumatic stress disorder (PTSD)? Results from a large longitudinal study of referred children with and without ADHD. *The World Journal of Biological Psychiatry, 15*(1), 49–55.

Biederman, J., & Pliszka, S. R. (2008). Modafinil improves symptoms of attention-deficit/hyperactivity disorder across subtypes in children and adolescents. *Journal of Pediatrics, 152*(3), 394–399.

Biederman, J., Seidman, L. J., Petty, C. R., Fried, R., Doyle, A. E., Cohen, D. R., et al. (2008). Effects of stimulant medication on neuropsychological functioning in young adults with attention-deficit/hyperactivity disorder. *Journal of Clinical Psychiatry, 69*(7), 1150–1156.

Bijlenga, D., Jasperse, M., Gehlhaar, S. K., & Kooij, J. J. S. (2015, January). Objective QbTest and subjective evaluation of stimulant treatment in adult attention deficit-hyperactivity disorder. *European Psychiatry, 30*(1), 179–185.

Bijlenga, D., Ulberstad, F., Thorell, L. B., Christiansen, H., Hirsch, O., & Kooij, J. J. S. (2019 Oct). Objective assessment of attention-deficit/hyperactivity disorder in older adults compared with controls using the QbTest. *International Journal of Geriatric Psychiatry, 34*(10), 1526–1533.

Bijlenga, D., Van der Heijden, K. B., Breuk, M., Van Someren, E. J., Lie, M. E., Boonstra, A. M., et al. (2013). Associations between sleep characteristics, seasonal depressive symptoms, lifestyle, and ADHD symptoms in adults. *Journal of Attention Disorders, 17*(3), 261–275.

Bijlenga, D., Van Someren, E. J., Gruber, R., Bron, T. I., Kruithof, I. F., Spanbroek, E. C., & Kooij, J. J. (2013, December). Body temperature, activity and melatonin profiles in adults with attention-deficit/hyperactivity disorder and delayed sleep: A case-control study. *Journal of Sleep Research, 22*(6), 607–616.

Bijlenga, D., Vroege, J. A., Stammen, A. J. M., Breuk, M., Boonstra, M., Van der Rhee, K., & et al. (2017). *Prevalence of sexual dysfunctions and other sexual disorders in adults with attention-deficit/hyperactivity disorder compared to the general population.*

Bilodeau, M., Simon, T., Beauchamp, M. H., Lesperance, P., Dubreucq, S., Doree, J. P., et al. (2014). Duloxetine in adults with ADHD: A randomized, placebo-controlled pilot study. *Journal of Attention Disorders, 18*, 169–175.

Birnbaum, H. G., Kessler, R. C., Lowe, S. W., Secnik, K., Greenberg, P. E., Leong, S. A., et al. (2005). Costs of attention deficit-hyperactivity disorder (ADHD) in the US: Excess costs of persons with ADHD and their family members in 2000. *Current Medical Research and Opinion, 21*(2), 195–206.

Blick, S. K., & Keating, G. M. (2007). Lisdexamfetamine. *Paediatric Drugs, 9*(2), 129–135. discussion 136-128.

Bloch, M. H., & Qawasmi, A. (2011). Omega-3 fatty acid supplementation for the treatment of children with attention-deficit/hyperactivity disorder symptomatology: systematic review and meta-analysis. *Journal of the American Academy of Child and Adolescent Psychiatry, 50*, 991–1000.

Blocher, D., Henkel, K., Retz, W., Retz-Junginger, P., Thome, J., & Rosler, M. (2001). Symptoms from the spectrum of attention-deficit/hyperactivity disorder (ADHD) in sexual delinquents. *Fortschritte der Neurologie-Psychiatrie, 69*(10), 453–459.

Blockmans, D., Persoons, P., Van Houdenhove, B., & Bobbaers, H. (2006). Does methylphenidate reduce the symptoms of chronic fatigue syndrome? *American Journal of Medicine, 119*(2), 167.e123–167.e130.

Blom, J. D., & Kooij, J. J. S. (2012). De ADD psychose: Behandeling met antipsychotica en methylfenidaat? *Tijdschrift voor Psychiatrie, 54*(1), 89–93.

Blum, K., Sheridan, P. J., Wood, R. C., Braverman, E. R., Chen, T. J., & Comings, D. E. (1995). Dopamine D2 receptor gene variants: Association and linkage studies in impulsive-addictive-compulsive behaviour. *Pharmacogenetics, 5*(3), 121–141.

Boere-Boonekamp, M. M., LíHoir, M. P., Beltman, M., Bruil, J., Dijkstra, N., & Engelberts, A. C. (2008). Overweight and obesity in preschool children (0-4 years): Behaviour and views of parents, in Dutch. *Ned Tijdschr voor Geneeskd, 152*(6), 324–330.

Boonstra, A. M., Kooij, J. J. S., Oosterlaan, J., Sergeant, J. A., & Buitelaar, J. K. (2007). Hyperactive night and day? Actigraphy studies in adult ADHD: Baseline comparison and the effect of methylphenidate. *Sleep, 30*(4), 433–442.

Boonstra, A. M., Oosterlaan, J., Sergeant, J. A., & Buitelaar, J. K. (2005). Executive functioning in adult ADHD: A meta-analytic review. *Psychological Medicine, 35*(8), 1097–1108.

Boonstra, A. M., Sergeant, J. A., & Kooij, J. J. S. (1999, October). Attention deficit hyperactivity disorder, een typische kinderstoornis... Of toch niet? *De Psycholoog, 34*(10), 442–447.

Botting, N., Powls, A., Cooke, R. W., & Marlow, N. (1997). Attention deficit hyperactivity disorders and other psychiatric outcomes in very low birthweight children at 12 years. *Journal of Child Psychology and Psychiatry, 38*(8), 931–941.

Briscoe-Smith, A. M., & Hinshaw, S. P. (2006). Linkages between child abuse and attention-deficit/hyperactivity disorder in girls: Behavioral and social correlates. *Child Abuse and Neglect, 30*(11), 1239–1255.

Bro, S. P., Kjaersgaard, M. I., Parner, E. T., Sørensen, M. J., Olsen, J., Bech, B. H., et al. (2015, January). Adverse pregnancy outcomes after exposure to methylphenidate or atomoxetine during pregnancy. *Clinical Epidemiology, 29*(7), 139–147.

Bron, T. I., Bijlenga, D., Boonstra, A. M., Breuk, M., Pardoen, W. F., Beekman, A. T., & Kooij, J. J. S. (2014, April). OROS-methylphenidate efficacy on specific executive functioning deficits in adults with ADHD: A randomized, placebo-controlled cross-over study. *European Neuropsychopharmacology, 24*(4), 519–528.

Bron, T. I., Bijlenga, D., Breuk, M., Michielsen, M., Beekman, A. T. F., & Kooij, J. J. S. (2017, Submitted). *Risk factors for adverse driving outcomes in Dutch adults with ADHD and controls.*

Bron, T. I., Bijlenga, D., Kasander, M. V., Spuijbroek, A. T., Beekman, A. T., & Kooij, J. J. S. (2013, June). Long-term relationship between methylphenidate and tobacco consumption and nicotine craving in adults with ADHD in a prospective cohort study. *European Neuropsychopharmacology, 23*(6), 542–554.

Bron, T. I., Bijlenga, D., Verduijn, J., Penninx, B. W., Beekman, A. T., & Kooij, J. J. S. (2016, June). Prevalence of ADHD symptoms across clinical stages of major depressive disorder. *Journal of Affective Disorders, 197*, 29–35.

Brown, T. E. (1996). *Brown attention-deficit disorder scales. Manual.* The Psychological Corporation.

Brown, T. E. (Ed.). (2000). *Attention-deficit disorders and comorbidities in children, adolescents, and adults.* American Psychiatric Publishing, Inc..

Brue, A. W., & Oakland, T. D. (2002). Alternative treatments for attention-deficit/hyperactivity disorder: Does evidence support their use? *Alternative Therapies in Health & Medicine, 8*(1), 68–70. 72-64.

Brue, A. W., Oakland, T. D., & Evans, R. A. (2001). The use of a dietary supplement combination and an essential fatty acid as an alternative and complementary treatment for children with attention-deficit/hyperactivity disorder. *Scientific Review of Alternative Medicine, 5*(4), 187–194.

Bruni, O., Alonso-Alconada, D., Besag, F., Biran, V., Braam, W., Cortese, S., Moavero, R., et al. (2015, March). Current role of melatonin in pediatric neurology: clinical recommendations. *European Journal of Paediatric Neurology, 19*(2), 122–33. https://doi.org/10.1016/j.ejpn.2014.12.007. Epub 2014 Dec 17. PMID: 25553845.

Bryer, J. B., Nelson, B. A., Miller, J. B., & Krol, P. A. (1987). Childhood sexual and physical abuse as factors in adult psychiatric illness. *American Journal of Psychiatry, 144*(11), 1426–1430.

Buhagiar, K., & Cassar, J. (2007). Methylphenidate augmentation of fluvoxamine for treatment-resistant depression: A case report and review literature. *Türk Psikiyatri Dergisi, 18*(2), 179–183.

Buitelaar, J. K. (2001, August 4). Discussie over attention deficit-hyperactivity disorder (ADHD): Feiten, meningen en emoties. *Nederlands Tijdschrift voor Geneeskunde, 145*(31), 1485–1489.

Buitelaar, J. K. (2002). Epidemiological aspects: What have we learned over the last decade? In S. Sandberg (Ed.), *Hyperactivity and attention disorders of childhood* (2nd ed., pp. 30–64). Cambridge University Press.

Buitelaar, J. K., Danckaerts, M., Gillberg, C., Zuddas, A., Becker, K., Bouvard, M., et al. (2004). A prospective, multicenter, open-label assessment of atomoxetine in non-North American children and adolescents with ADHD. *European Child & Adolescent Psychiatry, 13*(4), 249–257.

Buitelaar, J. K., & Kooij, J. J. S. (2000). Attention deficit hyperactivity disorder (ADHD): Etiology, diagnosis and treatment. (in Dutch). *Nederlands Tijdschrift voor Geneeskunde, 144*(36), 1716–1723.

Buitelaar, N. J., Posthumus, J. A., & Buitelaar, J. K. (2015, May 20). ADHD in childhood and/or adulthood as a risk factor for domestic violence or intimate partner violence: A systematic review. *Journal of Attention Disorders.*

Bumb, J. M., Mier, D., Noelte, I., Schredl, M., Kirsch, P., Hennig, O., et al. (2016, July). Associations of pineal volume, chronotype and symptom severity in adults with attention deficit hyperactivity disorder and healthy controls. *European Neuropsychopharmacology, 26*(7), 1119–1126.

Busch, B. (2007). Polyunsaturated fatty acid supplementation for ADHD? Fishy, fascinating, and far from clear. *Journal of Developmental and Behavioral Pediatrics, 28*(2), 139–144.

Bush, G., Frazier, J. A., Rauch, S. L., Seidman, L. J., Whalen, P. J., Jenike, M. A., et al. (1999). Anterior cingulate cortex dysfunction in attention-deficit/hyperactivity disorder revealed by fMRI and the Counting Stroop. *Biological Psychiatry, 45*(12), 1542–1552.

Butterfield, M. E., Saal, J., Young, B., & Young, J. L. (2016). Supplementary guanfacine hydrochloride as a treatment of attention deficit hyperactivity disorder in adults: A double blind, placebo-controlled study. *Psychiatry Research, 236*, 136–141.

Caci, H., Robert, P., & Boyer, P. (2004, April). Novelty seekers and impulsive subjects are low in morningness. *European Psychiatry, 19*(2), 79–84. https://doi.org/10.1016/j.eurpsy.2003.09.007. PMID: 15051106.

Caci, H., Mattei, V., Bayle, F. J., Nadalet, L., Dossios, C., Robert, P., et al. (2005). Impulsivity but not venturesomeness is related to morningness. *Psychiatry Research, 134*(3), 259–265.

Cairncross, M., & Miller, C. J. (2020). The effectiveness of mindfulness-based therapies for ADHD: A meta-analytic review. *Journal of Attention Disorders, 24*(5), 627–643. https://doi.org/10.1177/1087054715625301. Epub 2016 Feb 2.

Calarge, C., Farmer, C., DiSilvestro, R., & Arnold, L. E. (2010). Serum ferritin and amphetamine response in youth with attention-deficit/hyperactivity disorder. *Journal of Child and Adolescent Psychopharmacology, 20*(6), 495–502.

Campbell, B. C., & Eisenberg, D. (2007). Obesity, attention deficit-hyperactivity disorder and the dopaminergic reward system. *Collegium Antropologicum, 31*(1), 33–38.

Canu, W. H., & Carlson, C. L. (2003). Differences in heterosocial behavior and outcomes of ADHD-symptomatic subtypes in a college sample. *Journal of Attention Disorders, 6*(3), 123–133.

Cappuccio, F. P., Taggart, F. M., Kandala, N. B., Currie, A., Peile, E., Stranges, S., et al. (2008). Meta-analysis of short sleep duration and obesity in children and adults. *Sleep, 31*(5), 619–626.

Capusan, A. J., Kuja-Halkola, R., Bendtsen, P., Viding, E., McCrory, E., Marteinsdottir, I., et al. (2016, September). Childhood maltreatment and attention deficit hyperactivity disorder symptoms in adults: A large twin study. *Psychol Med, 46*(12), 2637–2646.

Carlson, G. A., Loney, J., Salisbury, H., Kramer, J. R., & Arthur, C. (2000). Stimulant treatment in young boys with symptoms suggesting childhood mania: A report from a longitudinal study. *Journal of Child and Adolescent Psychopharmacology, 10*(3), 175–184.

Carlson, P. J., Merlock, M. C., & Suppes, T. (2004). Adjunctive stimulant use in patients with bipolar disorder: Treatment of residual depression and sedation. *Bipolar Disorders, 6*(5), 416–420.

Carpentier, P. J. (2002). Olie op de golven, olie op het vuur: ADHD en verslaving. In *Handboek Verslaving*. Bohn Stafleu van Loghum.

Carpentier, P. J. (2007). Farmacotherapie bij ADHD met verslaving. *Psyfar, nascholingstijdschrift over psychofarmacologie, 2*(4), 46–48.

Carpentier, P.J., & Levin, F.R. (2017, March/April). Pharmacological Treatment of ADHD in Addicted Patients: What Does the Literature Tell Us? *Harvard Review of Psychiatry, 25*(2),

50–64. https://doi.org/10.1097/HRP.0000000000000122. PMID: 28272130; PMCID: PMC5518741.

Carrillo-Vico, A., Guerrero, J. M., Lardone, P. J., & Reiter, R. J. (2005). A review of the multiple actions of melatonin on the immune system. *Endocrine, 27*(2), 189–200.

Castellanos, F. X. (2002). Anatomic magnetic resonance imaging studies of attention-deficit/ hyperactivity disorder. *Dialogues in Clinical Neuroscience, 4*(4), 444–448.

Castellanos, F. X., Giedd, J. N., Berquin, P. C., Walter, J. M., Sharp, W., Tran, T., et al. (2001). Quantitative brain magnetic resonance imaging in girls with attention-deficit/hyperactivity disorder. *Archives of General Psychiatry, 58*(3), 289–295.

Castellanos, F. X., Lee, P. P., Sharp, W., Jeffries, N. O., Greenstein, D. K., Clasen, L. S., et al. (2002). Developmental trajectories of brain volume abnormalities in children and adolescents with attention-deficit/hyperactivity disorder. *Journal of the American Medical Association, 288*(14), 1740–1748.

Castellanos, F. X., & Tannock, R. (2002). Neuroscience of attention-deficit/hyperactivity disorder: The search for endophenotypes. *Nature Reviews. Neuroscience, 3*, 617–628.

Castells, X., Ramos-Quiroga, J. A., Bosch, R., et al. (2011). Amphetamines for Attention Deficit Hyperactivity Disorder (ADHD) in adults. *Cochrane Database of Systematic Reviews, 6*, CD007813.

Cath, D. C., Ran, N., Smit, J. H., Van Balkom, A. J., & Comijs, H. C. (2008). Symptom overlap between autism spectrum disorder, generalized social anxiety disorder and obsessive-compulsive disorder in adults: A preliminary case-controlled study. *Psychopathology, 41*(2), 101–110.

Caye, A., Rocha, T. B., Anselmi, L., Murray, J., Menezes, A. M., Barros, F. C., et al. (2016, July 1). Attention-deficit/hyperactivity disorder trajectories from childhood to young adulthood: Evidence from a birth cohort supporting a late-onset syndrome. *JAMA Psychiatry, 73*(7), 705–712.

Chamberlain, S. R., Del Campo, N., Dowson, J., Muller, U., Clark, L., Robbins, T. W., et al. (2007). Atomoxetine improved response inhibition in adults with attention deficit/hyperactivity disorder. *Biological Psychiatry, 62*(9), 977–984.

Chan, E., Rappaport, L. A., & Kemper, K. J. (2003). Complementary and alternative therapies in childhood attention and hyperactivity problems. *Journal of Developmental & Behavioral Pediatrics, 24*(1), 4–8.

Chan, E., Zhan, C., & Homer, C. J. (2002). Health care use and costs for children with attention-deficit/hyperactivity disorder: National estimates from the medical expenditure panel survey. *Archives of Pediatrics and Adolescent Medicine, 156*(5), 504–511.

Chandra, S., Biederman, J., & Faraone, S. V. (2021 Jan). Assessing the validity of the age at onset criterion for diagnosing ADHD in *DSM-5*. *Journal of Attention Disorders, 25*(2), 143–153.

Chang, Z., D'Onofrio, B. M., Quinn, P. D., Lichtenstein, P., & Larsson, H. (2016, December 15). Medication for attention-deficit/hyperactivity disorder and risk for depression: A nationwide longitudinal cohort *study. Biological Psychiatry, 80*(12), 916–922.

Chao, C. Y., Gau, S. S., Mao, W. C., Shyu, J. F., Chen, Y. C., & Yeh, C. B. (2008). Relationship of attention-deficit-hyperactivity disorder symptoms, depressive/anxiety symptoms, and life quality in young men. *Psychiatry and Clinical Neurosciences, 62*(4), 421–426.

Chen, M. H., Pan, T. L., Hsu, J. W., Huang, K. L., Su, T. P., Li, C. T., et al. (2016, November). Attention-deficit hyperactivity disorder comorbidity and antidepressant resistance among patients with major depression: A nationwide longitudinal study. *European Neuropsychopharmacology, 26*(11), 1760–1767.

Cherkasova, M. V., French, L. R., Syer, C. A., Cousins, L., Galina, H., Ahmadi-Kashani, Y., et al. (2016, October 1). Efficacy of cognitive behavioral therapy with and without medication for adults with ADHD. *Journal of Attention Disorders*.

Christakou, A., Murphy, C. M., Chantiluke, K., Cubillo, A. I., Smith, A. B., Giampietro, V., et al. (2013). Disorder-specific functional abnormalities during sustained attention in youth with Attention Deficit Hyperactivity Disorder (ADHD) and with autism. *Molecular Psychiatry, 18*(2), 236–244.

Christiansen, H., Oades, R. D., Psychogiou, L., Hauffa, B. P., & Sonuga-Barke, E. J. (2010, July). Does the cortisol response to stress mediate the link between expressed emotion and oppositional behavior in Attention-Deficit/Hyperactivity-Disorder (ADHD)? *Behavioral and Brain Functions, 15*(6), 45.

Clemow, D. B., & Walker, D. J. (2014, September). The potential for misuse and abuse of medications in ADHD: a review. *Postgraduate Medicine, 126*(5), 6–81. https://doi.org/10.3810/pgm.2014.09.2801. PMID: 25295651.

Colter, A. L., Cutler, C., & Meckling, K. A. (2008). Fatty acid status and behavioural symptoms of attention deficit hyperactivity disorder in adolescents: A case-control study. *Nutrition Journal, 14*(7), 8.

Compernolle, T. (1993). Adolescenten en volwassenen met een ADHD vallen tussen de wal van de kinderpsychiatrie en het schip van de volwassen psychiatrie. In J. K. Buitelaar (Ed.), *Diagnostiek en behandeling van ADHD: Aandachtstekortstoornis met hyperactiviteit* (pp. 107–118). Stichting Onderwijs en Voorlichting.

Conners, C. K., Erhardt, D., & Sparrow, E. (1999). *Conners Adult ADHD Rating Scales (CAARS). Technical Manual.* Multi Health Systems Inc..

Connor, D. F., & Steingard, R. J. (2004). New formulations of stimulants for attention-deficit hyperactivity disorder: Therapeutic potential. *CNS Drugs, 18*(14), 1011–1030.

Conway, J., Wong, K. K., OíConnell, C., & Warren, A. E. (2008). Cardiovascular risk screening before starting stimulant medications and prescribing practices of Canadian physicians: Impact of the Health Canada advisory. *Pediatrics, 122*(4), e828–e834.

Coogan, A. N., & McGowan, N. M. (2017, September). A systematic review of circadian function, chronotype and chronotherapy in attention deficit hyperactivity disorder. *Attention Deficit Hyperactivity Disorder, 9*(3), 129–47. https://doi.org/10.1007/s12402-016-0214-5.

Cooke, T., & So, T. Y. (2016). Attention deficit hyperactive disorder and occurrence of tic disorders in children and adolescents-what is the verdict. *Current Pediatric Reviews, 12*(3), 230–238.

Copinschi, G., Leproult, R., & Spiegel, K. (2014). The important role of sleep in metabolism. *Frontiers of Hormone Research, 42*, 59–72.

Corkum, P., Tannock, R., Moldofsky, H., Hogg-Johnson, S., & Humphries, T. (2001). Actigraphy and parental ratings of sleep in children with attention-deficit/hyperactivity disorder (ADHD). *Sleep, 24*(3), 303–312.

Corominas-Roso, M., Palomar, G., Ferrer, R., Real, A., Nogueira, M., Corrales, M., et al. (2015, March 17). Cortisol response to stress in adults with attention deficit hyperactivity disorder. *The International Journal of Neuropsychopharmacology, 18*(9), pyv027.

Cortese, S., Azoulay, R., Castellanos, F. X., Chalard, F., Lecendreux, M., Chechin, D., et al. (2012). Brain iron levels in attention-deficit/hyperactivity disorder: A pilot MRI study. *The World Journal of Biological Psychiatry, 13*(3), 223–231.

Cortese, S., Ferrin, M., Brandeis, D., Holtmann, M., Aggensteiner, P., Daley, D., et al. (2016, June). Neurofeedback for attention-deficit/hyperactivity disorder: Meta-analysis of clinical and neuropsychological outcomes from randomized controlled trials. *Journal of the American Academy of Child and Adolescent Psychiatry, 55*(6), 444–455.

Cortese, S., Isnard, P., Frelut, M. L., Michel, G., & Quantin, L. (2007). Association between symptoms of attention-deficit/hyperactivity disorder and bulimic behaviors in a clinical sample of severely obese adolescents. *International Journal of Obesity, 31*(2), 340–346.

Cortese, S., Kelly, C., Chabernaud, C., Proal, E., Di Martino, A., Milham, M. P., & Castellanos, F. X. (2012, October). Toward systems neuroscience of ADHD: A meta-analysis of 55 fMRI studies. *The American Journal of Psychiatry, 169*(10), 1038–1055.

Cortese, S., Vincenzi, B. (2012). Obesity and ADHD: clinical and neurobiological implications. *Current Topics in Behavioral Neurosciences*, 9, 199–218. https://doi.org/10.1007/7854_2011_154. PMID: 21845534.

Cortese, S., Konofal, E., Bernardina, B. D., Mouren, M. C., & Lecendreux, M. (2009). Sleep disturbances and serum ferritin levels in children with attention-deficit/hyperactivity disorder. *European Child & Adolescent Psychiatry, 18*(7), 393–399.

Cortese, S., Konofal, E., Dalla Bernardina, B., Mouren, M. C., & Lecendreux, M. (2008). Does excessive daytime sleepiness contribute to explaining the association between obesity and ADHD symptoms? *Medical Hypotheses, 70*(1), 12–16.

Cortese, S., Konofal, E., Lecendreux, M., Arnulf, I., Mouren, M. C., Darra, F., et al. (2005). Restless legs syndrome and attention-deficit/hyperactivity disorder: A review of the literature. *Sleep, 28*(8), 1007–1013.

Cortese, S., Moreira-Maia, C. R., St Fleur, D., Morcillo-Peñalver, C., Rohde, L. A., & Faraone, S. V. (2016, January). Association between ADHD and obesity: A systematic review and meta-analysis. *The American Journal of Psychiatry, 173*(1), 34-43.

Cortese, S., & Tessari, L. (2017, January). Attention-Deficit/Hyperactivity Disorder (ADHD) and obesity: Update 2016. *Current Psychiatry Reports, 19*(1), 4.

Coulter, M. K., & Dean, M. E. (2007). Homeopathy for attention deficit/hyperactivity disorder or hyperkinetic disorder. *Cochrane Database of Systematic Reviews, 17*(4), CD005648.

Cox, D. J., Humphrey, J. W., Merkel, R. L., Penberthy, J. K., & Kovatchev, B. (2004). Controlled-release methylphenidate improves attention during on-road driving by adolescents with attention-deficit/hyperactivity disorder. *Journal of the American Board of Family Practice, 17*(4), 235–239.

Cox, D. J., Merkel, R. L., Moore, M., Thorndike, F., Muller, C., & Kovatchev, B. (2006). Relative benefits of stimulant therapy with OROS methylphenidate versus mixed amphetamine salts extended release in improving the driving performance of adolescent drivers with attention-deficit/hyperactivity disorder. *Pediatrics, 118*(3), e704–e710.

Cox, D. J., Merkel, R. L., Penberthy, J. K., Kovatchev, B., & Hankin, C. S. (2004). Impact of methylphenidate delivery profiles on driving performance of adolescents with attention-deficit/hyperactivity disorder: A pilot study. *Journal of the American Academy of Child and Adolescent Psychiatry, 43*(3), 269–275.

Cox, D. J., Punja, M., Powers, K., Merkel, R., Burket, R., Moore, M., et al. (2006a). Manual transmission enhances attention and driving performance of ADHD adolescent males: Pilot study. *Journal of Attention Disorders, 10*(2), 212–216.

Cox, D. J., Punja, M., Powers, K., Merkel, R., Burket, R., Moore, M., et al. (2006b). Manual transmission enhances attention and driving performance of ADHD adolescent males: Pilot study. *Journal of Attention Disorders, 10*(2), 212–216.

Crosbie, J., Perusse, D., Barr, C. L., & Schachar, R. J. (2008). Validating psychiatric endophenotypes: Inhibitory control and attention deficit hyperactivity disorder. *Neuroscience and Biobehavioral Reviews, 32*(1), 40–55.

Da Silva, M. A., & Louza, M. (2008). Case of a 67-year-old woman diagnosed with ADHD successfully treated with methylphenidate. *Journal of Attention Disorders, 11*(6), 623.

Dalsgaard, S., Mortensen, P. B., Frydenberg, M., & Thomsen, P. H. (2013, April). Long-term criminal outcome of children with attention deficit hyperactivity disorder. *Criminal Behaviour and Mental Health, 23*(2), 86–98.

Dalsgaard, S., Østergaard, S. D., Leckman, J. F., Mortensen, P. B., & Pedersen, M. G. (2015, May 30). Mortality in children, adolescents, and adults with attention deficit hyperactivity disorder: A nationwide cohort study. *Lancet, 385*(9983), 2190–2196.

Daviss, W. B., Birmaher, B., Diler, R. S., Mintz, J., & Spencer, T. J. (2008). Does pharmacotherapy for attention-deficit/hyperactivity disorder predict risk of later major depression? Treatment of adult ADHD and comorbid depression. *Journal of Child and Adolescent Psychopharmacology, 18*(3), 257–264.

De Carvalho, T. D., Wajnsztejn, R., De Abreu, L. C., Marques Vanderlei, L. C., Godoy, M. F., Adami, F., et al. (2014, April). Analysis of cardiac autonomic modulation of children with attention deficit hyperactivity disorder. *Neuropsychiatric Disease and Treatment, 11*(10), 613–618.

De Crescenzo, F., Cortese, S., Adamo, N., & Janiri, L. (2017). Pharmacological and non-pharmacological treatment of adults with ADHD: A meta-review. *BMC Psychiatry*. in press.

De Ridder, T., Bruffearts, R., Danckaerts, M., Bonnewyn, A., & Demyttenaere, K. (2008). The prevalence of ADHD in the Belgian general adult population: An epidemiological explanatory study, in Dutch. *Tijdschrift voor Psychiatrie, 50*(8), 499–508.

De Zeeuw, P., Mandl, R. C., Hulshoff Pol, H. E., Van Engeland, H., & Durston, S. (2012, August). Decreased frontostriatal microstructural organization in attention deficit/hyperactivity disorder. *Human Brain Mapping, 33*(8), 1941–1951.

Dekker, M. C., & Koot, H. M. (2003). DSM-IV disorders in children with borderline to moderate intellectual disability. II: Child and family predictors. *Journal of the American Academy of Child and Adolescent Psychiatry, 42*(8), 923–931.

Demontis, D., Walters, R. K., Martin, J., Mattheisen, M., Als, T. D., Agerbo, E., Baldursson, G., Belliveau, R., Bybjerg-Grauholm, J., Bækvad-Hansen, M., Cerrato, F., Chambert, K., Churchhouse, C., Dumont, A., Eriksson, N., Gandal, M., Goldstein, J. I., Grasby, K. L., Grove, J., … Neale, B. M. (2019 January). Discovery of the first genome-wide significant risk loci for attention deficit/hyperactivity disorder. *Nature Genetics, 51*(1), 63–75.

Dideriksen, D., Pottegård, A., Hallas, J., Aagaard, L., & Damkier, P. (2013, February). First trimester in utero exposure to methylphenidate. *Basic & Clinical Pharmacology & Toxicology, 112*(2), 73–76.

Dodson, W. W. (1999). *The prevalence and treatment of sleep disorders in adults with Attention Deficit/Hyperactivity Disorder.* Presented at the american psychiatric association annual convention, Washington DC.

Dolder, C. R., Davis, L. N., & McKinsey, J. (2010). Use of psychostimulants in patients with dementia. *The Annals of Pharmacotherapy, 44*(10), 1624–1632.

Donfrancesco, R., Parisi, P., Vanacore, N., Martines, F., Sargentini, V., & Cortese, S. (2013). Iron and ADHD: Time to move beyond serum ferritin levels. *Journal of Attention Disorders, 17*(4), 347–357. https://doi.org/10.1177/1087054711430712. Epub 2012 Jan 30.

Donnelly, M., Haby, M. M., Carter, R., Andrews, G., & Vos, T. (2004). Cost-effectiveness of dexamphetamine and methylphenidate for the treatment of childhood attention deficit hyperactivity disorder. *The Australian and New Zealand Journal of Psychiatry, 38*(8), 592–601.

Dopfel, R. P., Schulmeister, K., & Schernhammer, E. S. (2007). Nutritional and lifestyle correlates of the cancer-protective hormone melatonin. *Cancer Detection and Prevention, 31*(2), 140–148.

Dorani, F., Bijlenga, D., & Kooij, J. J. S. (2017, Submitted). *Premenstrual dysphoric disorder in women with ADHD.*

Dougherty, D. D., Bonab, A. A., Spencer, T. J., Rauch, S. L., Madras, B. K., & Fischman, A. J. (1999). Dopamine transporter density in patients with attention-deficit hyperactivity disorder. *Lancet, 354*(9196), 2132–2133.

Dowson, J. H. (2008). Characteristics of adults with attention-deficit/hyperactivity disorder and past conduct disorder. *Acta Psychiatrica Scandinavica, 117*(4), 299–305.

Doyle, A. E., Faraone, S. V., Seidman, L. J., Willcutt, E. G., Nigg, J. T., Waldman, I. D., et al. (2005). Are endophenotypes based on measures of executive functions useful for molecular genetic studies of ADHD? *Journal of Child Psychology and Psychiatry, 46*(7), 774–803.

Doyle, A. E., Willcutt, E. G., Seidman, L. J., Biederman, J., Chouinard, V. A., Silva, J., & Faraone, S. V. (2005, June). Attention-deficit/hyperactivity disorder endophenotypes. *Biological Psychiatry, 57*(11), 1324–35. https://doi.org/10.1016/j.biopsych.2005.03.015. PMID: 15950005.

Dresel, S., Krause, J., Krause, K. H., LaFougere, C., Brinkbaumer, K., Kung, H. F., et al. (2000). Attention deficit hyperactivity disorder: Binding of [99mTc]TRODAT-1 to the dopamine transporter before and after methylphenidate treatment. *European Journal of Nuclear Medicine, 27*(10), 1518–1524.

Dubois, L., Girard, M., Potvin Kent, M., Farmer, A., & Tatone-Tokuda, F. (2008). Breakfast skipping is associated with differences in meal patterns, macronutrient intakes and overweight among pre-school children. *Public Health Nutrition, 18*, 1–10.

Dueñas, J. L., Lete, I., Bermejo, R., Arbat, A., Perez-Campos, E., Martinez-Salmean, J., et al. (2011). Prevalence of premenstrual syndrome and premenstrual dysphoric disorder in a representative cohort of Spanish women of fertile age. *European Journal of Obstetrics & Gynecology and Reproductive Biology, 156*(1), 72–77.

Durst, R., & Rebaudengo-Rosca, P. (1997). Attention deficit hyperactivity disorder, facilitating alcohol and drug abuse in an adult. *Harefuah, 132*(9), 618–622. 680.

Durston, S., Pol, H. E., Schnack, H. G., Buitelaar, J. K., Steenhuis, M. P., Minderaa, R. B., et al. (2004). Magnetic resonance imaging of boys with attention-deficit/hyperactivity disorder and their unaffected siblings. *Child & Adolescent Social Work Journal, 21*(1), 332–340.

Edebol, H., Helldin, L., & Norlander, T. (2013, April). Measuring adult attention deficit hyperactivity disorder using the quantified behavior test plus. *Psychiatry Journal, 2*(1), 48–62.

Einat, T., & Einat, A. (2008). Learning disabilities and delinquency: A study of Israeli prison inmates. *International Journal of Offender Therapy and Comparative Criminology, 52*(4), 416–434.

Elia, J., Ambrosini, P., & Berrettini, W. (2008). ADHD characteristics: I. Concurrent co-morbidity patterns in children & adolescents. *Child and Adolescent Psychiatry and Mental Health, 2*(1), 15.

Elia, J., Borcherding, B. G., Rapoport, J. L., & Keysor, C. S. (1991). Methylphenidate and dextro-amphetamine treatments of hyperactivity: Are there true nonresponders? *Psychiatry Research, 36*(2), 141–155.

Elliott, R., Sahakian, B. J., Matthews, K., Bannerjea, A., Rimmer, J., & Robbins, T. W. (1997, May). Effects of methylphenidate on spatial working memory and planning in healthy young adults. *Psychopharmacology, 131*(2), 196–206.

Epstein, J. N., Johnson, D. E., & Conners, C. K. (2001). *CAADID. The Conner's adult ADHD diagnostic interview for DSM-IV*. MHS Inc.

Epstein, J. N., & Kollins, S. H. (2006). Psychometric properties of an adult ADHD diagnostic interview. *Journal of Attention Disorders, 9*(3), 504–514.

Faber, A., Van Agthoven, M., Kalverdijk, L. J., Tobi, H., De Jong-van den Berg, L. T., Annemans, L., et al. (2008). Long-acting methylphenidate-OROS in youths with attention-deficit hyperactivity disorder suboptimally controlled with immediate-release methylphenidate: A study of cost effectiveness in the Netherlands. *CNS Drugs, 22*(2), 157–170.

Fang, X., Massetti, G. M., Ouyang, L., Grosse, S. D., & Mercy, J. A. (2010, November). Attention-deficit/hyperactivity disorder, conduct disorder, and young adult intimate partner violence. *Archives of General Psychiatry, 67*(11), 1179–1186.

Faraone, S. V. (2000). Attention deficit hyperactivity disorder in adults: Implications for theories of diagnosis. *Current Directions in Psychological Science, 9*, 33–36.

Faraone, S. V. (2005). The scientific foundation for understanding attention-deficit/hyperactivity disorder as a valid psychiatric disorder. *European Child and Adolescent Psychiatry, 14*(1), 1–10.

Faraone, S. V. (2008). Lisdexamfetamine dimesylate: The first long-acting prodrug stimulant treatment for attention deficit/hyperactivity disorder. *Expert Opinion on Pharmacotherapy, 9*(9), 1565–1574.

Faraone, S. V., Biederman, J., Morley, C.P., & Spencer, T. J. (2008, September). Effect of stimulants on height and weight: a review of the literature. *Journal of the American Academy of Child and Adolescent Psychiatry, 47*(9), 994–1009. https://doi.org/10.1097/CHI.ObO13e31817eOea7. PMID: 18580502.

Faraone, S. V., & Biederman, J. (2002). Efficacy of adderall for attention-deficit/hyperactivity disorder: A meta-analysis. *Journal of Attention Disorders, 6*(2), 69–75.

Faraone, S. V., & Biederman, J. (2005). What is the prevalence of adult ADHD? Results of a population screen of 966 adults. *Journal of Attention Disorders, 9*(2), 384–391.

Faraone, S. V., Biederman, J., Doyle, A., Murray, K., Petty, C., Adamson, J. J., et al. (2006). Neuropsychological studies of late onset and subthreshold diagnoses of adult attention-deficit/ hyperactivity disorder. *Biological Psychiatry, 60*(10), 1081–1087.

Faraone, S. V., Biederman, J., & Mick, E. (2006). The age-dependent decline of attention deficit hyperactivity disorder: A meta-analysis of follow-up studies. *Psychological Medicine, 36*(2), 159–165.

Faraone, S. V., Biederman, J., Spencer, T., Michelson, D., Adler, L., Reimherr, F., et al. (2005a). Efficacy of atomoxetine in adult attention-deficit/hyperactivity disorder: A drug-placebo response curve analysis. *Behavioral and Brain Functions, 1*, 16.

Faraone, S. V., Biederman, J., Spencer, T., Michelson, D., Adler, L., Reimherr, F., et al. (2005b). Atomoxetine and stroop task performance in adult attention-deficit/hyperactivity disorder. *Journal of Child and Adolescent Psychopharmacology, 15*(4), 664–670.

Faraone, S. V., Biederman, J., Spencer, T., Mick, E., Murray, K., Petty, C., et al. (2006). Diagnosing adult attention deficit hyperactivity disorder: Are late onset and subthreshold diagnoses valid? *American Journal of Psychiatry, 163*(10), 1720–1729.

Faraone, S. V., & Glatt, S. J. (2010, June). A comparison of the efficacy of medications for adult attention-deficit/hyperactivity disorder using meta-analysis of effect sizes. *Journal of Clinical Psychiatry, 71*(6), 754–63. https://doi.org/10.4088/JCP.08m04902pur. Epub 2009 Dec 29. PMID: 20051220.

Faraone, S. V., Glatt, S. J., & Tsuang, M. T. (2003, June). The genetics of pediatric-onset bipolar disorder. *Biological Psychiatry, 53*(11), 970–7. https://doi.org/10.1016/s0006-3223(02)01893-0. PMID: 12788242.

Faraone, S. V., Perlis, R. H., Doyle, A. E., Smoller, J. W., Goralnick, J. J., Holmgren, M. A., et al. (2005). Molecular genetics of attention-deficit/hyperactivity disorder. *Biological Psychiatry, 57*(11), 1313–1323.

Faraone, S. V., Sergeant, J., & Gillberg, C. (2003, June). The worldwide prevalence of ADHD: Is it an American condition? *World Psychiatry, 2*, 104–113. PMID: 16946911; PMCID: PMC1525089.

Faraone, S. V., Short, E. J., Biederman, J., Findling, R. L., Roe, C., & Manos, M. J. (2002). Efficacy of Adderall and methylphenidate in attention deficit hyperactivity disorder: A drug-placebo and drug-drug response curve analysis of a naturalistic study. *International Journal of Neuropsychopharmacology, 5*(2), 121–129.

Faraone, S. V., & Upadhyaya, H. P. (2007). The effect of stimulant treatment for ADHD on later substance abuse and the potential for medication misuse, abuse, and diversion. *Journal of Clinical Psychiatry, 68*(11), e28.

Fargason, R. E., Fobian, A. D., Hablitz, L. M., Paul, J. R., White, B. A., Cropsey, K. L., et al. (2017, March). Correcting delayed circadian phase with bright light therapy predicts improvement in ADHD symptoms: A pilot study. *Journal of Psychiatric Research, 6*(91), 105–110.

Fayyad, J., De Graaf, R., Kessler, R., Alonso, J., Angermeyer, M., Demyttenaere, K., et al. (2007). Cross-national prevalence and correlates of adult attention-deficit hyperactivity disorder. *British Journal of Psychiatry, 190*, 402–409.

Fayyad, J., Sampson, N. A., Hwang, I., Adamowski, T., Aguilar-Gaxiola, S., Al-Hamzawi, A., et al. (2017, March). WHO world mental health survey collaborators. The descriptive epidemiology of DSM-IV adult ADHD in the world health organization world mental health surveys. *Atten Defic Hyperact Disord, 9*(1), 47–65.

Ferdinand, R. F., Van der Ende, J., & Verhulst, F. C. (2004). Parent-adolescent disagreement regarding psychopathology in adolescents from the general population as a risk factor for adverse outcome. *Journal of Abnormal Psychology, 113*(198), 206.

Fernandez-Alvarez, E. (2002). Comorbid disorders associated with tics, in Spanish. *Revista de Neurologia, 34 Suppl, 1*(1), S122–S129.

Ferrer, M., Andión, Ó., Calvo, N., Ramos-Quiroga, J. A., Prat, M., Corrales, M., et al. (2017). Differences in the association between childhood trauma history and borderline personality disorder or attention deficit/hyperactivity disorder diagnoses in adulthood. *European Archives of Psychiatry and Clinical Neuroscience, 267*, 541–549. https://doi.org/10.1007/s00406-016-0733-2

Findling, R. L., Bukstein, O. G., Melmed, R. D., Lopez, F. A., Sallee, F. R., Arnold, L. E., et al. (2008). A randomized, double-blind, placebo-controlled, parallel-group study of methylphenidate transdermal system in pediatric patients with attention-deficit/hyperactivity disorder. *Journal of Clinical Psychiatry, 69*(1), 149–159.

Fisch, R. Z. (1985). Methylphenidate for medical in-patients. *International Journal of Psychiatry in Medicine, 15*(1), 75–79.

Fleming, J. P., Levy, L. D., & Levitan, R. D. (2005). Symptoms of attention deficit hyperactivity disorder in severely obese women. *Eating and Weight Disorders, 10*(1), e10–e13.

Fliers, E. A., Vasquez, A. A., Poelmans, G., Rommelse, N., Altink, M., Buschgens, C., et al. (2012). Genome-wide association study of motor coordination problems in ADHD identifies genes for brain and muscle function. *The World Journal of Biological Psychiatry, 13*(3), 211–222.

Flory, K., Molina, B. S., Pelham, W. E., Jr., Gnagy, E., & Smith, B. (2006). Childhood ADHD predicts risky sexual behavior in young adulthood. *Journal of Clinical Child and Adolescent Psychology, 35*(4), 571–577.

Fones, C. S., Pollack, M. H., Susswein, L., & Otto, M. (2000). History of childhood attention deficit hyperactivity disorder (ADHD) features among adults with panic disorder. *Journal of Affective Disorders, 58*(2), 99–106.

Fossati, A., Novella, L., Donati, D., Donini, M., & Maffei, C. (2002). History of childhood attention deficit/hyperactivity disorder symptoms and borderline personality disorder: A controlled study. *Comprehensive Psychiatry, 43*(5), 369–377.

Frampton, J. E. (2016, April). Lisdexamfetamine: A review in ADHD in adults. *CNS Drugs, 30*(4), 343–354.

Franke, A. G., Bagusat, C., Rust, S., Engel, A., & Lieb, K. (2014, November). Substances used and prevalence rates of pharmacological cognitive enhancement among healthy subjects. *European Archives of Psychiatry and Clinical Neuroscience, 264*(Suppl 1), S83–S90.

Franke, B., Neale, B. M., & Faraone, S. V. (2009). Genome-wide association studies in ADHD. *Human Genetics, 126*(1), 13–50.

Fredriksen, M., Halmoy, A., Faraone, S. V., & Haavik, J. (2013). Long-term efficacy and safety of treatment with stimulants and atomoxetine in adult ADHD: A review of controlled and naturalistic studies. *European Neuropsychopharmacology: The Journal of the European College of Neuropsychopharmacology, 23*(6), 508–527.

Fridman, M., Hodgkins, P. S., Kahle, J. S., & Erder, M. H. (2015, June). Predicted effect size of lisdexamfetamine treatment of attention deficit/hyperactivity disorder (ADHD) in European adults: Estimates based on indirect analysis using a systematic review and meta-regression analysis. *European Psychiatry, 30*(4), 521–527.

Fuermaier, A. B., Tucha, L., Evans, B. L., Koerts, J., De Waard, D., Brookhuis, K., et al. (2017, February). Driving and attention deficit hyperactivity disorder. *Journal of Neural Transmission (Vienna), 124*(Suppl 1), 55–67.

Fuermaier, A. B. M., Tucha, L., Koerts, J., Aschenbrenner, S., Kaunzinger, I., Hauser, J., et al. (2015). Cognitive impairment in adult ADHD – Perspective matters! *Neuropsychology, 29*(1), 45–58.

Furczyk, K., & Thome, J. (2014, September). Adult ADHD and suicide. *Atten Defic Hyperact Disord, 6*(3), 153–158.

Gadow, K. D., & Sverd, J. (2006). Attention deficit hyperactivity disorder, chronic tic disorder, and methylphenidate. *Advances in Neurology, 99*, 197–207.

Gadow, K. D., Sverd, J., Sprafkin, J., Nolan, E. E., & Grossman, S. (1999). Long-term methylphenidate therapy in children with comorbid attention-deficit hyperactivity disorder and chronic multiple tic disorder. *Archives of General Psychiatry, 56*(4), 330–336.

Gaïffas, A., Galéra, C., Mandon, V. & Bouvard, M.P. (2014, July). Attention-deficit/hyperactivity disorder in young French male prisoners. *Journal of Forensic Sciences, 59*(4), 1016-1019.

Gajos, J. M., & Beaver, K. M. (2016, October). The effect of omega-3 fatty acids on aggression: A meta-analysis. *Neuroscience & Biobehavioral Reviews, 69*:147–58. https://doi.org/10.1016/j.neubiorev.2016.07.017. Epub 2016 Jul 20. PMID: 27450580.

Galanter, C. A., Carlson, G. A., Jensen, P. S., Greenhill, L. L., Davies, M., Li, W., et al. (2003). Response to methylphenidate in children with attention deficit hyperactivity disorder and manic symptoms in the multimodal treatment study of children with attention deficit hyperactivity disorder titration trial. *Journal of Child and Adolescent Psychopharmacology, 13*(2), 123–136.

Gau, S. S., Kessler, R. C., Tseng, W. L., Wu, Y. Y., Chiu, Y. N., Yeh, C. B., et al. (2007). Association between sleep problems and symptoms of attention-deficit/hyperactivity disorder in young adults. *Sleep, 30*(2), 195–201.

Gaultney, J. F., Terrell, D. F., & Gingras, J. L. (2005). Parent-reported periodic limb movement, sleep disordered breathing, bedtime resistance behaviors, and ADHD. *Behavioral Sleep Medicine, 3*(1), 32–43.

Gezondheidsraad. (2006). Health Council of the Netherlands (In Dutch). *Nachtwerk en borst-kanker: Een oorzakelijk verband?* Advies Gezondheidsraad. Den Haag. www.gezond-heidsraad.nl.

Ghanizadeh, A. (2015). A systematic review of reboxetine for treating patients with attention deficit hyperactivity disorder. *Nordic Journal of Psychiatry, 69*, 241–248.

Ghirardi, L., Brikell, I., Kuja-Halkola, R., Freitag, C. M., Franke, B., Asherson, P., et al. (2017, February). The familial co-aggregation of ASD and ADHD: a registerbased cohort study. *Molecular Psychiatry, 23*(2), 257–62. https://doi.org/10.1038/mp.2017.17. Epub 2017 Feb 28. PMID: 28242872; PMCID: PMC5794881.

Gibbs, E. L., Kass, A. E., Eichen, D. M., Fitzsimmons-Craft, E. E., Trockel, M., & Wilfley, D. E. (2016, May–June). Attention-deficit/hyperactivity disorder-specific stimulant misuse, mood, anxiety, and stress in college-age women at high risk for or with eating disorders. *Journal of American College Health, 64*(4), 300–308.

Gibson, A. P., Bettinger, T. L., Patel, N. C., & Crismon, M. L. (2006). Atomoxetine versus stimulants for treatment of attention deficit/hyperactivity disorder. *Annals of Pharmaco-Therapy, 40*(6), 1134–1142.

Gilger, J. W., Pennington, B. F., & DeFries, J. C. (1992). A twin study of the etiology of comorbidity: Attention-deficit hyperactivity disorder and dyslexia. *Journal of the American Academy of Child and Adolescent Psychiatry, 31*(2), 343–348.

Gillberg, C. (2003). Deficits in attention, motor control, and perception: A brief review. *Archives of Disease in Childhood, 88*(10), 904–910.

Gillies, D., Sinn, J. Kh., Lad, S. S., Leach, M. J., & Ross, M. J. (2012, July 11). Polyunsaturated fatty acids (PUFA) for attention deficit hyperactivity disorder (ADHD) in children and adolescents *Cochrane Database of Systematic Reviews, 2012*(7):CD007986

Gilmore, A., & Milne, R. (2001). Methylphenidate in children with hyperactivity: Review and cost-utility analysis. *Pharmacoepidemiology and Drug Safety, 10*(2), 85–94.

Gimpel, G. A., Collett, B. R., Veeder, M. A., Gifford, J. A., Sneddon, P., Bushman, B., et al. (2005). Effects of stimulant medication on cognitive performance of children with ADHD. *Clinical Pediatrics, 44*(5), 405–411.

Ginsberg, Y., Hirvikoski, T., & Lindefors, N. (2010, December). Attention Deficit Hyperactivity Disorder (ADHD) among longer-term prison inmates is a prevalent, persistent and disabling disorder. *BMC Psychiatry, 22*(10), 112.155–112.160.

Ginsberg, Y., Långström, N., Larsson, H., & Lindefors, N. (2015, October). Long-term treatment outcome in adult male prisoners with attention-deficit/hyperactivity disorder: Three-year naturalistic follow-up of a 52-week methylphenidate trial. *Journal of Clinical Psychopharmacology, 35*(5), 535–543.

Gobbo, M. A., & Louzã, M. R. (2014, September). Influence of stimulant and non-stimulant drug treatment on driving performance in patients with attention deficit hyperactivity disorder: A systematic review. *European Neuropsychopharmacology, 24*(9), 1425–1443.

Goldberg, T. E., Bigelow, L. B., Weinberger, D. R., Daniel, D. G., & Kleinman, J. E. (1991, January). Cognitive and behavioral effects of the coadministration of dextroamphetamine and haloperidol in schizophrenia. *The American Journal of Psychiatry, 148*(1), 78–84.

Golubchik, P., Sever, J., Zalsman, G., Weizman, A., Martel, M. M., Nigg, J. T., et al. (2008). Methylphenidate in the treatment of female adolescents with co-occurrence of attention deficit/hyperactivity disorder and borderline personality disorder: A preliminary open-label trial. *International Clinical Psychopharmacology, 23*(4), 228–231.

Goossensen, M. A., Van de Glind, G., Carpentier, P. J., Wijsen, R. M. A., Van Duin, D., & Kooij, J. J. S. (2006). An intervention program for ADHD in patients with substance use disorders: Preliminary results of a field trial. *Journal of Substance Abuse Treatment, 30*(3), 253–259.

Gosselin, N., Mathieu, A., Mazza, S., Petit, D., Malo, J., & Montplaisir, J. (2006). Attentional deficits in patients with obstructive sleep apnea syndrome: An event-related potential study. *Clinical Neurophysiology, 117*(10), 2228–2235.

Gow, R. V., Sumich, A., Vallee-Tourangeau, F., Crawford, M. A., Ghebremeskel, K., Bueno, A. A., et al. (2013). Omega-3 fatty acids are related to abnormal emotion processing in adolescent boys with attention deficit hyperactivity disorder. *Prostaglandins, Leukotrienes, and Essential Fatty Acids, 88*, 419–429.

Greenfield, B., Hechtman, L., Stehli, A., & Wigal, T. (2014, September). Sexual maturation among youth with ADHD and the impact of stimulant medication. *European Child & Adolescent Psychiatry, 23*(9), 835–839.

Gross-Tsur, V., Manor, O., Van Der Meere, J., Joseph, A., & Shalev, R. S. (1997, January). Epilepsy and attention deficit hyperactivity disorder: Is methylphenidate safe and effective? *Journal of Pediatrics, 130*(1), 40–4. https://doi.org/10.1016/s0022-3476(97)70308-1. Corrected and republished in: *Journal of Pediatrics.* 1997 Apr;*130*(4), 670–4. PMID: 9003849.

Gu, Y., Xu, G., & Zhu, Y. (2018). A randomized controlled trial of mindfulness-based cognitive therapy for college students with ADHD. *Journal of Attention Disorders, 22*(4), 388–399. https://doi.org/10.1177/1087054716686183. Epub 2016 Dec 30.

Gucuyener, K., Erdemoglu, A. K., Senol, S., Serdaroglu, A., Soysal, S., & Kockar, A. I. (2003). Use of methylphenidate for attention-deficit hyperactivity disorder in patients with epilepsy or electroencephalographic abnormalities. *Journal of Child Neurology, 18*(2), 109–112.

Gudmundsdottir, B. G., Weyandt, L., & Ernudottir, G. B. (2020). Prescription stimulant misuse and ADHD symptomatology among college students in Iceland. *Journal of Attention Disorders, 24*(3), 384–401. https://doi.org/10.1177/1087054716684379. Epub 2016 Dec 25.

Guendelman, M. D., Ahmad, S., Meza, J. I., Owens, E. B., & Hinshaw, S. P. (2016). Childhood attention-deficit/hyperactivity disorder predicts intimate partner victimization in young women. *Journal of Abnormal Child Psychology, 44*(1), 155–166. https://doi.org/10.1007/s10802-015-9984-z

Guldberg-Kjär, T., & Johansson, B. (2009). Old people reporting childhood AD/HD symptoms: Retrospectively self-rated AD/HD symptoms in a population-based Swedish sample aged 65-80. *Nordic Journal of Psychiatry, 63*(5), 375–382.

Gunning, W. B. (1992). *A controlled trial of clonidine in hyperkinetic children.* Erasmus Universiteit. Proefschrift.

Hah, M., & Chang, K. (2005). Atomoxetine for the treatment of attention-deficit/hyperactivity disorder in children and adolescents with bipolar disorders. *Journal of Child and Adolescent Psychopharmacology, 15*(6), 996–1004.

Halperin, J. M., Berwid, O. G., & O'Neill, S. (2014, October). Healthy body, healthy mind? The effectiveness of physical activity to treat ADHD in children. *Child and Adolescent Psychiatric Clinics of North America, 23*(4), 899–936.

Hammerness, P. G., Karampahtsis, C., Babalola, R., & Alexander, M. E. (2015, April). Attention-deficit/hyperactivity disorder treatment: What are the long-term cardiovascular risks? *Expert Opinion on Drug Safety, 14*(4), 543–551.

Hardan, A., & Sahl, R. (1997). Psychopathology in children and adolescents with developmental disorders. *Research in Developmental Disabilities, 18*(5), 369–382.

Harpold, T., Biederman, J., Gignac, M., Hammerness, P., Surman, C., Potter, A., et al. (2007). Is oppositional defiant disorder a meaningful diagnosis in adults? Results from a large sample of adults with ADHD. *Journal of Nervous and Mental Disease, 195*(7), 601–605.

Hartmann, T. (2010). *The Edison gene. ADHD and the gift of the hunter child.* Park Street Press.

Hebebrand, J., Dempfle, A., Saar, K., Thiele, H., Herpertz-Dahlmann, B., Linder, M., et al. (2006). A genome-wide scan for attention-deficit/hyperactivity disorder in 155 German sib-pairs. *Molecular Psychiatry, 11*(2), 196–205.

Hennig, T., Jaya. E. S., Koglin, U., & Lincoln, T. M. (2016, April). Associations of attention-deficit/hyperactivity and other childhood disorders with psychotic experiences and disorders in adolescence. *European Child & Adolescent Psychiatry, 26*(4), 421–31. https://doi.org/:10.1007/s00787-016-0904-8. Epub 2016 Sep 13. PMID: 27623819.

Hennig, T., Jaya, E. S., & Lincoln, T. M. (2017). Bullying Mediates Between Attention-Deficit/ Hyperactivity Disorder in Childhood and Psychotic Experiences in Early Adolescence. *Schizophrenia Bulletin, 43*(5), 1036–1044. https://doi.org/10.1093/schbul/sbw139.

Hennig, T., Jaya, E. S., Koglin, U., Lincoln, T. M. (2017 April). Associations of attention-deficit/ hyperactivity and other childhood disorders with psychotic experiences and disorders in adolescence. *European Child & Adolescent Psychiatry, 26*(4), 421–431. https://doi.org/10.1007/ s00787-016-0904-8. Epub 2016 Sep 13. PMID: 27623819.

Henrichs, J., & Bogaerts, S. (2012, June). Correlates of posttraumatic stress disorder in forensic psychiatric outpatients in the Netherlands. *Journal of Traumatic Stress, 25*(3), 315-322.

Herpers, P. C., & Buitelaar, J. K. (1996). De validiteit en betrouwbaarheid van de diagnose ADHD bij volwassenen. *Tijdschrift voor Psychiatrie, 38*(11), 809–821.

Hesdorffer, D. C., Ludvigsson, P., Olafsson, E., Gudmundsson, G., Kjartansson, O., & Hauser, W. A. (2004). ADHD as a risk factor for incident unprovoked seizures and epilepsy in children. *Archives of General Psychiatry, 61*(7), 731–736.

Hesslinger, B., Tebartz-van Elst, L., Mochan, F., & Ebert, D. (2003). Attention deficit hyperactivity disorder in adults – early vs. late onset in a retrospective study. *Psychiatry Research, 119*, 217–223.

Hill, S. M., Belancio, V. P., Dauchy, R. T., Xiang, S., Brimer, S., Mao, L., et al. (2015, June). Melatonin: An inhibitor of breast cancer. *Endocrine-Related Cancer, 22*(3), R183–R204.

Hill, S. M., Cheng, C., Yuan, L., Mao, L., Jockers, R., Dauchy, B., et al. (2013, February). Age-related decline in melatonin and its MT1 receptor are associated with decreased sensitivity to melatonin and enhanced mammary tumor growth. *Current Aging Science, 6*(1), 125–133.

Hinney, A., Scherag, A., Jarick, I., Albayrak, Ö., Pütter, C., Pechlivanis, S., et al. (2011). Psychiatric GWAS Consortium: ADHD subgroup. Genome-wide association study in German patients with attention deficit/hyperactivity disorder. *American Journal of Medical Genetics. Part B, Neuropsychiatric Genetics, 156B*(8), 888–897.

Hinshaw, S. P., Owens, E. B., Sami, N., & Fargeon, S. (2006). Prospective follow-up of girls with attention-deficit/hyperactivity disorder into adolescence: Evidence for continuing cross-domain impairment. *Journal of Consulting and Clinical Psychology, 74*(3), 489–499.

Holtkamp, K., Konrad, K., Muller, B., Heussen, N., Herpertz, S., Herpertz-Dahlmann, B., et al. (2004). Overweight and obesity in children with Attention-deficit/hyperactivity disorder. *International Journal of Obesity and Related Metabolic Disorders, 28*(5), 685–689.

Hooberman, D., & Stern, T. A. (1984). Treatment of attention deficit and borderline personality disorders with psychostimulants: Case report. *Journal of Clinical Psychiatry, 45*(10), 441–442.

Hoogman, M., Bralten, J., Hibar, D. P., Mennes, M., Zwiers, M. P., Schweren, L. S. J., et al. (2017, February). Subcortical brain volume differences in participants with attention deficit hyperactivity disorder in children and adults: A cross-sectional mega-analysis. *The Lancet Psychiatry, 4*(4), 310–319.

Huber, M., Kirchler, E., Niederhofer, H., & Gruber, L. (2007, May). Neuropsychiatric bases of the methylphenidate-therapy of the attention deficit/hyperactivity disorder (ADHD). *Fortschritte der Neurologie-Psychiatrie, 75*(5), 275–284.

Huizink, A. C., van Lier, P. A., & Crijnen, A. A. (2009). Attention deficit hyperactivity disorder symptoms mediate early-onset smoking. *European Addiction Research, 15*(1), 1–9.

Huss, M., Chen, W., & Ludolph, A. G. (2016). Guanfacine extended release: A new pharmacological treatment option in Europe. *Clinical Drug Investigation, 36*, 1–25.

Huss, M., Poustka, F., Lehmkuhl, G., Lehmkuhl, U., Kollins, S. H., Wilens, T. E., et al. (2008). No increase in long-term risk for nicotine use disorders after treatment with methylphenidate in children with attention-deficit/hyperactivity disorder (ADHD): Evidence from a non-randomised retrospective study. *Journal of Neural Transmission, 115*(2), 335–339.

Hynd, G. W., Hern, K. L., Novey, E. S., Eliopulos, D., Marshall, R., Gonzalez, J. J., et al. (1993). Attention deficit-hyperactivity disorder and asymmetry of the caudate nucleus. *Journal of Child Neurology, 8*(4), 339–347.

Ilieva, I. P., & Farah, M. J. (2013, October). Enhancement stimulants: perceived motivational and cognitive advantages. *Front Neurosciences, 7*:198. https://doi.org/10.3389/fnins.2013.00198. PMID: 24198755; PMCID: PMC3813924.

Ilieva, I. P., & Farah, M. J. (2019). Attention, motivation, and study habits in users of unprescribed ADHD Medication. *Journal of Attention Disorders, 23*(2), 149–162. https://doi.org/10.1177/1087054715591849. Epub 2015 Aug 19. PMID: 26290484.

Imeraj, L., Antrop, I., Roeyers, H., Deschepper, E., Bal, S., & Deboutte, D. (2011, August). Diurnal variations in arousal: A naturalistic heart rate study in children with ADHD. *European Child & Adolescent Psychiatry, 20*(8), 381–392.

Isaksson, J., Nilsson, K. W., & Lindblad, F. (2013, July 22). Early psychosocial adversity and cortisol levels in children with attention-deficit/hyperactivity disorder. *European Child & Adolescent Psychiatry, 22*(7), 425–432.

Isaksson, J., Nilsson, K. W., Nyberg, F., Hogmark, A., & Lindblad, F. (2012, November). Cortisol levels in children with attention-deficit/hyperactivity disorder. *Journal of Psychiatric Research, 46*(11), 1398–1405.

Jasinski, D. R., Faries, D. E., Moore, R. J., Schuh, L. M., & Allen, A. J. (2008). Abuse liability assessment of atomoxetine in a drug-abusing population. *Drug and Alcohol Dependence, 95*(1–2), 140–146.

Jastrowski, K. E., Berlin, K. S., Sato, A. F., & Davies, W. H. (2007). Disclosure of attention-deficit/hyperactivity disorder may minimize risk of social rejection. *Psychiatry, 70*(3), 274–282.

Jensen, C. M., Amdisen, B. L., Jørgensen, K. J., & Arnfred, S. M. (2016, March). Cognitive behavioural therapy for ADHD in adults: Systematic review and meta-analyses. *Attention Deficit Hyperactivity Disorder, 8*(1), 3–11.

Jeste, S. S., Frohlich, J., & Loo, S. K. (2015, April). Electrophysiological biomarkers of diagnosis and outcome in neurodevelopmental disorders. *Curr Opin Neurol, 28*(2), 110–6. 2013 July, *17*(5), 384-92.

Juneja, M., Jain, R., Singh, V., & Mallika, V. (2010). Iron deficiency in Indian children with attention deficit hyperactivity disorder. *Indian Pediatrics, 47*(11), 955–958.

Kafka, M. (2012). Axis I psychiatric disorders, paraphilic sexual offending and implications for pharmacological treatment. *The Israel Journal of Psychiatry and Related Sciences, 49*(4), 255–261.

Kafka, M. P., & Hennen, J. (2000). Psychostimulant augmentation during treatment with selective serotonin reuptake inhibitors in men with paraphilia-related disorders: A case series. *Journal of Clinical Psychiatry, 61*(9), 664–670.

Kafka, M. P., & Hennen, J. (2002). A DSM-IV Axis I comorbidity study of males (n = 120) with paraphilias and paraphilia-related disorders. *Sexual Abuse, 14*(4), 349–366.

Kafka, M. P., & Prentky, R. A. (1998). Attention-deficit/hyperactivity disorder in males with paraphilias and paraphilia-related disorders: A comorbidity study. *Journal of Clinical Psychiatry, 59*(7), 388–396.

Kakizaki, M., Inoue, K., Kuriyama, S., Sone, T., Matsuda-Ohmori, K., Nakaya, N., et al. (2008). Sleep duration and the risk of prostate cancer: The Ohsaki Cohort Study. *British Journal of Cancer, 99*(1), 176–178.

Kan, C. C., Buitelaar, J. K., & van der Gaag, R. J. (2008). Autism spectrum disorders in adults, in Dutch. *Nederlands Tijdschrift voor Geneeskunde, 152*(24), 1365–1369.

Katon, W., & Raskind, M. (1980). Treatment of depression in the medically ill elderly with methylphenidate. *The American Journal of Psychiatry, 137*(8), 963–965.

Kaufmann, M. W., Cassem, N., Murray, G., & MacDonald, D. (1984). The use of methylphenidate in depressed patients after cardiac surgery. *The Journal of Clinical Psychiatry, 45*(2), 82–84.

Kay, G. G., Michaels, M. A., & Pakull, B. (2009). Simulated driving changes in young adults with ADHD receiving mixed amphetamine salts extended release and atomoxetine. *Journal of Attention Disorders, 12*(4), 316–329.

Kayumov, L., Lowe, A., Rahman, S. A., Casper, R. F., & Shapiro, C. M. (2007). Prevention of melatonin suppression by nocturnal lighting: Relevance to cancer. *European Journal of Cancer Prevention, 16*(4), 357–362.

Keijsers, G. P. J., Minnen, A., & Hoogduin, C. A. L. (2004). *Protocollaire behandelingen in de ambulante geestelijke gezondheidszorg II*. Bohn Stafleu, Van Loghum.

Kelly, A. M., Margulies, D. S., & Castellanos, F. X. (2007). Recent advances in structural and functional brain imaging studies of attention-deficit/hyperactivity disorder. *Current Psychiatry Reports, 9*(5), 401–407.

Kelly, K., Ramundo, P., & Hallowell, E. M. (2006). *You mean I am not lazy, stupid or crazy?! The classic self-help book for adults with ADHD: Scribner*.

Kessler, R. C. (2007). *Comorbidity patterns in a community sample of adults with ADHD: Results from the National Comorbidity Survey Replication*. Paper presented at the APA 160th Annual Meeting.

Kessler, R. C., Adler, L. E., Ames, M., Barkley, R. A., Birnbaum, H., Greenberg, P., et al. (2005). The prevalence and effects of adult attention deficit/hyperactivity disorder on work performance in a nationally representative sample of workers. *Journal of Occupational and Environmental Medicine, 47*(6), 565–572.

Kessler, R. C., Adler, L., Berkley, R., Biederman, J., Conners, C. K., Demler, O., et al. (2006). The prevalence and correlates of adult ADHD in the United States: Results from the national comorbidity survey replication. *American Journal of Psychiatry, 163*(4), 716–723.

Kessler, R. C., Adler, L. A., Gruber, M. J., Sarawate, C. A., Spencer, T., & Van Brunt, D. L. (2007). Validity of the world health organization adult ADHD self-report scale (ASRS) Screener in a representative sample of health plan members. *International Journal of Methods in Psychiatric Research, 16*(2), 52–65.

Kessler, R. C., Lane, M., Stang, P. E., & Van Brunt, D. L. (2009, January). The prevalence and workplace costs of adult attention deficit hyperactivity disorder in a large manufacturing firm. *Psychological Medicine, 39*(1), 137–147.

Kessler, R. C., Lane, M., Stang, P. E., Van Brunt, D. L., & Trott, G. E. (2008). The prevalence and workplace costs of adult attention deficit hyperactivity disorder in a large manufacturing firm. *Psychological Medicine, 21*(1), 1–11.

Khoury, B., Lecomte, T., Fortin, G., Masse, M., Therien, P., Bouchard, V., et al. (2013, August). Mindfulness-based therapy: A comprehensive meta-analysis. *Clinical Psychology Review, 33*(6), 763–771.

King, S., Griffin, S., Hodges, Z., Weatherly, H., Asseburg, C., Richardson, G., et al. (2006). A systematic review and economic model of the effectiveness and cost-effectiveness of methylphenidate, dexamphetamine and atomoxetine for the treatment of attention deficit hyperactivity disorder in children and adolescents. *Health Technology Assessment, 10*(23), iii–iv. xiii-146.

Klöppel, S., Stonnington, C. M., Chu, C., Draganski, B., Scahill, R. I., Rohrer, J. D., et al. (2008, March). Automatic classification of MR scans in Alzheimer's disease. *Brain, 131*(Pt 3), 681–689.

Knell, E. R., & Comings, D. E. (1993). Tourette's syndrome and attention-deficit hyperactivity disorder: Evidence for a genetic relationship. *Journal of Clinical Psychiatry, 54*(9), 331–337.

Knivsberg, A. M., & Andreassen, A. B. (2008). Behaviour, attention and cognition in severe dyslexia. *Nordic Journal of Psychiatry, 62*(1), 59–65.

Knutson, K. L., & Van Cauter, E. (2008). Associations between sleep loss and increased risk of obesity and diabetes. *Annals of the New York Academy of Sciences, 1129*, 287–304.

Kollins, S. H., English, J. S., Itchon-Ramos, N., Chrisman, A. K., Dew, R., et al. (2014, February). A pilot study of lis-dexamfetamine dimesylate (LDX/SPD489) to facilitate smoking cessation in nicotine-dependent adults with ADHD. *Journal of Attention Disorders, 18*(2), 158–168.

Kollins, S. H. (2008, September). ADHD, substance use disorders, and psychostimulant treatment: current literature and treatment guidelines. *Journal of Attention Disorders, 12*(2), 115–25. https://doi.org/10.1177/1087054707311654. Epub 2008 Jan 11. PMID: 18192623.

Kollins, S. H., McClernon, F., & Fuemmeler, B. F. (2005, October). Association between smoking and attention-deficit/hyperactivity disorder symptoms in a population-based sample of young adults. *Archives of General Psychiatry, 62*(10), 1142–47. https://doi.org/10.1001/archpsyc.62.10.1142. PMID: 16203959.

Kollins, S. H., MacDonald, E. K., Rush, C, R. (2001, March). Assessing the abuse potential of methylphenidate in nonhuman and human subjects: a review. *Pharmacology Biochemistry and Behavior, 68*(3), 611–627. https://doi.org/10.1016/s0091-3057(01)00464-6. PMID: 11325419.

Konagai, C., Yanagimoto, K., Hayamizu, K., Han, L., Tsuji, T., & Koga, Y. (2013). Effects of krill oil containing n-3 polyunsaturated fatty acids in phospholipid form on human brain function: A randomized controlled trial in healthy elderly volunteers. *Clinical Interventions in Aging, 8,* 1247–1257.

Konofal, E., Lecendreux, M., Arnulf, I., & Mauren, M. C. (2004). Iron deficiency in children with attention-deficit/hyperactivity disorder. *Archives of Pediatrics & Adolescent Medicine, 158*(12), 1113–1115.

Konofal, E., Lecendreux, M., Bouvard, M. P., & Mouren-Simeoni, M. C. (2001). High levels of nocturnal activity in children with attention-deficit hyperactivity disorder: A video analysis. *Psychiatry and Clinical Neurosciences, 55*(2), 97–103.

Konofal, E., Lecendreux, M., Deron, J., Marchand, M., Cortese, S., Zaïm, M., et al. (2008). Effects of iron supplementation on attention deficit hyperactivity disorder in children. *Pediatric Neurology, 38*(1), 20–26.

Konstenius, M., Jayaram-Lindström, N., Guterstam, J., Beck, O., Philips, B., & Franck, J. (2014, March). Methylphenidate for attention deficit hyperactivity disorder and drug relapse in criminal offenders with substance dependence: A 24-week randomized placebo-controlled trial. *Addiction, 109*(3), 440–449.

Kooij, J. J. S. (2001). *Eetproblemen bij volwassenen met ADHD.* Interne publicatie PsyQ, psychomedische programma's.

Kooij, J. J. S. (2002). *Seksuele problemen bij 120 volwassenen met ADHD.* Interne publicatie PsyQ, psychomedische programma's.

Kooij, J. J. S. (2003a). ADHD bij volwassenen. In *Inleiding in diagnostiek en behandeling, 2e druk.* Swets & Zeitlinger Publishers.

Kooij, J. J. S. (2003b). Na de diagnose. *Impulsief, 1,* 2–5.

Kooij, J. J. S. (2006). *ADHD in adults. Clinical studies on assessment and treatment.* Proefschrift, Radboud University Nijmegen, Nijmegen.

Kooij, J. J. S. (2010, 2e druk). *Over medicatie voor volwassenen met ADHD.* : Kenniscentrum ADHD bij volwassenen, PsyQ en Impuls.

Kooij, J. J., Aeckerlin, L. P., Buitelaar, J. K. (2001). Functioneren, comorbiditeit en behandeling van 141 volwassenen met aandachtstekort-hyperactiviteitstoornis (ADHD) op een algemene polikliniek Psychiatrie [Functioning, comorbidity and treatment of 141 adults with attention deficit hyperactivity disorder (ADHD) at a psychiatric outpatient department]. *Nederlands Tijdschrift voor Geneeskunde, 145*(31), 1498–501. Dutch. PMID: 11512422.

Kooij, J. J. S., & Bijlenga, D. (2013). The circadian rhythm in adult attention-deficit/hyperactivity disorder: Current state of affairs. *Expert Review of Neurotherapeutics, 13*(10), 1107–1116.

Kooij, J. J. S., & Bijlenga, D. (2014, December 10). High prevalence of self-reported photophobia in adult ADHD. *Frontiers in Neurology, 5,* 256.

Kooij, J. J. S., Boonstra, A. M., Huijbrechts, I., & Buitelaar, J. K. (2006). Coexistence with borderline and antisocial personality disorder, and role of childhood sexual abuse in adults with ADHD. Proefschrift, *ADHD in adults. Clinical studies on assessment and treatment,* Radboud University Nijmegen, Nijmegen.

Kooij, J. J. S., Boonstra, A. M., Vermeulen, S. H., Heister, A. G., Burger, H., Buitelaar, J. K., et al. (2008). Response to methylphenidate in adults with ADHD is associated with a polymorphism in SLC6A3 (DAT1). *American Journal of Medical Genetics. Part B, Neuropsychiatric Genetics, 147B*(2), 201–208.

Kooij, J. J. S., Boonstra, A. M., Willemsen-Swinkels, S. H. N., Bekker, E. M., De Noord, I., & Buitelaar, J. K. (2008). Reliability, validity, and utility of instruments for self-report and informant report regarding symptoms of Attention-Deficit/Hyperactivity Disorder (ADHD) in adult patients. *Journal of Attention Disorders, 11*(4), 445–458.

Kooij, J. J. S., Buitelaar, J. K., Van den Oord, E. J., Furer, J. W., Rijnders, C. A. T., & Hodiamont, P. P. G. (2005). Internal and external validity of attention-deficit hyperactivity disorder in a population-based sample of adults. *Psychological Medicine, 35*(6), 817–827.

Kooij, J. J. S., Buitelaar, J. K., & Van Tilburg, W. (1999). Voorstel voor diagnostiek en behandeling van aandachtstekortstoornis met hyperactiviteit (ADHD) op volwassen leeftijd. *Tijdschrift voor Psychiatrie, 41*(6), 349–358.

Kooij, J. J. S., Burger, H., Boonstra, A. M., Van der Linden, P. D., Kalma, L. E., & Buitelaar, J. K. (2004). Efficacy and safety of methylphenidate in 45 adults with attention-deficit/hyperactivity disorder. A randomized placebo-controlled double-blind cross-over trial. *Psychological Medicine, 34*(6), 973–982.

Kooij, J. J. S., & Francken, M. H. (2007a). *Diagnostic interview for ADHD (DIVA) in adults.* Downloaden via www.divacenter.eu.

Kooij, J. J. S., & Francken, M. H. (2007b). (Diagnostisch Interview voor ADHD (DIVA) bij volwassenen, in Dutch). Gratis te downloaden in verschillende talen via www.divacenter.eu.

Kooij, J. J. S., & Francken, M. H. (2007c). *Diagnostisch Interview voor ADHD (DIVA 2.0).* Te downloaden via www.divacenter.eu.

Kooij, J. J. S., Goekoop, J. G., & Gunning, W. B. (1996). Aandachtstekortstoornis met hyperactiviteit op volwassen leeftijd; implicaties voor diagnostiek en behandeling. *Nederlands Tijdschrift voor Geneeskunde, 140*(37), 1848–1851.

Kooij, J. J., Michielsen, M., Kruithof, H., & Bijlenga, D. (2016, December). ADHD in old age: A review of the literature and proposal for assessment and treatment. *Expert Review of Neurotherapeutics, 16*(12), 1371–1381.

Kooij, J. J. S., Middelkoop, H. A. M., Van Gils, K., & Buitelaar, J. K. (2001). The effect of stimulants on nocturnal motor activity and sleep quality in adults with ADHD: An open-label case-control study. *Journal of Clinical Psychiatry, 62*(12), 952–956.

Koutsouleris, N., Meisenzahl, E. M., Davatzikos, C., Bottlender, R., Frodl, T., Scheuerecker, J., et al. (2009, July). Use of neuroanatomical pattern classification to identify subjects in at-risk mental states of psychosis and predict disease transition. *Archives of General Psychiatry, 66*(7), 700–712.

Kraguljac, N. V., White, D. M., Hadley, J. A., Visscher, K., Knight, D., Ver Hoef, L., et al. (2015, November). Abnormalities in large scale functional networks in unmedicated patients with schizophrenia and effects of risperidone. *Neuroimage Clin, 22*(10), 146–158.

Krause, K. H., Dresel, S. H., Krause, J., Kung, H. F., & Tatsch, K. (2000). Increased striatal dopamine transporter in adult patients with attention deficit hyperactivity disorder: Effects of methylphenidate as measured by single photon emission computed tomography. *Neuroscience Letters, 285*(2), 107–110.

Krause, K. H., Dresel, S. H., Krause, J., la Fougere, C., & Ackenheil, M. (2003). The dopamine transporter and neuroimaging in attention deficit hyperactivity disorder. *Neuroscience & Biobehavioral Reviews, 27*(7), 605–613.

Krause, K. H., Krause, J., & Trott, G. E. (1998). Hyperkinetic syndrome (attention deficit/hyperactivity disorder) in adulthood. *Nervenarzt, 69*(7), 543–556.

Kumar, R. (2008). Approved and investigational uses of modafinil: An evidence-based review. *Drugs, 68*(13), 1803–1839.

Kuntsi, J., Eley, T. C., Taylor, A., Hughes, C., Asherson, P., Caspi, A., et al. (2004). Co-occurrence of ADHD and low IQ has genetic origins. *American Journal of Medical Genetics. Part B, Neuropsychiatric Genetics, 124B*(1), 41–47.

Lahey, B. B., Applegate, B., McBurnett, K., Biederman, J., Greenhill, L., Hynd, G. W., et al. (1994, November). DSM-IV field trials for attention deficit hyperactivity disorder in children and adolescents. *The American Journal of Psychiatry, 151*(11), 1673–1685.

Lakhan, S. E., & Vieira, K. F. (2008). Nutritional therapies for mental disorders. *Nutrition Journal, 7*, 2.

Lange, K. W., Hauser, J., Lange, K. M., Makulska-Gertruda, E., Takano, T., Takeuchi, Y., et al. (2014, December). Utility of cognitive neuropsychological assessment in attention-deficit/hyperactivity disorder. *Atten Defic Hyperact Disord, 6*(4), 241–248.

Lavretsky, H., Reinlieb, M., St Cyr, N., Siddarth, P., Ercoli, L. M., & Senturk, D. (2015). Citalopram, methylphenidate, or their combination in geriatric depression: A randomized, double-blind, placebo-controlled trial. *The American Journal of Psychiatry, 172*(6), 561–569.

Le, H. H., Hodgkins, P., Postma, M. J., et al. (2014). Economic impact of childhood/adolescent ADHD in a European setting: The Netherlands as a reference case. *European Child & Adolescent Psychiatry, 23*(7), 587–598. https://doi.org/10.1007/s00787-013-0477-8

Lecendreux, M., Konofal, E., Bouvard, M., Falissard, B., & Mouren-Simeoni, M. C. (2000). Sleep and alertness in children with ADHD. *Journal of Child Psychology and Psychiatry, 41*(6), 803–812.

Leckman, J. F., Bloch, M. H., Scahill, L., & King, R. A. (2006). Tourette syndrome: The self under siege. *Journal of Child Neurology, 21*(8), 642–649.

Leibenluft, E., Cohen, P., Gorrindo, T., Brook, J. S., & Pine, D. S. (2006). Chronic versus episodic irritability in youth: A community-based, longitudinal study of clinical and diagnostic associations. *Journal of Child and Adolescent Psychopharmacology, 16*(4), 456–466.

Leibson, C. L., Katusic, S. K., Barbaresi, W. J., Ransom, J., & O'Brien, P. C. (2001, January 3). Use and costs of medical care for children and adolescents with and without attention-deficit/hyperactivity disorder. *JAMA, 285*(1), 60–66.

Levin, F. R., Mariani, J. J., Specker, S., Mooney, M., Mahony, A., Brooks, D. J., et al. (2015, June). Extended-release mixed amphetamine salts vs placebo for comorbid adult attention-deficit/hyperactivity disorder and cocaine use disorder: A randomized clinical trial. *JAMA Psychiatry, 72*(6), 593–602.

Levin, F. R., & Upadhyaya, H. P. (2007). Diagnosing ADHD in adults with substance use disorder: DSM-IV criteria and differential diagnosis. *Journal of Clinical Psychiatry, 68*(7), e18.

Levitan, R. D., Jain, U. R., & Katzman, M. A. (1999). Seasonal affective symptoms in adults with residual attention-deficit hyperactivity disorder. *Comprehensive Psychiatry, 40*(4), 261–267.

Levitan, R. D., Masellis, M., Lam, R. W., Muglia, P., Basile, V. S., Jain, U., et al. (2004). Childhood inattention and dysphoria and adult obesity associated with the dopamine D4 receptor gene in overeating women with seasonal affective disorder. *Neuropsychopharmacology, 29*(1), 179–186.

Lewy, A. J. (2007). Melatonin and human chronobiology. *Cold Spring Harber Symposia on Quantitative Biology, 72*, 623–636.

Lewy, A. J., Ahmed, S., Jackson, J. M., & Sack, R. L. (1992). Melatonin shifts human circadian rhythms according to a phase-response curve. *Chronobiology International, 9*(5), 380–392.

Lewy, A. J., Emens, J., Jackman, A., & Yuhas, K. (2006a). Circadian uses of melatonin in humans. *Chronobiology International, 23*(1–2), 403–412. https://doi.org/10.1080/07420520500545862. PMID: 16687313.

Lewy, A. J., Lefler, B. J., Emens, J. S., & Bauer, V. K. (2006b, May). The circadian basis of winter depression. *Proceedings of the National Academy of Sciences of USA, 103*(19), 7414–9. https://doi.org/10.1073/pnas.0602425103. Epub 2006 Apr 28. PMID: 16648247; PMCID: PMC1450113.

Lewy, A. J., Rough, J. N., Songer, J. B., Mishra, N., Yuhas, K., & Emens, J. S. (2007). The phase shift hypothesis for the circadian component of winter depression. *Dialogues of Clinical Neurosciences, 9*(3), 291–300.

Lichtenstein, P., Halldner, L., Zetterqvist, J., Sjölander, A., Serlachius, E., Fazel, S., et al. (2012, November 22). Medication for attention deficit-hyperactivity disorder and criminality. *The New England Journal of Medicine, 367*(21), 2006–2014.

Lim, L., Chantiluke, K., Cubillo, A. I., Smith, A. B., Simmons, A., Mehta, M. A., & Rubia, K. (2014, September). Disorder-specific grey matter deficits in attention deficit hyperactivity disorder relative to autism spectrum disorder. *Psychological Medicine, 17*, 1–12.

Lindenmayer, J. P., Nasrallah, H., Pucci, M., James, S., & Citrome, L. (2013, July). A systematic review of psychostimulant treatment of negative symptoms of schizophrenia: Challenges and therapeutic opportunities. *Schizophrenia Research, 147*(2-3), 241–252.

Linnet, K. M., Dalsgaard, S., Obel, C., Wisborg, K., Henriksen, T. B., Rodriguez, A., et al. (2003). Maternal lifestyle factors in pregnancy risk of attention deficit hyperactivity disorder and associated behaviors: Review of the current evidence. *American Journal of Psychiatry, 160*(6), 1028–1040.

Lissoni, P., Resentini, M., Mauri, R., Esposti, D., Esposti, G., Rossi, D., et al. (1986). Effects of tetrahydrocannabinol on melatonin secretion in man. *Hormone and Metabolic Research, 18*(1), 77–78.

Liu, L. L., Li, B. M., Yang, J., & Wang, Y. W. (2008). Does dopaminergic reward system contribute to explaining comorbidity obesity and ADHD? *Medical Hypotheses, 70*(6), 1118–1120.

Loo, S. K., & Barkley, R. A. (2005). Clinical utility of EEG in attention deficit hyperactivity disorder. *Applied Neuropsychology, 12*(2), 64–76.

Loo, S. K., Cho, A., Hale, T. S., McGough, J., McCracken, J., & Smalley, S. L. (2013, July). Characterization of the theta to beta ratio in ADHD: Identifying potential sources of heterogeneity. *Journal of Attention Disorders, 17*(5), 384–392.

Lou, H. C., Henriksen, L., Bruhn, P., Borner, H., & Nielsen, J. B. (1989). Striatal dysfunction in attention deficit and hyperkinetic disorder. *Archives of Neurology, 46*(1), 48–52.

Loughman, A., Bowden, S. C., & D'Souza, W. J. (2017, February). Self and informant report ratings of psychopathology in genetic generalized epilepsy. *Epilepsy & Behavior, 67*, 13–19.

Louik, C., Kerr, S., Kelley, K. E., & Mitchell, A. A. (2015, February). Increasing use of ADHD medications in pregnancy. *Pharmacoepidemiology and Drug Safety, 24*(2), 218–220.

Lovecchio, F., & Kashani, J. (2006). Isolated atomoxetine (Strattera) ingestions commonly result in toxicity. *The Journal of Emergency Medicine, 31*(3), 267–268.

Lu, A. T., Ogdie, M. N., Jarvelin, M. R., Moilanen, I. K., Loo, S. K., McCracken, J. T., et al. (2008). Association of the cannabinoid receptor gene (CNR1) with ADHD and post-traumatic stress disorder. *American Journal of Medical Genetics Part B Neuropsychiatric Genetics, 147B*(8), 1488–1494.

Luo, S. X., & Levin, F. R. (2017, March). Towards precision addiction treatment: New findings in co-morbid substance use and attention-deficit hyperactivity disorders. *Current Psychiatry Reports, 19*(3), 14.

Lyall, K., Croen, L., Daniels, J., Fallin, M. D., Ladd-Acosta, C., Lee, B. K., Park, B. Y., et al. (2017). The changing epidemiology of autism spectrum disorders. *Annual Review of Public Health, 38*, 81–102.

Lydon, E., & El-Mallakh, R. S. (2006). Naturalistic long-term use of methylphenidate in bipolar disorder. *Journal of Clinical Psychopharmacology, 26*(5), 516–518.

Maia, C. R., Stella, S. F., Mattos, P., Polanczyk, G. V., Polanczyk, C. A., & Rohde, L. A. (2015, January–March). The Brazilian policy of withholding treatment for ADHD is probably increasing health and social costs. *Revista Brasileira de Psiquiatria, 37*(1), 67–70.

Maibing, C. F., Pedersen, C. B., Benros, M. E., Mortensen, P. B., Dalsgaard, S., & Nordentoft, M. (2015, July). Risk of schizophrenia increases after all child and adolescent psychiatric disorders: A nationwide study. *Schizophrenia Bulletin, 41*(4), 963–970.

Man, K. K., Coghill, D., Chan, E. W., Lau, W. C., Hollis, C., Liddle, E., et al. (2016, November 15). Methylphenidate and the risk of psychotic disorders and hallucinations in children and adolescents in a large health system. *Translational Psychiatry, 6*(11), e956.

Maneeton, N., Maneeton, B., Srisurapanont, M., & Martin, S. D. (2011, December). Bupropion for adults with attention-deficit hyperactivity disorder: Meta-analysis of randomized, placebo-controlled trials. *Psychiatry and Clinical Neurosciences, 65*(7), 611–617.

Maneeton, N., Maneeton, B., Suttajit, S., et al. (2014). Exploratory meta-analysis on lisdexamfetamine versus placebo in adult ADHD. *Drug Design, Development and Therapy, 8*, 1685–1693.

Mannuzza, S., Klein, R. G., Bessler, A., Malloy, P., & Hynes, M. E. (1997, September). Educational and occupational outcome of hyperactive boys grown up. *Journal of the American Academy of Child and Adolescent Psychiatry, 36*(9), 1222–1227.

Mannuzza, S., Klein, R. G., Bessler, A., Malloy, P., & LaPadula, M. (1998). Adult psychiatric status of hyperactive boys grown up. *American Journal of Psychiatry, 155*(4), 493–498.

Mannuzza, S., Klein, R. G., & Moulton, J. L., 3rd. (2008). Lifetime criminality among boys with attention deficit hyperactivity disorder: A prospective follow-up study into adulthood using official arrest records. *Psychiatry Research, 160*(3), 237–246.

Manor, I., Rozen, S., Zemishlani, Z., Weizman, A., & Zalsman, G. (2011). When does it end? Attention-deficit/hyperactivity disorder in the middle aged and older populations. *Clinical Neuropharmacology, 34*(4), 148–154.

Marchese, M., Koren, G., & Bozzo, P. (2015, September). Is it safe to breastfeed while taking methylphenidate? *Canadian Family Physician, 61*(9), 765–766.

Martinez-Badía, J., & Martinez-Raga, J. (2005, December 22). Who says this is a modern disorder? The early history of attention deficit hyperactivity disorder. *World Journal of Psychiatry, 5*(4), 379–386.

Martinez-Raga, J., Ferreros, A., Knecht, C., De Alvaro, R., & Carabal, E. (2017, March). Attention-deficit hyperactivity disorder medication use: Factors involved in prescribing, safety aspects and outcomes. *Therapeutic Advances in Drug Safety, 8*(3), 87–99.

Marzocchi, G. M., Oosterlaan, J., Zuddas, A., Cavolina, P., Geurts, H., Redigolo, D., et al. (2008). Contrasting deficits on executive functions between ADHD and reading disabled children. *Journal of Child Psychology and Psychiatry, 49*(5), 543–552.

Masi, G., Perugi, G., Toni, C., Millepiedi, S., Mucci, M., Bertini, N., et al. (2006). Attention-deficit hyperactivity disorder-bipolar comorbidity in children and adolescents. *Bipolar Disorders, 8*(4), 373–381.

Matheson, L., Asherson, P., Wong, I. C., Hodgkins, P., Setyawan, J., Sasane, R., et al. (2013, May 21). Adult ADHD patient experiences of impairment, service provision and clinical management in England: A qualitative study. *BMC Health Services Research, 13*, 184.

Matza, L. S., Paramore, C., & Prasad, M. (2005, June). A review of the economic burden of ADHD. *Cost Eff Resour Alloc, 9*(3), 5.

Mayes, S. D., Calhoun, S. L., Bixler, E. O., Vgontzas, A. N., Mahr, F., Hillwig-Garcia, J., et al. (2008). ADHD subtypes and comorbid anxiety, depression, and oppositional-defiant disorder: Differences in sleep problems. *Journal of Pediatric Psychology, 34*(3), 328–337.

Mazza, S., Pepin, J. L., Naegele, B., Plante, J., Deschaux, C., & Levy, P. (2005). Most obstructive sleep apnoea patients exhibit vigilance and attention deficits on an extended battery of tests. *The European Respiratory Journal, 25*(1), 75–80.

McElroy, S. L., Hudson, J. I., Mitchell, J. E., Wilfley, D., Ferreira-Cornwell, M. C., et al. (2015, March). Efficacy and safety of lisdexamfetamine for treatment of adults with moderate to severe binge-eating disorder: A randomized clinical trial. *JAMA Psychiatry, 72*(3), 235–246.

McIntyre, R. S., Alsuwaidan, M., Soczynska, J. K., Szpindel, I., Bilkey, T. S., Almagor, D., et al. (2013, September). The effect of lisdexamfetamine dimesylate on body weight, metabolic parameters, and attention deficit hyperactivity disorder symptomatology in adults with bipolar I/II disorder. *Human Psychopharmacology, 28*(5), 421–427.

McLeer, S. V., Callaghan, M., Henry, D., & Wallen, J. (1994). Psychiatric disorders in sexually abused children. *Journal of the American Academy of Child and Adolescent Psychiatry, 33*(3), 313–319.

Medori, R., Ramos-Quiroga, J. A., Casas, M., Kooij, J. J. S., Niemela, A., Trott, G. E., et al. (2008). A randomized, placebo-controlled trial of three fixed dosages of prolonged-release OROS methylphenidate in adults with attention-deficit/hyperactivity disorder. *Biological Psychiatry, 63*(10), 981–989.

Merikangas, K. R., Akiskal, H. S., Angst, J., Greenberg, P. E., Hirschfeld, R. M., Petukhova, M., et al. (2007). Lifetime and 12-month prevalence of bipolar spectrum disorder in the National Comorbidity Survey replication. *Archives of General Psychiatry, 64*(5), 543–552.

Merkx, M. J., Schippers, G. M., Koeter, M. J., Vuijk, P. J., Oudejans, S., De Vries, C. C., et al. (2007). Allocation of substance use disorder patients to appropriate levels of care: Feasibility of matching guidelines in routine practice in Dutch treatment centres. *Addiction, 102*(3), 466–474.

Merry, S. N., & Andrews, L. K. (1994). Psychiatric status of sexually abused children 12 months after disclosure of abuse. *Journal of the American Academy of Child and Adolescent Psychiatry, 33*(7), 939–944.

Mersch, P. P., Middendorp, H. M., Bouhuys, A. L., Beersma, D. G., & Van den Hoofdakker, R. H. (1999). The prevalence of seasonal affective disorder in the Netherlands: A prospective and retrospective study of seasonal mood variation in the general population. *Biological Psychiatry, 45*(8), 1013–1022.

Meyer, B. J., Byrne, M. K., Collier, C., Parletta, N., Crawford, D., Winberg, P. C., et al. (2015). Baseline omega-3 index correlates with aggressive and attention deficit disorder behaviours in adult prisoners. *PLoS One, 10,* e0120220.

Michielsen, M., de Kruif, J. T., Comijs, H. C., Van Mierlo, S., Semeijn, E. J., Beekman, A. T., et al. (2018, October 29). The burden of ADHD in older adults: A qualitative study. *Journal of Attention Disorders, 22*(6), 591–600. https://doi.org/10.1177/1087054715610001

Michielsen, M., Kleef, D., Bijlenga, D., Zwennes, C., Dijkhuizen, K., Smulders, J., Hazewinkel, A., Beekman, A. T. F., & Kooij, J. J. S. (2020 June). Response and side effects using stimulant medication in older adults with ADHD: An observational archive study. *Journal of Attention Disorders, 8,* 1087054720925884.

Michielsen, M., Semeijn, E., Comijs, H. C., Van de Ven, P., Beekman, A. T., Deeg, D. J., & Kooij, J. J. S. (2012, October). Prevalence of attention-deficit hyperactivity disorder in older adults in the Netherlands. *The British Journal of Psychiatry, 201*(4), 298–305.

Mick, E., & Faraone, S. V. (2008). Genetics of attention deficit hyperactivity disorder. *Child and Adolescent Psychiatric Clinics of North America, 17*(2), 261–284. vii-viii.

Mick, E., Neale, B., Middleton, F. A., McGough, J. J., & Faraone, S. V. (2008). Genome-wide association study of response to methylphenidate in 187 children with attention-deficit/hyperactivity disorder. *American Journal of Medical Genetics. Part B, Neuropsychiatric Genetics, 147B*(8), 1412–1418.

Middelkoop, H. A. M., Van Gils, K., & Kooij, J. J. S. (1997). Adult attention-deficit hyperactivity disorder (ADHD): Actimetric evaluation of nocturnal motor activity and subjective sleep characteristics. *Dutch Society of Sleep-Wake Research, 8,* 87–89.

Milberger, S., Biederman, J., Faraone, S. V., Guite, J., & Tsuang, M. T. (1997). Pregnancy, delivery and infancy complications and attention deficit hyperactivity disorder: Issues of gene-environment interaction. *Biological Psychiatry, 41*(1), 65–75.

Milioni, A. L., Chaim, T. M., Cavallet, M., De Oliveira, N. M., Annes, M., Dos Santos, B., et al. (2014, October 30). High IQ May 'Mask' the diagnosis of ADHD by compensating for deficits in executive functions in treatment-naïve adults with ADHD. *Journal of Attention Disorders.*

Miller, C. J., Flory, J. D., Miller, S. R., Harty, S. C., Newcorn, J. H., & Halperin, J. M. (2008). Childhood attention-deficit/hyperactivity disorder and the emergence of personality disorders in adolescence: A prospective follow-up study. *Journal of Clinical Psychiatry, 69*(9), 1477–1484.

Millichap, J. G. (2008). Etiologic classification of attention-deficit/hyperactivity disorder. *Pediatrics, 121*(2), e358–e365.

Millichap, J. G., & Yee, M. M. (2012). The diet factor in attention-deficit/hyperactivity disorder. *Pediatrics, 129*(2), 330–337.

Millstein, R. B., Wilens, T. E., Biederman, J., & Spencer, T. J. (1997). Presenting ADHD symptoms and subtypes in clinically referred adults with ADHD. *Journal of Attention Disorders, 2*(3), 159–166.

Minde, K., Eakin, L., Hechtman, L., Ochs, E., Bouffard, R., Greenfield, B., et al. (2003, May). The psychosocial functioning of children and spouses of adults with ADHD. *Journal of Child Psychology and Psychiatry, 44*(4), 637–646.

Minzenberg, M. J., & Carter, C. S. (2008). Modafinil: A review of neurochemical actions and effects on cognition. *Neuropsychopharmacology, 33*(7), 1477–1502.

Mitchell, R. B., Nañez, G., Wagner, J. D., & Kelly, J. (2003, March). Dog bites of the scalp, face, and neck in children. *Laryngoscope, 13*(3), 492–495.

Moffitt, T. E., Houts, R., Asherson, P., Belsky, D. W., Corcoran, D. L., & Hammerle, M. (2015, October). Is adult ADHD a Childhood-Onset Neurodevelopmental Disorder? Evidence from a four-decade longitudinal cohort study. *The American Journal of Psychiatry, 172*(10), 967–977.

Mogavero, F., Jager, A., & Glennon, J. C. (2016, August). Clock genes, ADHD and aggression. *Neuroscience & Biobehavioral Reviews, 91*:51–68. https://doi.org/10.1016/j.neubiorev.2016.11.002. Epub 9. PMID: 27836462.

Mohr-Jensen, C., & Steinhausen, H. C. (2016, August). A meta-analysis and systematic review of the risks associated with childhood attention-deficit hyperactivity disorder on long-term outcome of arrests, convictions, and incarcerations. *Clinical Psychology Review, 48*, 32–42.

Mooney, M. E., Herin, D. V., Specker, S., Babb, D., Levin, F. R., & Grabowski, J. (2015, August). Pilot study of the effects of lisdexamfetamine on cocaine use: A randomized, double-blind, placebo-controlled trial. *Drug and Alcohol Dependence, 1(153)*, 94–103.

Moser, M., Schaumberger, K., Schernhammer, E., & Stevens, R. G. (2006). Cancer and rhythm. *Cancer Causes & Control, 17*(4), 483–487.

Mota, J., Fidalgo, F., Silva, R., Ribeiro, J. C., Santos, R., Carvalho, J., et al. (2008). Relationships between physical activity, obesity and meal frequency in adolescents. *Annals of Humam Biology, 35*(1), 1–10.

Mouridsen, S. E., Rich, B., & Isager, T. (2008). Psychiatric disorders in adults diagnosed as children with atypical autism. A case control study. *Journal of Neural Transmission, 115*(1), 135–138.

Mulligan, A., Anney, R. J., OfRegan, M., Chen, W., Butler, L., Fitzgerald, M., et al. (2009). Autism symptoms in Attention-Deficit/Hyperactivity Disorder: A familial trait which correlates with conduct, oppositional defiant, language and motor disorders. *Journal of Autism and Developmental Disorders, 39*(2), 197–209.

Multidisciplinaire Richtlijn Depressie. (2013, derde revisie). *Richtlijn voor de diagnostiek, behandeling en begeleiding van volwassen patiënten met een depressieve stoornis*. Trimbos-instituut.

Murphy, K. R. (1995). Empowering the adult with ADD. In K. G. Nadeau (Ed.), *A comprehensive guide to attention deficit disorder in adults: Research, diagnosis, and treatment* (pp. 135–145). Brunner/Mazel, Inc..

Murphy, K., & Barkley, R. A. (1996). Prevalence of DSM-IV symptoms of ADHD in adult licensed drivers: Implications for clinical diagnosis. *Journal of Attention Disorders, 3*, 147–161.

Murphy, K. R., Barkley, R. A., & Bush, T. (2002). Young adults with attention deficit hyperactivity disorder: Subtype differences in comorbidity, educational, and clinical history. *Journal of Nervous and Mental Disease, 190*(3), 147–157.

Mwangi, B., Ebmeier, K. P., Matthews, K., & Douglas Steele, J. (2012, May). Multi-centre diagnostic classification of individual structural neuroimaging scans from patients with major depressive disorder. *Brain, 135*(Pt 5), 1508–1521.

Nadeau, K. G. (1999). *Aandacht, een kopzorg? Een gids voor volwassenen met concentratieproblemen*. Pearson Assessment and Information.

Nadeau, K. G. (1994). Survival guide for college students with ADD or LD. New York: Magination Press.

Narayan, S., & Hay, J. (2004). Cost effectiveness of methylphenidate versus AMP/DEX mixed salts for the first-line treatment of ADHD. *Expert Review of Pharmacoeconomics & Outcomes Research, 4*(6), 625–634.

Naseem, S., Chaudhary, B., & Collop, N. (2001). Attention deficit hyperactivity disorder in adults and obstructive sleep apnea. *Chest, 119*(1), 294–296.

Neale, B. M., Medland, S. E., Ripke, S., Asherson, P., Franke, B., Lesch, K. P., et al. (2010, September). Meta-analysis of genome-wide association studies of attention-deficit/hyperactivity disorder. *Journal of the American Academy of Child and Adolescent Psychiatry, 49*(9), 884–897.

Neuman, R. J., Lobos, E., Reich, W., Henderson, C. A., Sun, L. W., & Todd, R. D. (2007). Prenatal smoking exposure and dopaminergic genotypes interact to cause a severe ADHD subtype. *Biological Psychiatry, 61*(12), 1320–1328.

Newcorn, J. H., Kratochvil, C. J., Allen, A. J., Casat, C. D., Ruff, D. D., Moore, R. J., et al. (2008). Atomoxetine and osmotically released methylphenidate for the treatment of attention deficit hyperactivity disorder: Acute comparison and differential response. *American Journal of Psychiatry, 165*(6), 721–730.

Nichols, S. A., McLeod, J. S., Holder, R. L., & McLeod, H. S. (2009). Screening for dyslexia, dyspraxia and Meares-Irlen syndrome in higher education. *Dyslexia, 15*(1), 42–60.

Nickel, M. K. T., Tritt, K., Mitterlehner, F. O., Leiberich, P., Nickel, C., Lahmann, C., et al. (2004). Sexual abuse in childhood and youth as psychopathologically relevant life occurrence: Cross-sectional survey. *Croatian Medical Journal, 45*(4), 483–489.

Nielsen, P. R., Benros, M. E., & Dalsgaard, S. (2017, March). Associations between autoimmune diseases and attention-deficit/hyperactivity disorder: A nationwide study. *Journal of the American Academy of Child and Adolescent Psychiatry, 56*(3), 234–240.e1.

Nooshinfar, E., Safaroghli-Azar, A., Bashash, D., & Akbari, M. E. (2017, January). Melatonin, an inhibitory agent in breast cancer. *Breast Cancer, 24*(1), 42–51.

Nuijten, M., Blanken, P., Van de Wetering, B., Nuijen, B., Van den Brink, W., & Hendriks, V. M. (2016, May 28). Sustained-release dexamfetamine in the treatment of chronic cocaine-dependent patients on heroin-assisted treatment: A randomised, double-blind, placebo-controlled trial. *Lancet, 387*(10034), 2226–2234.

NVvP (Nederlandse Vereniging voor Psychiatrie). (2015). *Richtlijn ADHD bij volwassenen. Deel I Diagnostiek en Medicamenteuze behandeling.*

Oner, P., Dirik, E. B., Taner, Y., Caykoylu, A., & Anlar, O. (2007). Association between low serum ferritin and restless legs syndrome in patients with attention deficit hyperactivity disorder. *Tohoku Journal of Experimental Medicine, 213*(2), 269–276.

Oner, P., Oner, O., Azik, F. M., Cop, E., & Munir, K. M. (2012, May 17). Ferritin and hyperactivity ratings in attention deficit hyperactivity disorder. *Pediatrics International, 54*(5), 688–692. https://doi.org/10.1111/j.1442-200X.2012.03664.x

Oner, O., Oner, P., Bozkurt, O. H., Odabas, E., Keser, N., Karadag, H., & Kizilgün, M. (2010). Effects of zinc and ferritin levels on parent and teacher reported symptom scores in attention deficit hyperactivity disorder. *Child Psychiatry and Human Development, 41*(4), 441–447.

Oosterloo, M., Lammers, G. J., Overeem, S., De Noord, I., & Kooij, J. J. S. (2006). Possible confusion between primary hypersomnia and adult attention-deficit/hyperactivity disorder. *Psychiatry Research, 143*(2-3), 293–297.

Opler, L. A., Frank, D. M., & Ramirez, P. M. (2001, June). Psychostimulants in the treatment of adults with psychosis and attention deficit disorder. *Annals of the New York Academy of Sciences, 931*, 297–301.

Ornoy, A., & Spivak, A. (2019 Jul 9). Cost effectiveness of optimal treatment of ADHD in Israel: A suggestion for national policy. *Health Economics Review, 9*(1), 24.

Otasowie, J., Castells, X., Ehimare, U. P., & Smith, C. H. (2014). Tricyclic antidepressants for attention deficit hyperactivity disorder (ADHD) in children and adolescents. *Cochrane Database of Systematic Reviews, 2*, CD006997.

Ouyang, L., Fang, X., Mercy, J., Perou, R., & Grosse, S. D. (2008). Attention-deficit/ hyperactivity disorder symptoms and child maltreatment: A population-based study. *Journal of Pediatrics, 153*(6), 851–856.

Paine, S. J., Gander, P. H., & Travier, N. (2006). The epidemiology of morningness/eveningness: Influence of age, gender ethnicity, and socioeconomic factors in adults (30-49 years). *Journal of Biological Rhythms, 21*(1), 68–76.

Pallanti, S., & Salerno, L. (2015, March 22). Raising attention to attention deficit hyperactivity disorder in schizophrenia. *World J Psychiatry, 5*(1), 47–55.

Palumbo, D., Spencer, T., Lynch, J., Co-Chien, H., & Faraone, S. V. (2004). Emergence of tics in children with ADHD: Impact of once-daily OROS methylphenidate therapy. *Journal of Child and Adolescent Psychopharmacology, 14*(2), 185–194.

Pandi-Perumal, S. R., Srinivasan, V., Spence, D. W., & Cardinali, D. P. (2007). Role of the melatonin system in the control of sleep: Therapeutic implications. *CNS Drugs, 21*(12), 995–1018.

Panzer, A., & Viljoen, M. (1997). The validity of melatonin as an oncostatic agent. *Journal of Pineal Research, 22*(4), 184–202.

Parisi, P., Villa, M. P., Donfrancesco, R., Miano, S., Paolino, M. C., & Cortese, S. (2012). Could treatment of iron deficiency both improve ADHD and reduce cardiovascular risk during treatment with ADHD drugs? *Medical Hypotheses, 79*(2), 246–249.

Patrick, R. P., & Ames, B. N. (2015, January). Vitamin D and the omega-3 fatty acids control serotonin synthesis and action, part 2: relevance for ADHD, bipolar disorder, schizophrenia, and impulsive behavior. *FASEB Journal, 29*(6), 2207–22. https://doi.org/10.1096/fj.14-268342. Epub 2015 Feb 24. PMID: 25713056.

Pelham, W. E., Jr., Greenslade, K. E., Vodde-Hamilton, M., Murphy, D. A., Greenstein, J. J., Gnagy, E. M., et al. (1990). Relative efficacy of long-acting stimulants on children with attention deficit-hyperactivity disorder: A comparison of standard methylphenidate, sustained-release methylphenidate, sustained-release dextroamphetamine, and pemoline. *Pediatrics, 86*(2), 226–237.

Pelsser, L. M., Frankena, K., Toorman, J., Savelkoul, H. F., Dubois, A. E., Pereira, R. R., et al. (2011). Effects of a restricted elimination diet on the behaviour of children with attention-deficit hyperactivity disorder (INCA study): A randomised controlled trial. *Lancet, 377*(9764), 494–503.

Pelsser, L. M., Frankena, K., Toorman, J., Savelkoul, H. F., Pereira, R. R., & Buitelaar, J. K. (2009). A randomised controlled trial into the effects of food on ADHD. *European Child and Adolescent Psychiatry, 18*(1), 12–19.

Pennington, B. F., & Ozonoff, S. (1996). Executive functions and developmental psychopathology. *Journal of Child Psychology and Psychiatry, 37*(1), 51–87.

Peralta, V., Campos, M. S., De Jalon, E. G., & Cuesta, M. J. (2010, May). DSM-IV catatonia signs and criteria in first-episode, drug-naive, psychotic patients: Psychometric validity and response to antipsychotic medication. *Schizophrenia Research, 118*(1–3), 168–175.

Peralta, V., De Jalón, E. G., Campos, M. S., Basterra, V., Sanchez-Torres, A., & Cuesta, M. J. (2011, June). Risk factors, pre-morbid functioning and episode correlates of neurological soft signs in drug-naive patients with schizophrenia-spectrum disorders. *Psychological Medicine, 41*(6), 1279–1289.

Perroud, N., Hasler, R., Golay, N., Zimmermann, J., Prada, P., Nicastro, R., et al. (2016, June 14). Personality profiles in adults with attention deficit hyperactivity disorder (ADHD). *BMC Psychiatry, 16*, 199.

Pettersson, R., Söderström, S., & Nilsson, K. W. (2017). Diagnosing ADHD in adults: An examination of the discriminative validity of neuropsychological tests and diagnostic assessment instruments. *Journal of Attention Disorders, 22*(11), 1019–1031. https://doi.org/10.1177/1087054715618788. Epub 2015 Dec 17.

Pettersson, R., Söderström, S., & Nilsson, K. W. (2018). Diagnosing ADHD in adults: An examination of the discriminative validity of neuropsychological tests and diagnostic assessment instruments. *Journal of Attention Disorders, 22*(11), 1019–1031. https://doi.org/10.1177/1087054715618788. Epub 2015 Dec 17.

Phelps, J., Angst, J., Katzow, J., & Sadler, J. (2008). Validity and utility of bipolar spectrum models. *Bipolar Disorders, 10*(1 Pt 2), 179–193.

Philipsen, A., Jans, T., Graf, E., Matthies, S., Borel, P., Colla, M., et al. (2015a). Effects of group psychotherapy, individual counseling, methylphenidate, and placebo in the treatment of adult attention-deficit/hyperactivity disorder: A randomized clinical trial. *JAMA Psychiatry, 72*, 1199–1210.

Philipsen, A., Jans, T., Graf, E., Matthies, S., Borel, P., Colla, M., et al. (2015b, December). Comparison of Methylphenidate and Psychotherapy in Adult ADHD Study (COMPAS) consortium. Effects of group psychotherapy, individual counseling, methylphenidate, and placebo in the treatment of adult attention-deficit/hyperactivity disorder: A randomized clinical trial. *JAMA Psychiatry, 72*(12), 1199–1210.

Philipsen, A., Lam, A. P., Breit, S., Lücke, C., Müller, H. H., & Matthies, S. (2017). Early maladaptive schemas in adult patients with attention deficit hyperactivity disorder. *Attention Deficit Hyperactivity Disorder, 9*(2), 101–111. https://doi.org/10.1007/s12402-016-0211-8. Epub 2016 Dec 23.

Philipsen, A., Limberger, M. F., Lieb, K., Feige, B., Kleindienst, N., Ebner-Priemer, U., et al. (2008). Attention-deficit hyperactivity disorder as a potentially aggravating factor in borderline personality disorder. *British Journal of Psychiatry, 192*(2), 118–123.

Pierce, D., Dixon, C. M., Wigal, S. B., & McGough, J. J. (2008). Pharmacokinetics of methylphenidate transdermal system (MTS): Results from a laboratory classroom study. *Journal of Child and Adolescent Psychopharmacology, 18*(4), 355–364.

Poltavski, D., & Petros, T. (2006). Effects of transdermal nicotine on attention in adult non-smokers with and without attentional deficits. *Physiology & Behavior, 87*(3), 614–624.

Poncin, Y., Sukhodolsky, D. G., McGuire, J., & Scahill, L. (2007). Drug and non-drug treatments of children with ADHD and tic disorders. *European Child and Adolescent Psychiatry, 16*(*Suppl 1*), 78–88.

Posey, D. J., & McDougle, C. J. (2007). Guanfacine and guanfacine extended release: treatment for ADHD and related disorders. *CNS Drugs Reviews, 13*(4), 465–74. https://doi.org/10.1111/j.1527-3458.2007.00026.x. PMID: 18078429; PMCID: PMC6494159.

Prada, P., Hasler, R., Baud, P., Bednarz, G., Ardu, S., Krejci, I., Nicastro, R., et al. (2014, June 30). Distinguishing borderline personality disorder from adult attention deficit/hyperactivity disorder: A clinical and dimensional perspective. *Psychiatry Research, 217*(1–2), 107–114.

Prada, P., Nicastro, R., Zimmermann, J., Hasler, R., Aubry, J. M., & Perroud, N. (2015, September). Addition of methylphenidate to intensive dialectical behaviour therapy for patients suffering from comorbid borderline personality disorder and ADHD: A naturalistic study. *Attention Deficit Hyperactivity Disorder, 7*(3), 199–209.

Prince, J. B., Wilens, T. E., Biederman, J., Spencer, T. J., Millstein, R., Polisner, D. A., et al. (2000). A controlled study of nortriptyline in children and adolescents with attention deficit hyperactivity disorder. *Journal of Child and Adolescent Psychopharmacology, 10*, 193–204.

Qin, L. Q., Li, J., Wang, Y., Wang, J., Xu, J. Y., & Kaneko, T. (2003). The effects of nocturnal life on endocrine circadian patterns in healthy adults. *Life Sciences, 73*(19), 2467–2475.

Quinn, P., & Nadeau, K. (2004). *ADHD bij vrouwen. (1e druk ed.).* Harcourt Assessment BV.

Quinn, P., & Wigal, S. (2004). Perceptions of girls and ADHD: Results from a national survey. *MedGenMed, Medscape General Medicine, 6*(2), 2.

QuintilesIMS. (2016). *Xtrend.*

Ramos-Quiroga, J. A., Bosch, R., Castells, X., Valero, S., Nogueira, M., Gomez, N., et al. (2008). Effect of switching drug formulations from immediate-release to extended-release OROS methylphenidate: A chart review of Spanish adults with attention-deficit hyperactivity disorder. *CNS Drugs, 22*(7), 603–611.

Ramos-Quiroga J. A., Nasillo V., Richarte V., Corrales M., Palma F., Ibáñez P., et al. (2019, August). Criteria and Concurrent Validity of DIVA 2.0: A Semi-Structured Diagnostic Interview for Adult ADHD. *Journal of Attention Disorders, 23*(10), 1126–35. https://doi.org/10.1177/1087054716646451. Epub 2016 Apr 28. PMID: 27125994.

Ramos-Quiroga, J. A., Nasillo, V., Richarte, V., Corrales, M., Palma, F., Ibáñez, P., et al. (2019a). Criteria and concurrent validity of DIVA 2.0: A semi-structured diagnostic interview for adult ADHD. *Journal of Attention Disorders, 23*(10), 1126–1135. https://doi.org/10.1177/1087054716646451. Epub 2016 Apr 28.

Ramos-Quiroga, J. A., Nasillo, V., Richarte, V., Corrales, M., Palma, F., Ibáñez, P., et al. (2019b). Criteria and concurrent validity of DIVA 2.0: A semi-structured diagnostic interview for adult ADHD. *Journal of Attention Disorders, 23*(10), 1126–1135. https://doi.org/10.1177/1087054716646451. Epub 2016 Apr 28.

Ramsay, J. R. (2007). Current Status of Cognitive-behavioral Therapy as a Psychosocial Treatment for Adult Attention-Deficit/Hyperactivity Fisorder. *Current Psychiatry Reports, 9*(5), 427–433.

Ramsay, J. R., & Rostain, A. L. (2008). *Cognitive-behavioral therapy for adult ADHD: An integrative psychosocial and medical approach.* Routledge.

Rapoport, J. L., & Inoff-Germain, G. (2002). Responses to methylphenidate in Attention-Deficit/Hyperactivity Disorder and normal children: Update. *Journal of Attention Disorders, 6*(Suppl 1), S57–S60.

Rasmussen, K., Almvik, R., & Levander, S. (2001). Attention deficit hyperactivity disorder, reading disability, and personality disorders in a prison population. *The Journal of the American Academy of Psychiatry and the Law, 29*(2), 186–193.

Ratey, J. J., Hallowell, E. M., & Miller, A. C. (1995). Relationship dilemmas for adults with ADD: The biology of intimacy. In K. G. Nadeau (Ed.), *A comprehensive guide to attention deficit disorder in adults: Research, diagnosis, and treatment* (pp. 218–235). Brunner/Mazel, Inc..

Ravishankar, V., Chowdappa, S. V., Benegal, V., & Muralidharan, K. (2016, December). The efficacy of atomoxetine in treating adult attention deficit hyperactivity disorder (ADHD): A meta-analysis of controlled trials. *Asian Journal of Psychiatry, 24*, 53–58.

Raz, S., & Dan, O. (2015, February 2). Behavioral and neural correlates of facial versus nonfacial stimuli processing in adults with ADHD: An ERP study. *Neuropsychology, 29*(5), 726–738.

Raz, R., & Gabis, L. (2009). Essential fatty acids and attention-deficit-hyperactivity disorder: A systematic review. *Developmental Medical Child Neurology, 22*, 22.

Raz, S., & Leykin, D. (2015, June). Psychological and cortisol reactivity to experimentally induced stress in adults with ADHD. *Psychoneuroendocrinology, 10*(60), 7–17.

Reh, V., Schmidt, M., Lam, L., Schimmelmann, B. G., Hebebrand, J., Rief, W., & Christiansen, H. (2015). Behavioral assessment of core ADHD symptoms using the QbTest. *Journal of Attention Disorders, 19*(12), 1034–1045. https://doi.org/10.1177/1087054712472981. Epub 2013 Feb 4.

Reiersen, A. M., Constantino, J. N., Volk, H. E., & Todd, R. D. (2007). Autistic traits in a population-based ADHD twin sample. *Journal of Child Psychology and Psychiatry, 48*(5), 464–472.

Reimer, B., DíAmbrosio, L. A., Coughlin, J. F., Fried, R., & Biederman, J. (2007). Task-induced fatigue and collisions in adult drivers with attention deficit hyperactivity disorder. *Traffic Injury Prevention, 8*(3), 290–299.

Reimherr, F. W., Marchant, B. K., Strong, R. E., Hedges, D. W., Adler, L., Spencer, T. J., et al. (2005). Emotional dysregulation in adult ADHD and response to atomoxetine. *Biological Psychiatry, 58*(2), 125–131.

Robin, A. L. (2002). The impact of ADHD on marriage. *The ADHD Report, 10*(3), 9–14. Guilford Publications Inc.

Rodriguez, A., Miettunen, J., Henriksen, T. B., Olsen, J., Obel, C., & Taanila, A. (2008). Maternal adiposity prior to pregnancy is associated with ADHD symptoms in offspring: Evidence from three prospective pregnancy cohorts. *International Journal of Obesity, 32*(3), 550–557.

Roesch, B., Corcoran, M. E., Fetterolf, J., Haffey, M., Martin, P., Preston, P., et al. (2013). Pharmacokinetics of coadministered guanfacine extended release and lisdexamfetamine dimesylate. *Drugs in R&D, 13*, 119–128.

Roessner, V., Banaschewski, T., Uebel, H., Becker, A., & Rothenberger, A. (2004). Neuronal network models of ADHD - lateralization with respect to interhemispheric connectivity reconsidered. *European Child and Adolescent Psychiatry, 13*(Suppl 1), 171–179.

Rommelse, N. N., Altink, M. E., Martin, N. C., Buschgens, C. J., Buitelaar, J. K., Sergeant, J. A., et al. (2008). Neuropsychological measures probably facilitate heritability research of ADHD. *Archives of Clinical Neuropsychology, 15*, 15.

Ronald, A., Simonoff, E., Kuntsi, J., Asherson, P., & Plomin, R. (2008). Evidence for overlapping genetic influences on autistic and ADHD behaviours in a community twin sample. *Journal of Child Psychology and Psychiatry, 49*(5), 535–542.

Ronkainen, H., Vakkuri, O., & Kauppila, A. (1986). Effects of physical exercise on the serum concentration of melatonin in female runners. *Acta Obstetrica Gynecologica Scandinavica, 65*(8), 827–829.

Rosenberg, P. B., Lanctôt, K. L., Drye, L. T., Herrmann, N., Scherer, R. W., Bachman, D. L., et al. (2013). Safety and efficacy of methylphenidate for apathy in Alzheimer's disease: A randomized, placebo-controlled trial. *The Journal of Clinical Psychiatry, 74*(8), 810–816.

Rosler, M., Retz, W., Yaqoobi, K., Burg, E., & Retz-Junginger, P. (2008). Attention deficit/ hyperactivity disorder in female offenders: Prevalence, psychiatric comorbidity and psychosocial implications. *European Archives of Psychiatry and Clinical Neuroscience, 19*, 19.

Rostain, A. L. (2008). Attention-deficit/hyperactivity disorder in adults: Evidence-based recommendations for management. *Postgraduate Medicine, 120*(3), 27–38.

Rubia, K., Alegria, A., & Brinson, H. (2014a, May). Imaging the ADHD brain: Disorder-specificity, medication effects and clinical translation. *Expert Review of Neurotherapeutics, 14*(5), 519–538.

Rubia, K., Alegria, A. A., & Brinson, H. (2014b, February 24). Brain abnormalities in attention-deficit hyperactivity disorder: A review. *Revista de Neurologia, 58*(S01), S3–S18.

Ruchkin, V., Koposov, R. A., Koyanagi, A., & Stickley, A. (2016, October 12). Suicidal behavior in juvenile delinquents: The role of ADHD and other comorbid psychiatric disorders. *Child Psychiatry and Human Development*.

Rucklidge, J. J., Brown, D. L., Crawford, S., & Kaplan, B. J. (2006). Retrospective reports of childhood trauma in adults with ADHD. *Journal of Attention Disorders, 9*(4), 631–641.

Rucklidge, J. J., Frampton, C. M., Gorman, B., & Boggis. (2014). A. Vitamin-mineral treatment of attention-deficit hyperactivity disorder in adults: Double-blind randomised placebo-controlled trial. *The British Journal of Psychiatry, 204*, 306–315.

Rucklidge, J. J., Johnstone, J., Gorman, B., Boggis, A., & Frampton, C. M. (2014). Moderators of treatment response in adults with ADHD treated with a vitamin-mineral supplement. *Progress in Neuro-Psychopharmacology & Biological Psychiatry, 50*, 163–171.

Rudo-Hutt, A. S. (2015, February). Electroencephalography and externalizing behavior: A meta-analysis. *Biological Psychology, 105*, 1–19.

Rush, C. R., Higgins, S. T., Vansickel, A. R., Stoops, W. W., Lile, J. A., & Glaser, P. E. (2005). Methylphenidate increases cigarette smoking. *Psychopharmacology, 181*(4), 781–789.

Rybak, Y. E., McNeely, H. E., Mackenzie, B. E., Jain, U. R., & Levitan, R. D. (2006). An open trial of light therapy in adult attention-deficit/hyperactivity disorder. *Journal of Clinical Psychiatry, 67*(10), 1527–1535.

Rybak, Y. E., McNeely, H. E., Mackenzie, B. E., Jain, U. R., & Levitan, R. D. (2007, November-December). Seasonality and circadian preference in adult attention-deficit/hyperactivity disorder: clinical and neuropsychological correlates. *Comprehensive Psychiatry, 48*(6), 562–71. https://doi.org/10.1016/j.comppsych.2007.05.008. Epub 2007 Aug 20. PMID: 17954143.

Rylander, M., & Verhulst, S. (2013). Vitamin D insufficiency in psychiatric inpatients. *Journal of Psychiatric Practice, 19*, 296–300.

Sabzichi, M., Samadi, N., Mohammadian, J., Hamishehkar, H., Akbarzadeh, M., & Molavi, O. (2016, September). Sustained release of melatonin: A novel approach in elevating efficacy of tamoxifen in breast cancer treatment. *Colloids and Surfaces. B, Biointerfaces, 1*(145), 64–71.

Sadeh, A., Pergamin, L., & Bar-Haim, Y. (2006). Sleep in children with attention-deficit hyperactivity disorder: A meta-analysis of polysomnographic studies. *Sleep Medicine Reviews, 10*(6), 381–398.

Sadock, B. J., Sadock, V. A., & Ruiz, P. (2009). *Kaplan & sadockís comprehensive textbook of psychiatry*. Lippincott, Williams & Wilkins.

Sáez-Francàs, N., Alegre, J., Calvo, N., Antonio Ramos-Quiroga, J., Ruiz, E., Hernández-Vara, J., et al. (2012, December 30). Attention-deficit hyperactivity disorder in chronic fatigue syndrome patients. *Psychiatry Research, 200*(2–3), 748–753.

Safren, S. A. (2006). Cognitive-behavioral Approaches to ADHD Treatment in Adulthood. *Journal of Clinical Psychiatry, 67*(Suppl 8), 46–50.

Safren, S. A., Otto, M. W., Sprich, S., Winett, C. L., Wilens, T. E., & Biederman, J. (2005). Cognitive-behavioral therapy for ADHD in medication-treated adults with continued symptoms. *Behaviour Research and Therapy, 43*(7), 831–842.

Safren, S. A., Sprich, S., Perlman, T., & Otto, M. (2006a). *Behandelgids ADHD bij volwassenen. Cliëntenwerkboek. Een programma voor cognitieve gedragstherapie*. Nieuwezijds B.V.

Safren, S. A., Sprich, S., Perlman, T., & Otto, M. (2006b). *Behandelgids ADHD bij volwassenen. Therapeutenhandleiding*. Nieuwezijds B.V.

Sahakian, B. J., & Morein-Zamir, S. (2015, April) Pharmacological cognitive enhancement: treatment of neuropsychiatric disorders and lifestyle use by healthy people. *Lancet Psychiatry, 2*(4), 357–62. https://doi.org/10.1016/S2215-0366(15)00004-8. Epub 2015 Mar 31. PMID: 26360089.

Salgado, C. A., Bau, C. H., Grevet, E. H., Fischer, A. G., Victor, M. M., Kalil, K. L., et al. (2009). Inattention and hyperactivity dimensions of ADHD are associated with different personality profiles. *Psychopathology, 42*(2), 108–112.

Sandberg, S. (1996). *Hyperactivity disorders of childhood* (1st ed.). Cambridge University Press.

Sandberg, S. (2002). *Hyperactivity and attention disorders of childhood* (2nd ed.). Cambridge University Press.

Sangal, R. B., Owens, J., Allen, A. J., Sutton, V., Schuh, K., & Kelsey, D. (2006). Effects of atomoxetine and methylphenidate on sleep in children with ADHD. *Sleep, 29*(12), 1573–1585.

Sari Gokten, E., Saday Duman, N., Soylu, N., & Uzun, M. E. (2016, December). Effects of attention-deficit/hyperactivity disorder on child abuse and neglect. *Child Abuse & Neglect, 62*, 1–9.

Satterfield, J. H., Faller, K. J., Crinella, F. M., Schell, A. M., Swanson, J. M., & Homer, L. D. (2007). A 30-year prospective follow-up study of hyperactive boys with conduct problems: Adult criminality. *Journal of the American Academy of Child and Adolescent Psychiatry, 46*(5), 601–610.

Sawni, A. (2008). Attention-deficit/hyperactivity disorder and complementary/alternative medicine. *Adolescent Medicine: State of the Art Reviews, 19*(2), 313–326. xi.

Scheffer, R. E., Kowatch, R. A., Carmody, T., & Rush, A. J. (2005). Randomized, placebo-controlled trial of mixed amphetamine salts for symptoms of comorbid ADHD in pediatric bipolar disorder after mood stabilization with divalproex sodium. *American Journal of Psychiatry, 162*(1), 58–64.

Schelleman, H., Bilker, W. B., Kimmel, S. E., Daniel, G. W., Newcomb, C., Guevara, J. P., et al. (2012). Methylphenidate and risk of serious cardiovascular events in adults. *The American Journal of Psychiatry, 169*, 178–185.

Schernhammer, E. S., & Hankinson, S. E. (2005). Urinary melatonin levels and breast cancer risk. *Journal of the National Cancer Institute, 97*(14), 1084–1087.

Schernhammer, E. S., Kroenke, C. H., Laden, F., & Hankinson, S. E. (2006). Night work and risk of breast cancer. *Epidemiology, 17*(1), 108–111.

Schmid, Y., Hysek, C. M., Preller, K. H., Bosch, O. G., Bilderbeck, A. C., Rogers, R. D., et al. (2015, January). Effects of methylphenidate and MDMA on appraisal of erotic stimuli and intimate relationships. *European Neuropsychopharmacology, 25*(1), 17–25.

Schredl, M., Alm, B., & Sobanski, E. (2007). Sleep quality in adult patients with attention deficit hyperactivity disorder (ADHD). *European Archives of Psychiatry and Clinical Neuroscience., 257*(3), 164–168. https://doi.org/10.1007/s00406-006-0703-1. Epub 2006 Nov 25.

Schubiner, H., Tzelepis, A., Milberger, S., Lockhart, N., Kruger, M., Kelley, B. J., et al. (2000). Prevalence of attention-deficit/hyperactivity disorder and conduct disorder among substance abusers. *Journal of Clinical Psychiatry, 61*(4), 244–251.

Schuijers, F., & Kooij, J. J. S. (2007). *ADHD'ers voor elkaar. Lotgenotenproject.* Vereniging Impuls.

Scott, J. G., Giørtz Pedersen, M., Erskine, H. E., Bikic, A., Demontis, D., McGrath, J. J., & Dalsgaard, S. (2017, May). Mortality in individuals with disruptive behavior disorders diagnosed by specialist services – A nationwide cohort study. *Psychiatry Research, 251*, 255–260.

Seelen, M. L., & Blom, M. B. J. (2009). *Quality of response in bipolar II patients treated with moodstabilisers and stimulants for comorbid ADHD, in Dutch.* Interne publicatie PsyQ, psycho-medische programma's.

Seidman, L. J. (2006). Neuropsychological functioning in people with ADHD across the life-span. *Clinical Psychology Review, 26*(4), 466–485.

Seidman, L. J., Valera, E. M., & Makris, N. (2005). Structural brain imaging of attention-deficit/ hyperactivity disorder. *Biological Psychiatry, 57*(11), 1263–1272.

Semeijn, E. J., Korten, N. C., Comijs, H. C., Michielsen, M., Deeg, D. J., Beekman, A. T., & Kooij, J. J. S. (2015, September). No lower cognitive functioning in older adults with attention-deficit/ hyperactivity disorder. *International Psychogeriatrics, 27*(9), 1467–1476.

Semiz, U. B., Basoglu, C., Oner, O., & Munir, K. M. (2008). Effects of diagnostic comorbidity and dimensional symptoms of attention-deficit-hyperactivity disorder in men with antisocial personality disorder. *The Australian and New Zealand Journal of Psychiatry, 42*(5), 405–413.

Sentissi, O., Navarro, J. C., De Oliveira, H., Gourion, D., Bourdel, M. C., Bayle, F. J., et al. (2008). Bipolar disorders and quality of life: The impact of attention deficit/hyperactivity disorder and substance abuse in euthymic patients. *Psychiatry Research, 161*(1), 36–42.

Serrallach, B., Groß, C., Bernhofs, V., Engelmann, D., Benner, J., Gündert, N., et al. (2016, July 15). Neural biomarkers for dyslexia, ADHD, and ADD in the auditory cortex of children. *Frontiers in Neuroscience, 10*, 324.

Shah, N. R., Jones, J. B., Aperi, J., Shemtov, R., Karne, A., & Borenstein, J. (2008). Selective serotonin reuptake inhibitors for premenstrual syndrome and premenstrual dysphoric disorder: A meta-analysis. *Obstetrics and Gynecology, 111*(5), 1175–1182.

Sheehan, D. V., Harrett-Sheehan, K., & Raj, B. A. (1996). The measurement of disability. *International Clinical Psychopharmacology, 11*(Suppl 3), 89–95.

Sherman, D. K., McGue, M. K., & Iacono, W. G. (1997). Twin concordance for attention deficit hyperactivity disorder: A comparison of teachers' and mothers' reports. *American Journal of Psychiatry, 154*(4), 532–535.

Simon, V., Czobor, P., Bálint, S., Mészáros, A., & Bitter, I. (2009, March). Prevalence and correlates of adult attention-deficit hyperactivity disorder: Meta-analysis. *The British Journal of Psychiatry, 194*(3), 204–211.

Simon, N., Rolland, B., & Karila, L. (2015). Methylphenidate in adults with attention deficit hyperactivity disorder and substance use disorders. *Current Pharmaceutical Design, 21*(23), 3359–3366.

Simonoff, E. (2007). Hyperactivity disorders in children with mental retardation. In *People with hyperactivity: Understanding and managing their problems* (pp. 202–227). Mac Keith Press.

Simpson, D., & Plosker, G. L. (2004). Atomoxetine: A review of its use in adults with attention deficit hyperactivity disorder. *Drugs, 64*(2), 205–222.

Singh, M. K., DelBello, M. P., Kowatch, R. A., & Strakowski, S. M. (2006). Co-occurrence of bipolar and attention-deficit hyperactivity disorders in children. *Bipolar Disorders, 8*(6), 710–720.

Skirrow, C., & Asherson, P. (2013, May). Emotional lability, comorbidity and impairment in adults with attention-deficit hyperactivity disorder. *Journal of Affective Disorders, 147*(1–3), 80–86.

Sliwinski, T., Rozej, W., Morawiec-Bajda, A., Morawiec, Z., Reiter, R., & Blasiak, J. (2007). Protective action of melatonin against oxidative DNA damage-Chemical inactivation versus base-excision repair. *Mutation Research, 634*(1-2), 220–227.

Smits, M. G., Nagtegaal, E. E., Van der Heijden, J., Coenen, A. M., & Kerkhof, G. A. (2001). Melatonin for chronic sleep onset insomnia in children: A randomized placebo-controlled trial. *Journal of Child Neurology, 16*(2), 86–92.

Snyder, J. A. (2015, July 7). The link BETWEEN ADHD and the risk of sexual victimization among college women: Expanding the lifestyles/routine activities framework. *Violence Against Women, 21*(11), 1364–1384.

Soderstrom, H., Nilsson, T., Sjodin, A. K., Carlstedt, A., & Forsman, A. (2005). The childhood-onset neuropsychiatric background to adulthood psychopathic traits and personality disorders. *Comprehensive Psychiatry, 46*(2), 111–116.

Soendergaard, H. M., Thomsen, P. H., Pedersen, P., Pedersen, E., Poulsen, A. E., Nielsen, J. M., et al. (2015, March). Education, occupation and risk-taking behaviour among adults with attention-deficit/hyperactivity disorder. *Danish Medical Journal, 61*(3), A5032.

Solanto, M. V., Arnsten, A. F. T., & Castellanos, F. X. (Eds.). (2001). *Stimulant drugs and ADHD: Basic and clinical neuroscience.*: p xii, 410. Oxford University Press.

Solanto, M. V., Marks, D. J., Mitchell, K. J., Wasserstein, J., & Kofman, M. D. (2008). Development of a new psychosocial treatment for adult ADHD. *Journal of Attention Disorders, 11*(6), 728–736.

Solhkhah, R., Wilens, T. E., Daly, J., Prince, J. B., Van Patten, S. L., & Biederman, J. (2005). Bupropion SR for the treatment of substance-abusing outpatient adolescents with attention-deficit/hyperactivity disorder and mood disorders. *Journal of Child and Adolescent Psychopharmacology, 15*(5), 777–786.

Sonuga-Barke, E. J. (2002). Psychological heterogeneity in AD/HD – a dual pathway model of behaviour and cognition. *Behavioural Brain Research, 130*, 29–36.

Sonuga-Barke, E., Bitsakou, P., & Thompson, M. (2010, April). Beyond the dual pathway model: Evidence for the dissociation of timing, inhibitory, and delay-related impairments in attention-deficit/hyperactivity disorder. *Journal of the American Academy of Child and Adolescent Psychiatry, 49*(4), 345–355.

Sonuga-Barke, E. J., Brandeis, D., Cortese, S., Daley, D., Ferrin, M., Holtmann, M., et al. (2013, March). Nonpharmacological interventions for ADHD: Systematic review and meta-analyses of randomized controlled trials of dietary and psychological treatments. *The American Journal of Psychiatry, 170*(3), 275–289.

Spencer, T. J. (2007). *Adult ADHD and comorbidity in a clinically referred sample.* Paper presented at the APA, San Diego.

Spencer, T. J., Adler, L. A., McGough, J. J., Muniz, R., Jiang, H., & Pestreich, L. (2007). Adult ADHD Research Group. Efficacy and safety of dexmethylphenidate extended-release capsules in adults with attention-deficit/hyperactivity disorder. *Biological Psychiatry, 61*(12), 1380–1387.

Spencer, T., Biederman, J., Wilens, T., Doyle, R., Surman, C., Prince, J., et al. (2005). A large, double-blind, randomized clinical trial of methylphenidate in the treatment of adults with attention-deficit/hyperactivity disorder. *Biological Psychiatry, 57*(5), 456–463.

Spencer, T., Coffey, B., & Biederman, J. (1997). *Chronic tics in adults with ADHD.* Paper presented at the Annual Meeting of the American Academy of Child and Adult Psychiatry.

Spencer, A. E., Marin, M. F., Milad, M. R., Spencer, T. J., Bogucki, O. E., Pope, A. L., et al. (2017, February). Abnormal fear circuitry in attention deficit hyperactivity disorder: A controlled magnetic resonance imaging study. *Psychiatry Research, 10*(262), 55–62.

Spencer, T. J., Wilens, T. E., Biederman, J., Weisler, R. H., Read, S. C., & Pratt, R. (2006). Efficacy and safety of mixed amphetamine salts extended release (Adderall XR) in the management of attention-deficit/hyperactivity disorder in adolescent patients: A 4-week, randomized, double-blind, placebo-controlled, parallel-group study. *Clinical Therapy, 28*(2), 266–279.

Spencer, T., Wilens, T., Biederman, J., Wozniak, J., & Harding-Crawford, M. (2000). Attention-deficit/hyperactivity disorder with mood disorders. In T. E. Brown (Ed.), *Attention-deficit disorders and comorbidities in children, adolescents, and adults* (pp. 79–124). American Psychiatric Publishing, Inc..

Stahlberg, O., Soderstrom, H., Rastam, M., & Gillberg, C. (2004, July). Bipolar disorder, schizophrenia, and other psychotic disorders in adults with childhood onset AD/HD and/or autism spectrum disorders. *Journal of Neural Transmission (Vienna), 111*(7), 891–902.

Stein, M. A., & McGough, J. J. (2008). The pharmacogenomic era: Promise for personalizing attention deficit hyperactivity disorder therapy. *Child and Adolescent Psychiatric Clinics of North America, 17*(2), 475–490. xi–xii.

Stergiakouli, E., Hamshere, M., Holmans, P., Langley, K., Zaharieva, I., Psychiatric GWAS Consortium, et al. (2012). Investigating the contribution of common genetic variants to the risk and pathogenesis of ADHD. *The American Journal of Psychiatry, 69*(2), 186–194.

Stevenson, J., Buitelaar, J., Cortese, S., Ferrin, M., Konofal, E., Lecendreux, M., et al. (2014, May). Research review: The role of diet in the treatment of attention-deficit/hyperactivity disorder--an appraisal of the evidence on efficacy and recommendations on the design of future studies. *J Child Psychol Psychiatry, 55*(5), 416–427.

Stickley, A., Koyanagi, A., Ruchkin, V., & Kamio, Y. (2016, January). Attention-deficit/hyperactivity disorder symptoms and suicide ideation and attempts: Findings from the Adult Psychiatric Morbidity Survey 2007. *Journal of Affective Disorders, 1*(189), 321–328.

Strang, J. F., Kenworthy, L., Dominska, A., Sokoloff, J., Kenealy, L. E., Berl, M., et al. (2014, November). Increased gender variance in autism spectrum disorders and attention deficit hyperactivity disorder. *Archives of Sexual Behavior, 43*(8), 1525–1533.

Strohl, M. P. (2011, March). Bradley's Benzedrine studies on children with behavioral disorders. *The Yale Journal of Biology and Medicine, 84*(1), 27–33.

Stroux, D., Shushakova, A., Geburek-Höfer, A. J., Ohrmann, P., Rist, F., & Pedersen, A. (2016). Deficient interference control during working memory updating in adults with ADHD:

An event-related potential study. *Clinical Neurophysiology, 127*(1), 452–463. https://doi.org/10.1016/j.clinph.2015.05.021. *Epub 2015 Jun 3*.

Sugaya, L., Hasin, D. S., Olfson, M., Lin, K. H., Grant, B. F., & Blanco, C. (2012, August). Child physical abuse and adult mental health: A national study. *Journal of Traumatic Stress, 25*(4), 384–392.

Swanson, J., Arnold, L. E., Kraemer, H., Hechtman, L., Molina, B., Hinshaw, S., et al. (2008). Evidence, interpretation, and qualification from multiple reports of long-term outcomes in the Multimodal Treatment study of Children with ADHD (MTA): Part I: Executive summary. *Journal of Attention Disorders, 12*(1), 4–14.

Swanson, J. M., & Hechtman, L. (2005). Using long-acting stimulants: Does it change ADHD treatment outcome? *Canadian Child and Adolescent Psychiatric Reviews, 14*(Supplement 1), 2–3.

Swanson, E. N., Owens, E. B., & Hinshaw, S. P. (2014, May). Pathways to self-harmful behaviors in young women with and without ADHD: A longitudinal examination of mediating factors. *Journal of Child Psychology and Psychiatry, 55*(5), 505–515.

Swensen, A., Birnbaum, H. G., Ben Hamadi, R., Greenberg, P., Cremieux, P. Y., & Secnik, K. (2004). Incidence and costs of accidents among attention-deficit/hyperactivity disorder patients. *Journal of Adolescent Health, 35*(4), e341–e349.

Szobot, C. M., Shih, M. C., Schaefer, T., Junior, N., Hoexter, M. Q., Fu, Y. K., et al. (2008). Methylphenidate DAT binding in adolescents with attention-deficit/hyperactivity disorder comorbid with substance use disorder--a single photon emission computed tomography with [Tc(99m)]TRODAT-1 study. *NeuroImage, 40*(3), 1195–1201.

Tan, L. N., Wei, H. Y., Zhang, Y. D., Lu, A. L., & Li, Y. (2011). Relationship between serum ferritin levels and susceptibility to attention deficit hyperactivity disorder in children: A Meta analysis (Chinese). *Zhongguo Dang Dai Er Ke Za Zhi, 13*(9), 722–724.

Taylor, F. B., & Russo, J. (2001, April). Comparing guanfacine and dextroamphetamine for the treatment of adult attention-deficit/hyperactivity disorder. *Journal of Clinical Psychopharmacology, 21*(2), 223–8. https://doi.org/10.1097/00004714-200104000-00015. PMID: 11270920.

Ten Have, M., de Graaf, R., Van Dorsselaer, S., Verdurmen, J., van't Land, H., Vollebergh, W., et al. (2006). *Prevalentie van impulsstoornissen. Resultaten van the European Study of Epidemiology of Mental Disorders (ESEMeD)*. Trimbos Instituut.

Thoma, P., Edel, M. A., Suchan, B., & Bellebaum, C. (2015, January 30). Probabilistic reward learning in adults with Attention Deficit Hyperactivity Disorder--an electrophysiological study. *Psychiatry Research, 225*(1-2), 133–144.

Tillman, R., & Geller, B. (2006). Controlled study of switching from attention-deficit/hyperactivity disorder to a prepubertal and early adolescent bipolar I disorder phenotype during 6-year prospective follow-up: Rate, risk, and predictors. *Development and Psychopathology, 18*(4), 1037–1053.

Tomasi, D., & Volkow, N. D. (2012, March 1). Abnormal functional connectivity in children with attention-deficit/hyperactivity disorder. *Biological Psychiatry, 71*(5), 443–450.

Tonhajzerová, I., Ondrejka, I., Farský, I., Višňovcová, Z., Mešťaník, M., Javorka, M., et al. (2014). Attention deficit/hyperactivity disorder (ADHD) is associated with altered heart rate asymmetry. *Physiological Research, 63*(Suppl 4), S509–S519.

Toone, B. K., & der Linden, V. (1997). Attention deficit hyperactivity disorder or hyperkinetic disorder in adults. *British Journal of Psychiatry, 170*, 489–491.

Tordjman, S., Chokron, S., Delorme, R., Charrier, A., Bellissant, E., Jaafari, N., et al. (2017, April). Melatonin: Pharmacology, functions and therapeutic benefits. *Current Neuropharmacology, 15*(3), 434–443.

Triolo, S. J. (1999). *Attention deficit hyperactivity disorder in adulthood: A practitioner's handbook*. Brunner-Routledge.

Upadhyaya, H. P. (2008). Substance use disorders in children and adolescents with attention-deficit/hyperactivity disorder: Implications for treatment and the role of the primary care physician. *Primary Care Companion to the Journal of Clinical Psychiatry, 10*(3), 211–221.

Upadhyaya, H. P., Brady, K. T., & Wang, W. (2004). Bupropion SR in adolescents with comorbid ADHD and nicotine dependence: A pilot study. *Journal of the American Academy of Child and Adolescent Psychiatry, 43*(2), 199–205.

Urban, K. R., & Gao, W. J. (2014, May 13). Performance enhancement at the cost of potential brain plasticity: Neural ramifications of nootropic drugs in the healthy developing brain. *Frontiers in Systems Neuroscience, 8*, 38.

Valdizán Usón, J. R., Idiazábal Alecha, M., & A. (2008). Diagnostic and treatment challenges of chronic fatigue syndrome: Role of immediate-release methylphenidate. *Expert Review of Neurotherapeutics, 8*(6), 917–927.

Valera, E. M., Faraone, S. V., Biederman, J., Poldrack, R. A., & Seidman, L. J. (2005). Functional neuroanatomy of working memory in adults with attention-deficit/hyperactivity disorder. *Biological Psychiatry, 57*(5), 439–447.

Van Ameringen, M. (2008). Adult ADHD is common among patients in anxiety-disorders clinic. Paper presented at the *anxiety disorders association of America,* 28th annual meeting.

Van Ameringen, M., Mancini, C., Simpson, W., & Patterson, B. (2011 August). Adult attention deficit hyperactivity disorder in an anxiety disorders population. *CNS Neuroscience & Therapeutics, 17*(4), 221–6. https://doi.org/10.1111/j.1755-5949.2010.00148.x. Epub 2010 Apr 8. PMID: 20406249; PMCID: PMC6493806.

Van Berckelaer-Onnes, I. A. (2004). Zestig jaar autisme. *Nederlands Tijdschrift voor Geneeskunde, 148*(21), 1024–1030.

Van de Glind, G., Kooij, J. J. S., Van Duin, D., Goossensen, A., & Carpentier, P. J. (2004). *Protocol ADHD bij verslaving. Screening, diagnostiek en behandeling voor de ambulante en klinische verslavingszorg.* Trimbos Instituut.

Van de Glind, G., Van Emmerik-van Oortmerssen, K., Carpentier, P. J., Levin, F. R., Koeter, M. W., Barta, C., et al. (2013, September). The international ADHD in substance use disorders prevalence (IASP) study: Background, methods and study population. *International Journal of Methods in Psychiatric Research, 22*(3), 232–244.

Van de Putte, E. M. (2006). *Exploring chronic fatigue syndrome in adolescents.* Thesis, University of Utrecht, Utrecht.

Van der Feltz-Cornelis, C. M., & Aldenkamp, A. P. (2006). Effectiveness and safety of methylphenidate in adult attention deficit hyperactivity disorder in patients with epilepsy: An open treatment trial. *Epilepsy & Behaviour, 8*(3), 659–662.

Van der Heijden, K. B., Smits, M. G., & Gunning, W. B. (2006). Sleep hygiene and actigraphically evaluated sleep characteristics in children with ADHD and chronic sleep onset insomnia. *Journal of Sleep Research, 15*(1), 55–62.

Van der Heijden, K. B., Smits, M. G., Van Someren, E. J. W., & Gunning, W. B. (2005). Idiopathic chronic sleep onset insomnia in attention-deficit/hyperactivity disorder: A circadian rhythm sleep disorder. *Chronobiology International, 22*(3), 559–570.

Van der Heijden, K. B., Smits, M. G., Van Someren, E. J. W., Ridderinkhof, K. R., & Gunning, W. B. (2007). Effect of melatonin on sleep, behavior, and cognition in ADHD and chronic sleep-onset insomnia. *Journal of the American Academy of Child and Adolescent Psychiatry, 46*(2), 233–241.

Van der Kolk, A., Bouwmans, C. A., Schawo, S. J., Buitelaar, J. K., Van Agthoven, M., & Hakkaart-van Roijen, L. (2015, May 15). Association between societal costs and treatment response in children and adolescents with ADHD and their parents. A cross-sectional study in the Netherlands. *Springerplus, 4*, 224.

Van der Linden, G., Young, S., Ryan, P., & Toone, B. (2000). Attention deficit hyperactivity disorder in adults – Experience of the first National Health Service clinic in the United Kingdom. *Journal of Mental Health, 9*(5), 527–535.

Van Dijk, F., Lappenschaar, M., Kan, C., Verkes, R. J., & Buitelaar, J. K. (2011, December 30). Lifespan attention deficit/hyperactivity disorder and borderline personality disorder symptoms in female patients: A latent class approach. *Psychiatry Research, 190*(2–3), 327–334.

Van Dijk, F., Lappenschaar, M., Kan, C. C., Verkes, R. J., & Buitelaar, J. K. (2012, January). Symptomatic overlap between attention-deficit/hyperactivity disorder and borderline personality disorder in women: The role of temperament and character traits. *Comprehensive Psychiatry, 53*(1), 39–47.

Van Dijk, F., Schellekens, A., Van den Broek, P., Kan, C., Verkes, R. J., & Buitelaar, J. (2014, March 30). Do cognitive measures of response inhibition differentiate between attention deficit/hyperactivity disorder and borderline personality disorder? *Psychiatry Research, 215*(3), 733–739.

Van Emmerik-van Oortmerssen, K., Van de Glind, G., Van den Brink, W., Smit, F., Crunelle, C. L., Swets, M., et al. (2012, April 1). Prevalence of attention-deficit hyperactivity disorder in substance use disorder patients: A meta-analysis and meta-regression analysis. *Drug and Alcohol Dependence, 122*(1–2), 11–19.

Van Groenestijn, M. A. C., Akkerhuis, G. W., Kupka, R. W., Schneider, N., Nolen, W. A., & (Nederlandse vertaling). (2006). *SCID I. Gestructureerd Klinisch Interview voor DSM-IV as-I Stoornissen.* Swets Test Publishers.

Van Hulzen, K. J., Scholz, C. J., Franke, B., Ripke, S., Klein, M., McQuillin, A., et al. (2017). Genetic overlap between attention-deficit/hyperactivity disorder and bipolar disorder: Evidence from genome-wide association study meta-analysis. *Biological Psychiatry, 82*(9), 634–641. https://doi.org/10.1016/j.biopsych.2016.08.040. Epub 2016 Oct 18.

Van Reekum, R., & Links, P. S. (1994). N of 1 study: Methylphenidate in a patient with borderline personality disorder and attention deficit hyperactivity disorder. *Canadian Journal of Psychiatry, 39*(3), 186–187.

Van Reeth, O., Sturis, J., Byrne, M. M., Blackman, J. D., L'Hermite-Balériaux, M., Leproult, R., et al. (1994, June). Nocturnal exercise phase delays circadian rhythms of melatonin and thyrotropin secretion in normal men. *The American Journal of Physiology, 266*(6, Pt 1), E964–E974.

Van Veen, M. M., Kooij, J. J. S., Boonstra, A. M., Gordijn, M., & Van Someren, E. J. W. (2009). Disrupted circadian rhythm in adults with ADHD and chronic sleep onset insomnia. *Biological Psychiatry, 67*(11), 1091–1096.

Van Veen, M. M., Kooij, J. J. S., Boonstra, A. M., Gordijn, M., & Van Someren, E. J. W. (2010). Disrupted circadian rhythm in adults with ADHD and chronic sleep onset insomnia. *Biological Psychiatry, 67*(11), 1091–1096.

VanderDrift, L. E., Antshel, K. M., & Olszewski, A. K. (2017, May 1). Inattention and hyperactivity-impulsivity: Their detrimental effect on romantic relationship maintenance. *Journal of Attention Disorders.*

Vermeiren, R., De Clippele, A., & Deboutte, D. (2000). A descriptive survey of Flemish delinquent adolescents. *Journal of Adolescence, 23*(3), 277–285.

Verster, J. C., Bekker, E. M., De Roos, M., Minova, A., Eijken, E. J., Kooij, J. J. S., et al. (2008). Methylphenidate significantly improves driving performance of adults with attention-deficit hyperactivity disorder: A randomized crossover trial. *Journal of Psychopharmacology, 22*(3), 230–237.

Vgontzas, A. N., Bixler, E. O., & Chrousos, G. P. (2005). Sleep apnea is a manifestation of the metabolic syndrome. *Sleep Medicine Reviews, 9*(3), 211–224.

Viktorin, A., Rydén, E., Thase, M. E., Chang, Z., Lundholm, C., D'Onofrio, B. M., et al. (2017). The risk of treatment-emergent mania with methylphenidate in bipolar disorder. *The American Journal of Psychiatry, 174*(4), 341–348. https://doi.org/10.1176/appi.ajp.2016.16040467. Epub 2016 Oct 3.

Vogel, S. W., Bijlenga, D., Tanke, M., Bron, T. I., Van der Heijden, K. B., Swaab, H., Beekman, A. T., & Kooij, J. J. S. (2015, November). Circadian rhythm disruption as a link between attention-deficit/hyperactivity disorder and obesity? *Journal of Psychosomatic Research, 79*(5), 443–450.

Vogt, C., & Shameli, A. (2011). Assessments for attention-deficit hyperactivity disorder: Use of objective measurements. *The Psychiatrist, 35*, 380–383. https://doi.org/10.1192/pb.bp.110.032144

Volkow, N. D., Ding, Y. S., Fowler, J. S., Wang, G. J., Logan, J., Gatley, J. S., et al. (1995). Is methylphenidate like cocaine? Studies on their pharmacokinetics and distribution in the human brain. *Archives of General Psychiatry, 52*(6), 456–463.

Volkow, N. D., Fowler, J. S., Wang, G., Ding, Y., & Gatley, S. J. (2002). Mechanism of action of methylphenidate: Insights from PET imaging studies. *Journal of Attention Disorders, 6(Suppl 1)*, S31–S43.

Volkow, N. D., Fowler, J. S., Wang, G. J., & Swanson, J. M. (2004). Dopamine in drug abuse and addiction: Results from imaging studies and treatment implications. *Molecular Psychiatry, 9*(6), 557–569.

Volkow, N. D., Wang, G. J., Telang, F., Fowler, J. S., Logan, J., Childress, A. R., et al. (2008). Dopamine increases in striatum do not elicit craving in cocaine abusers unless they are coupled with cocaine cues. *NeuroImage, 39*(3), 1266–1273.

Vreugdenhil, C., Doreleijers, T. A., Vermeiren, R., Wouters, L. F., & Van den Brink, W. (2004). Psychiatric disorders in a representative sample of incarcerated boys in the Netherlands. *Journal of the American Academy of Child and Adolescent Psychiatry, 43*(1), 97–104.

Wagner, M. L., Walters, A. S., & Fisher, B. C. (2004). Symptoms of attention-deficit/hyperactivity disorder in adults with restless legs syndrome. *Sleep, 27*(8), 1499–1504.

Wang, S. M., Han, C., Lee, S. J., Jun, T. Y., Patkar, A. A., Masand, P. S., et al. (2017, January). Modafinil for the treatment of attention-deficit/hyperactivity disorder: A meta-analysis. *Journal of Psychiatric Research, 84*, 292–300.

Wang, L. J., Shyu, Y. C., Yuan, S. S., Yang, C. J., Yang, K. C., Lee, T. L., et al. (2016, January). Attention-deficit hyperactivity disorder, its pharmacotherapy, and the risk of developing bipolar disorder. *Journal of Psychiatric Research, 72*, 6–14.

Wang, L. J., Wu, C. C., Lee, S. Y. & Tsai, Y. F. (2014, August). Salivary neurosteroid levels and behavioural profiles of children with attention-deficit/hyperactivity disorder during six months of methylphenidate treatment. *Journal of Child and Adolescent Psychopharmacology, 24*(6), 336–340. (7), 425–432.

Waring, M. E., Lapane, K. L., Daviss, W. B., Birmaher, B., Diler, R. S., Mintz, J., et al. (2008). Overweight in children and adolescents in relation to attention-deficit/hyperactivity disorder: Results from a national sample. *Pediatrics, 122*(1), e1–e6.

Wasserstein, J., & Denckla, M. B. (2009). ADHD and learning disabilities in adults: Overlap with executive function. In T. E. Brown (Ed.), *ADHD comorbidities: Handbook for ADHD complications in children and adults*. American Psychiatric Publishing.

Weber, W., & Newmark, S. (2007). Complementary and alternative medical therapies for attention-deficit/hyperactivity disorder and autism. *Pediatric Clinics of North America, 54*(6), 983–1006. xii.

Weber, W., Van der Stoep, A., McCarty, R. L., Weiss, N. S., Biederman, J., & McClellan, J. (2008). Hypericum perforatum (St Johnís wort) for attention-deficit/hyperactivity disorder in children and adolescents: A randomized controlled trial. *Journal of the American Medical Association, 299*(22), 2633–2641.

Weertman, A., Arntz, A., & Kerkhofs, M. L. M. (2006). *SCID II. Gestructureerd Klinisch Interview voor DSM-IV as-II Persoonlijkheidsstoornissen*. Harcourt Test Publishers.

Weinstein, D., Staffelbach, D., & Biaggio, M. (2000). Attention-deficit hyperactivity disorder and posttraumatic stress disorder: Differential diagnosis in childhood sexual abuse. *Clinical Psychology Review, 20*(3), 359–378.

Weisfelt, M., Schrier, A. C., & de Leeuw, M. C. (2001). Hyperactive behavior in adults; possibly attention deficit/hyperactivity disorder (ADHD) (in Dutch). *Nederlands Tijdschrift voor Geneeskunde, 145*(31), 1481–1484.

Weisler, R. H., Biederman, J., Spencer, T. J., Wilens, T. E., Faraone, S. V., Chrisman, A. K., et al. (2006). Mixed amphetamine salts extended-release in the treatment of adult ADHD: A randomized, controlled trial. *CNS Spectrums, 11*(8), 625–639.

Weiss, G., & Hechtman, L. (1993). *Hyperactive children grown up. ADHD in children, adolescents and adults* (2nd ed.). Guilford Press.

Weiss, G., Hechtman, L., & Milroy, T. (1985). Psychiatric status of hyperactives as adults: A controlled prospective 15-year follow-up of 63 hyperactive children. *Journal of the American Academy of Child Psychiatry, 24*, 211–220.

Weiss, M., Hechtman, L. T., & Weiss, G. (1999). *ADHD in adulthood: A guide to current theory, diagnosis, and treatment*. The John Hopkins University Press.

Weiss, M., Safren, S. A., Solanto, M. V., Hechtman, L., Rostain, A. L., Ramsay, J. R., et al. (2008). Research forum on psychological treatment of adults with ADHD. *Journal of Attention Disorders, 11*(6), 642–651.

Weiss, M., Wasdell, M., et al. (2004). A post hoc Analysis of d-threo-Methylphenidate Hydrochloride (Focalin) versus d,l,-threo-Methylphenidate Hydrochloride (Ritalin). *Journal of the American Academy of Child and Adolescent Psychiatry, 43*(11), 1415–1421.

Westover, A. N., & Halm, E. A. (2012, June). Do prescription stimulants increase the risk of adverse cardiovascular events?: A systematic review. *BMC Cardiovascular Disorders, 9*;12:41. https://doi.org/10.1186/1471-2261-12-41. PMID: 22682429; PMCID: PMC3405448.

Wetterborg, D., Långström, N., Andersson, G., & Enebrink, P. (2015, October). Borderline personality disorder: Prevalence and psychiatric comorbidity among male offenders on probation in Sweden. *Comprehensive Psychiatry, 62*, 63–70.

Wilens, T. E. (2004a). Impact of ADHD and its treatment on substance abuse in adults. *Journal of Clinical Psychiatry, 65*(Suppl 3), 38–45. PMID: 15046534.

Wilens, T. E. (2004b, June). Attention-deficit/hyperactivity disorder and the substance use disorders: The nature of the relationship, subtypes at risk, and treatment issues. *Psychiatric Clinics of North America, 27*(2), 283–301. https://doi.org/10.1016/S0193-953X(03)00113-8. PMID: 15063998.

Wilens, T. E. (2007). The nature of the relationship between attention-deficit/hyperactivity disorder and substance use. *Journal of Clinical Psychiatry, 68*(Suppl 11), 4–8.

Wilens, T. E., Adler, L. A., Weiss, M. D., Michelson, D., Ramsey, J. L., Moore, R. J., et al. (2008). Atomoxetine treatment of adults with ADHD and comorbid alcohol use disorders. *Drug and Alcohol Dependence, 96*(1-2), 145–154.

Wilens, T. E., Biederman, J., Adamson, J. J., Henin, A., Sgambati, S., Gignac, M., et al. (2008). Further evidence of an association between adolescent bipolar disorder with smoking and substance use disorders: A controlled study. *Drug and Alcohol Dependence, 95*(3), 188–198.

Wilens, T. E., Biederman, J., Mick, E., Faraone, S. V., & Spencer, T. (1997). Attention deficit hyperactivity disorder (ADHD) is associated with early onset substance use disorders. *Journal of Nervous and Mental Disease, 185*(8), 475–482.

Wilens, T. E., Biederman, J., Spencer, T. J., & Frances, R. J. (1994). Comorbidity of attention-deficit hyperactivity and psychoactive substance use disorders. *Hospital and Community Psychiatry, 45*(5), 421–423. 435.

Wilens, T. E., Biederman, J., Wozniak, J., Gunawardene, S., Wong, J., & Monuteaux, M. (2003, July). Can adults with attention-deficit/hyperactivity disorder be distinguished from those with comorbid bipolar disorder? Findings from a sample of clinically referred adults. *Biological Psychiatry, 54*(1), 1–8. https://doi.org/10.1016/s0006-3223(02)01666-9. PMID: 12842302.

Wilens, T. E., & Decker, M. W. (2007). Neuronal nicotinic receptor agonists for the treatment of attention-deficit/hyperactivity disorder: Focus on cognition. *Biochemical Pharmacology, 7*, 7.

Wilens, T. E., Faraone, S. V., Biederman, J., & Gunawardene, S.(2003, January). Does stimulant therapy of attention-deficit/hyperactivity disorder beget later substance abuse? A metaanalytic review of the literature. *Pediatrics, 111*(1), 179–85. https://doi.org/10.1542/peds.111.1.179. PMID: 12509574.

Wilens, T. E., Haight, B. R., Horrigan, J. P., Hudziak, J. J., Rosenthal, N. E., Connor, D. F., et al. (2005). Bupropion XL in adults with attention-deficit/hyperactivity disorder: A randomized, placebo-controlled study. *Biological Psychiatry, 57*(7), 793–801.

Wilens, T. E., Kwon, A., Tanguay, S., Chase, R., Moore, H., Faraone, S. V., et al. (2005, July - September). Characteristics of adults with attention deficit hyperactivity disorder plus substance use disorder: The role of psychiatric comorbidity. *American Journal of Addictions, 14*(4), 319–327. https://doi.org/10.1080/10550490591003639. PMID: 16188712.

Wilens, T. E., Prince, J. B., Spencer, T. J., & Biederman, J. (2006). Stimulants and sudden death: What is a physician to do? *Pediatrics, 118*(3), 1215–1219.

Wilens, T. E., Prince, J. B., Spencer, T., Van Patten, S. L., Doyle, R., Girard, K., et al. (2003). An open trial of bupropion for the treatment of adults with attention-deficit/hyperactivity disorder and bipolar disorder. *Biological Psychiatry, 54*(1), 9–16.

Wilens, T. E., Spencer, T. J., Biederman, J., Girard, K., Doyle, R., Prince, J., et al. (2001). A controlled clinical trial of bupropion for attention deficit hyperactivity disorder in adults. *American Journal of Psychiatry, 158*(2), 282–288.

Wilens, T. E., Upadhyaya, H. P., Faraone, S. V., & Biederman, J. (2007). Impact of substance use disorder on ADHD and its treatment. *Journal of Clinical Psychiatry, 68*(8), e20.

Wilens, T. E., Verlinden, M. H., Adler, L. A., Wozniak, P. J., & West, S. A. (2006). ABT-089, a neuronal nicotinic receptor partial agonist, for the treatment of attention-deficit/hyperactivity disorder in adults: Results of a pilot study. *Biological Psychiatry, 59*(11), 1065–1070.

Wilens, T. E., Zusman, R. M., Hammerness, P. G., Podolski, A., Whitley, J., Spencer, T. J., et al. (2006). An open-label study of the tolerability of mixed amphetamine salts in adults with attention-deficit/hyperactivity disorder and treated primary essential hypertension. *Journal of Clinical Psychiatry, 67*(5), 696–702.

Wilens, T. E., et al. (1995). Pharmacotherpay of adult ADHD. In K. G. Nadeau (Ed.), *A comprehensive guide to attention deficit disorder in adults: Research - Diagnosis - Treatment* (pp. 168–190). Brunner/Mazel.

Willcutt, E. G., Pennington, B. F., Olson, R. K., Chhabildas, N., & Hulslander, J. (2005). Neuropsychological analyses of comorbidity between reading disability and attention deficit hyperactivity disorder: In search of the common deficit. *Developmental Neuropsychology, 27*(1), 35–78.

Williams, N. M., Franke, B., Mick, E., Anney, R. J., Freitag, C. M., Gill, M., et al. (2012). Genome-wide analysis of copy number variants in attention deficit hyperactivity disorder: The role of rare variants and duplications at 15q13.3. *The American Journal of Psychiatry, 169*(2), 195–204.

Willoughby, M. T., Curran, P. J., Costello, E. J., & Angold, A. (2000). Implications of early versus late onset of attention-deficit/hyperactivity disorder symptoms. *Journal of the American Academy of Child & Adolescent Psychiatry, 39*(12), 1512–1519.

Wingo, A. P., & Ghaemi, S. N. (2008). Frequency of stimulant treatment and of stimulant-associated mania/hypomania in bipolar disorder patients. *Psychopharmacology Bulletin, 41*(4), 37–47.

Winhusen, T. M., Somoza, E. C., Brigham, G. S., Liu, D. S., Green, C. A., Covey, L. S., et al. (2010, December). Impact of attention-deficit/hyperactivity disorder (ADHD) treatment on smoking cessation intervention in ADHD smokers: A randomized, double-blind, placebo-controlled trial. *The Journal of Clinical Psychiatry, 71*(12), 1680–1688.

Winkler, M., & Rossi, P. (2001). Borderline personality disorder and attention-deficit/hyperactivity disorder in adults. *Ptt: Personlichkeitsstorungen Theorie und Therapie, 5*(1), 39–48.

Winterstein, A. G., Gerhard, T., Shuster, J., Johnson, M., Zito, J. M., & Saidi, A. (2007). Cardiac safety of central nervous system stimulants in children and adolescents with attention-deficit/hyperactivity disorder. *Pediatrics, 120*(6), e1494–e1501.

Wirtz-Justice, A., Benedetti, F., & Terman, M. (2008). *Chronotherapeutics for affective disorders. A clinicianís manual for light and wake therapy.* Karger.

Witte, A. V., Kerti, L., Hermannstadter, H. M., Fiebach, J. B., Schreiber, S. J., Schuchardt, J. P., et al. (2014). Long-chain omega-3 fatty acids improve brain function and structure in older adults. *Cerebral Cortex, 24*, 3059–3068.

Wolf, U., Golombek, U., & Diefenbacher, A. (2006). Diagnosis and treatment of the attention-deficit/hyperactivity syndrome (ADHS) in adults with drug addiction in in-patient and out-patient setting. *Psychiatrische Praxis, 33*(5), 240–244.

Wood, D., Wender, P. H., & Reimherr, F. W. (1983). The prevalence of attention deficit disorder, residual type, or minimal brain dysfunction, in a population of male alcoholic patients. *American Journal of Psychiatry, 140*(1), 95–98.

Woods, S. P., Lovejoy, D. W., & Ball, J. D. (2002, February). Neuropsychological characteristics of adults with ADHD: A comprehensive review of initial studies. *The Clinical Neuropsychologist, 16*(1), 12–34.

Wozniak, J., Crawford, M. H., Biederman, J., Faraone, S. V., Spencer, T. J., Taylor, A., et al. (1999). Antecedents and complications of trauma in boys with ADHD: Findings from a longitudinal study. *Journal of the American Academy of Child and Adolescent Psychiatry, 38*(1), 48–55.

Wu, E. Q., Hodgkins, P., Ben-Hamadi, R., Setyawan, J., Xie, J., Sikirica, V., et al. (2012). Cost effectiveness of pharmacotherapies for attention-deficit hyperactivity disorder: A systematic literature review. *CNS Drugs, 26*(7), 581–600.

Wymbs, B. T., Dawson, A. E., Suhr, J. A., Bunford, N., & Gidycz, C. A. (2015, May 28). ADHD symptoms as risk factors for intimate partner violence perpetration and victimization. *Journal of Interpersonal Violence.*

Wymbs, B., Molina, B., Pelham, W., Cheong, J., Gnagy, E., Belendiuk, K., et al. (2012, July). Risk of intimate partner violence among young adult males with childhood ADHD. *Journal of Attention Disorders, 16*(5), 373–383.

Wynchank, D. S., Bijlenga, D., Lamers, F., Bron, T. I., Winthorst, W. H., Vogel, S. W., et al. (2016, October). ADHD, circadian rhythms and seasonality. *Journal of Psychiatric Research, 81*, 87–94.

Wynchank, D., Ten Have, M., Bijlenga, D., Penninx, B. W., Beekman, A. T., Lamers, F., de Graaf, R., & Kooij, J. J. S. (2018). The association between insomnia and sleep duration in adults with attention-deficit hyperactivity disorder: Results from a general population study. *Journal of Clinical Sleep Medicine, 14*(3), 349–357.

Yang, Z., Kelly, C., Castellanos, F. X., Leon, T., Milham, M. P., & Adler, L. A. (2016, August). Neural correlates of symptom improvement following stimulant treatment in adults with attention-deficit/hyperactivity disorder. *Journal of Child and Adolescent Psychopharmacology, 26*(6), 527–536.

Young, S., & Gudjonsson, G. H. (2006). ADHD symptomatology and its relationship with emotional, social and delinquency problems. *Psychology, Crime & Law, 12*(5), 463–471.

Young, G. S., Maharaj, N. J., & Conquer, J. A. (2004). Blood phospholipid fatty acid analysis of adults with and without attention deficit/hyperactivity disorder. *Lipids, 39*(2), 117–123.

Young, Z., Moghaddam, N. & Tickle, A. (2016, August 22). The efficacy of cognitive behavioral therapy for adults with ADHD: A systematic review and meta-analysis of randomized controlled trials. *J Atten Disord.*

Young, J. L., & Redmond, J. C. (2007). Fibromyalgia, chronic fatigue, and adult attention deficit hyperactivity disorder in the adult: A case study. *Psychopharmacology Bulletin, 40*(1), 118–126.

Young, S., Sedgwick, O., Fridman, M., Gudjonsson, G., Hodgkins, P., Lantigua, M., et al. (2015, September). Co-morbid psychiatric disorders among incarcerated ADHD populations: A meta-analysis. *Psychological Medicine, 45*(12), 2499–2510.

Young, S., Toone, B., & Tyson, C. (2003). Comorbidity and psychosocial profile of adults with attention deficit hyperactivity disorder. *Personality & Individual Differences, 35*(4), 743–755.

Yuen, K. M., & Pelayo, R. (1999). Sleep disorders and attention-deficit/hyperactivity disorder. *Journal of the American Medical Association, 281*(9), 797.

Zametkin, A. J., Nordahl, T. E., Gross, M., King, A. C., Semple, W. E., Rumsey, J., et al. (1990). Cerebral glucose metabolism in adults with hyperactivity of childhood onset. *New England Journal of Medicine, 323*(20), 1361–1366.

Zanarini, M. C., Frankenburg, F. R., Reich, D. B., Hennen, J., & Silk, K. R. (2005). Adult experiences of abuse reported by borderline patients and Axis II comparison subjects over six years of prospective follow-up. *The Journal of Nervous and Mental Disease, 193*(6), 412–416.

Zanarini, M. C., Williams, A. A., Lewis, R. E., Reich, R. B., Vera, S. C., Marino, M. F., et al. (1997). Reported pathological childhood experiences associated with the development of borderline personality disorder. *American Journal of Psychiatry, 154*(8), 1101–1106.

Zupancic, J., Miller, A., Raina, P., Lee, S., Klassen, A., & Olsen, L. (1998). Part 3: Economic evaluation of pharmaceutical and psychological/behavioural therapies for attention-deficit/hyperactivity disorde. In A. Miller, S. K. Lee, & P. Raina (Eds.), *Review of therapies for attention-deficit/hyperactivity disorder.* Canadian Coordinating Office for Health Technology Assessment.

Index

A
ADHD Europe, 227
ADHD groups, 195–198
ADHD Rating Scale, 106, 107
ADHD self-report scale (ASRS), 16
ADHD symptoms, 120
Adult ADHD Self-Report Screener
    (ASRSv1.1), 32
Aggressive behaviour, 198
Alcohol and cannabis use, 102–103
American Psychiatric Association (APA), 2
Amphetamines, 136
Antisocial personality disorder (ASP), 73
Anxiety disorder, 132, 137, 167
Atomoxetine, 124–126
Attention-deficit/hyperactivity disorder
    (ADHD), 1, 2
  acceptance process, 220–222
  addiction, 70–72
  additional information, 51
  adults, 3, 211
  age, 38
  anxiety, 68, 69
  attention problems, 23
  autism spectrum disorder, 79, 80
  benefits, 49
  binge-eating, 56
  biomarkers, 9, 10
  bipolar disorder, 65, 66
  boys and girls, 19
  chronic fatigue syndrome, 19
  combined presentation type, 37
  common comorbidities, 26, 27
  communication, 218
  comorbidity, 20, 53
  core symptoms, 23
  cost effectiveness, 29
  CPT, 12

  crime, 77, 78
  depression, 63
  diagnosis, 28
  diagnostics, 31
  driving, 41
  DSM criteria, 15–17, 33–36
  dysfunction, 40, 41
  dyslexia, 82
  family history, 51
  fashionable diagnosis, 52
  functional neuroimaging studies, 8, 9
  goal schedule, 208–209
  group participation rule, 212, 213
  health, 54–56
  history, 2
  hyper, 1
  hyperactivity, 24
  hyper-focus, 23
  impulsivity, 24, 25
  intelligence, 38–40
  late-onset, 17, 18
  life course, 28, 29, 218
  limitations, 49, 50
  medication, 217
  meeting, 213–217
  mood, 61–63
  morbidity, 28
  mortality, 28
  neural connectivity, 8
  neuroanatomy, 7, 8
  neurobiology, 4–7, 217
  neurophysiology, 10
  neuropsychology, 11, 51, 52, 66, 67
  new neuroimaging techniques, 9
  obesity, 57
  older people, 14
  partner, 46
  personality disorders, 72–76

Attention-deficit/hyperactivity disorder
    (ADHD) (*cont.*)
  PET studies, 8
  predominantly hyperactive/impulsive
    presentation type, 37
  predominantly inattentive presentation
    type, 37
  presentation type, 58
  prevalence, 12–14, 38
  prevention, men and women, 18
  problems, 26
  psychosis, 82, 83
  rating scale, 206
  relationship, 45, 46, 218
  reward system, 71
  screening, 31–33
  self-report, 206
  sex offenders, 78
  sexuality, 47
  skills
    distractions, 178
    E-mail and forms, 177
    financials, 177–178
    goals target, 175
    individual and group coaching, 170
    learning routines, 172
    noting activities, 173
    overscheduling, 176
    patient tips, 176
    planning and agenda
      management, 170
    planning time, 172
    procrastination, 178–179
    setting targets, 174–175
    task list, 174
    tips for patients, 171–172
    training, 223
    weekly schedule, 172, 173
  skipping breakfast, 56, 57
  sleep disorders, 58
  sleep duration, 61
  sleeping disorders, adults, 59, 60
  sleeping problems, 59
  SPECT studies, 8
  structure, 211
  suicidality, 67
  symptoms, 48, 49, 205
  tic disorders, 81
  tourette's, 81
  winter depression, 64, 65
  work, 42, 43
Autism Diagnostic Interview-Revised
    (ADI-R), 79

Autism Diagnostic Observation Schedule
    (ADOS), 79
Autism spectrum disorder (ASD), 79

B
Bipolar disorder, 99
Bipolar II disorder, 133
Body mass index (BMI), 56
B personality disorder, 104
British Association of Psychopharmacology
    (BAP), 100
Brown Attention Deficit Disorder Scale
    (BADDS), 32

C
Cannabinoid receptor (CNR1), 69
Chronic fatigue syndrome (CFS), 19
Coaching, 205–209
  aftercare, 186–187
  attitude and tasks of
    acceptance, 159
    active structuring, 158–159
    case management, 159–160
    changing role of, 160–161
    cooperation with doctor, 161
    cooperation with external
      organizations, 162
    digital coaching, 162
    individual coaching and group
      treatment relationship, 161
    information, 159
    learning practical skills, 160
    motivation, 159
    supporting, 160
  coach is too active, 179
  coach is too passive, 179–180
  coach overestimates, 180
  comorbid disorders, 151
  feeling of sharing and fellowship, 187
  indications for, 154–155
  motivation for treatment, 156–158
  patient characteristics, 181–182
  patient's comorbidity and social
    problems, 154
  practical goals, 151
  problems in treatment, 182–183
  psychosocial problems, 154
  rationale of, 152–154
  structure of
    dealing with being late, 164–165
    dealing with no-show, 165

duration and frequency of, 163
duration of treatment, 163
patient expectations, 162–163
setting targets, 164
treatment objectives, 163–164
use of session agenda, 163
tips for, 180
treatment structure
acceptance, 166–167
ADHD skills (*see* Attention-deficit/
hyperactivity disorder (ADHD))
comorbidity (*see* Comorbidity
coaching)
Cognitive behavioural therapy (CBT),
151, 168
differences, 152
inclusion criteria, 185
mindfulness, 184
organizational skills and self-esteem, 183
psycho-education, 185
relationship therapy, 185–186
schema therapy, 184
similarities, 152
Cognitive therapy, 120
Comorbidity coaching
anxiety disorder, 167
depression and bipolar disorder, 168
personality disorder, 169
reducing substance abuse, 167
seasonal affective disorder, 168–169
sleep phase, 169
Concerta, 100, 108, 113
Conduct disorder (CD), 65, 75
Conners Adult ADHD Rating Scale
(CAARS), 32, 62
Continuous performance tests (CPTs), 12, 107
Cortisol, 10
Cost effectiveness, 29

D
Depression and bipolar disorder, 168
Dexedrine spansule, 122
Dexmethylphenidate, 99, 121
Dextroamphetamine, 94, 96, 99, 100, 111,
119, 122, 123
Diagnostic Interview for ADHD (DIVA),
33, 86, 201
Diagnostic Interview for Social and
Communicative Disorders
(DISCO), 79
Dialectical Behavioural Therapy (DBT), 138
Digital coaching, 162

Digital medicine, 89–90
Dim Light Melatonin Onset (DLMO), 58, 59
Dopamine (DA), 94
Dopamine-5 receptor (DRD5), 6
Dopamine transporter (DAT), 8, 72, 94
DRD4 gene, 56
DSM criteria, 106
DSM-5 criteria, 31, 32
DSM-IV self-report questionnaire, 16
Dysfunction, Hyperkinetic Reaction of
Childhood (DSM-II), 2
Dyslexia, 82

E
Epidemiological research, 18
Equasym and Medikinet, 96, 113
Equasym XL, 100, 108, 114
Equasym XL 30, 113
ESEMeD study, 13
The European Network Adult ADHD, 227
Event-Related Potential (ERP), 10
EXEcutive functioning (EF), 11

F
FlexCare ADHD, 190
Fluoxetine, 124
Fronto-striatal system, 136

G
Gaming and exercise, 149
Genome wide association studies (GWAS), 6
Guanfacine, 100, 101
Guanfacine XR, 127

H
Harm avoidance, 74
Heart rate variability, 10
Hyperactivity, 22, 24
Hyper-focus, 23
Hyperthyroidism, 121

I
Individual coaching, 154
International Classification of Disease
(ICD), 2
Interpersonal psychotherapy (IPT), 168
Introductory group, 154

J
Juvenile Onset Bipolar Disorder (JOBD), 65
Juvenile onset form, 135

L
Learning routines, 172
Lisdexamphetamine, 122, 123
Long-acting bupropion, 127, 128
Long-acting guanfacine (Intuniv), 100
Longest-acting methylphenidate, 108

M
Marfan syndrome, 104
Medication, 205–209
Medikinet CR, 100, 108, 114
Melanocortin-4 receptor (MC4R), 57
Melatonin, 145
    resets clock, 146
    side effects and protective effects, 145
    sleep aid, 145–146
Metaphors, 116
Methylphenidate, 99, 104, 112, 119, 123,
        140, 183
Mindfulness based cognitive therapy
        (MBCT), 184
Minimal Brain Damage, 93
Minimum treatment, 194
Modiodal (modafinil), 100, 128, 129
Mood stabilizer, 133–136
Morbidity, 28
Multi Sleep Latency Test (MSLT), 58
Munich Chronotype Questionnaire, 141

N
National Comorbidity Survey Replication
        (NCS-R), 13, 53
Neuroimaging, 66
Nicotinergic drugs, 102
Noting activities, 173
Novelty seeking, 73, 74

O
Obsessive-compulsive disorder (OCD), 68, 80
Online psycho-education, 89–90
Oppositional defiant disorder (ODD), 65
Oros-methylphenidate/Concerta, 96, 129, 139
Outpatient and life course clinic
    ADHD groups, 195–197
    development of, 190

employees, 191–192
evaluation and impact
        measurement, 198–199
inclusion and exclusion criteria, 192
intake, 192–193
staff discussion, 193
starting, 190
systematic in-service training, 190
treatment range, 194, 198
Overdosing, 120
Overscheduling, 176

P
Patient tips, 176
Periodic Limb Movement Disorder
        (PLMD), 58
Personality disorder, 155, 169
Plannen, 22
Protocol ADHD bij verslaving, 3
Psycho-education, 166, 185
PsyQ, 189, 197

Q
QbTest, 107, 118

R
Randomized controlled trials (RCTs), 130
Reboxetine, 128
Restless Legs Syndrome (RLS), 58, 60
Ritalin or Medikinet, 100, 108
Routine Outcome Monitoring (ROM), 193

S
SCAN, 62
Schizophrenia, 104
Seasonal affective disorder, 168–169
Self-directedness, 74
Self-report questionnaire, 85–86, 201–204
Serotonin, 128
Sexual abuse, 48
Sheehan Disability Scale, 198
Short- and long-acting methylphenidate, 111
Short-acting Medikinet, 108
Short-acting methylphenidate, 100, 114,
        115, 136
Short-acting stimulants, 96
Sleep phase, 169
Sub-clinical mood disorder, 133
Super Brains app, 92, 95, 162

T
Tachycardia, 120
Task list, 174
Thrill seeking, 69
Traumatic sexual experiences, 48
Treatment
   alternative for ADHD, 148–149
   atomoxetine, 124–126
   combining stimulants
      and addiction, 138–140
      antidepressants, 132
      clinical dilemmas and
         experiences, 135–136
      cluster B personality disorder, 137–138
      low mood, 133
      mood stabilizer, 133–136
      psychosis, 136, 137
      and sexuality, 140
      therapy-resistant ADHD, 140
   contraindications for stimulants, 103–105
   delayed sleep phase disorder
      instructions to patient, 147
      light therapy for, 148
      melatonin (see Melatonin)
      melatonin for, 141–143
      out of phase, 141
      sleep hygiene, 143–145
      sleeping pattern, 141
   dextroamphetamine, 122, 123
   directive, 87
   educational, 87
   in elderly
      cardiovascular disease, 129
      depression and dementia, 131
      dexamphetamine, 129
      methylphenidate, 129–131
   goal-oriented, 87
   guanfacine XR, 127
   instruments for
      ADHD Rating Scale, 106, 107
      individual target symptom list, 107
      QbTest, 107
      symptom and side effects list, 106
   linking insight to action, 88
   long-acting bupropion, 127, 128
   medication
      alcohol and cannabis use, 102–103
      comorbid disorders, 99
      dopamine and norepinephrine
         agonists, 95
      dosage, 101
      functioning of stimulants, 98
      inhibition disorder, 95
      long-acting medication, 101
      nicotinergic drugs, 102

      off-label to adults, 95
      off-label, with the exception, 95
      registered and non-registered
         medications, 99
      registered medications versus off-label
         use, 101
      ritalin and dextroamphetamine, 95
      stimulants and addiction risk, 96–97
      stimulants and non stimulants, 99
      in the United States, 101
   methylphenidate to adults
      adjusting to long acting
         methylphenidate, 113–114
      cognitive functioning in healthy
         people, 112
      dexmethylphenidate, 121
      different methylphenidates, 113
      disadvantage of dosing, 108
      overdosing, 120
      physical conditions, 121–122
      short-acting methylphenidate, 114, 115
      short- and long-term
         effectiveness, 111–112
      side effects of, 119, 120
      treatment with stimulants, 116–119
      wearing off of methylphenidate, 110
   modiodal (modafinil), 128, 129
   practice-oriented: practical, 87
   pregnancy, lactation and
      stimulants, 123–124
   psycho-education
      acceptance of the diagnosis, 92
      brake fluid, 94
      dextroamphetamine, 94
      empowers the patient, 88
      family members, 89
      longitudinal population, 93
      online psycho-education, 89–90
      personal experience, 91
      short-acting medication, 92
      short sentences and closed
         questions, 91
      trendy diagnosis, 93
      untreated ADHD, 92
      Western invention, 93
   reboxetine, 128
   self-filled instruction manual, 124
   serotonin, 128
   side effects and duration of action, 105
   solution-focused, 87
   supportive, 88
   travelling abroad, 124
   tricyclic antidepressants, 128
Tricyclic antidepressants
      (TCAs), 128, 132

U
Ultra-short screening list, 85, 201

V
Velocardiofacial syndrome, 104
Vyvanse, 122

W
Weekly schedule, 172–174, 207–208

Wolff-Parkinson-White syndrome, 104
Working memory, 11
World Health Organization (WHO), 2, 32

Z
Zeitgebers, 141, 142